Designing Around People

Pat Langdon · Jonathan Lazar
Ann Heylighen · Hua Dong
Editors

Designing Around People

CWUAAT 2016

Springer

VI User Profiling and Visualising Inclusion

Another growth area for inclusive design has been in the use of personae and associated methodology for developing and understanding of users' lived experience. Kunur et al. use ethnographic design as a lead-in method of developing usage cases for automotive HMI for cars of the future. They argue for an agile and inexpensive process that can be employed in a technology design area traditionally closed to human centred design, and demonstrate its concept. A complementary paper by Morris and Mueller shows how good quality user data can be collected and used as a key element in developing wireless technology that is responsive to inclusion. In particular, the extension of user profiles to disability and wider capability ranges can be an effective tool to engage technology stakeholders.

Another type of user profiling is possible when objective data about user capabilities and performance; such as eye-tracking, are used to drive adaptive interfaces to better match cognitive demand and reduce occurrences for cognitive overload (Chakraborty et al.). This adaptive approach to inclusion is increasingly popular, has featured in past CWUAAT volumes, and relies critically on accurate objective profiling to avoid clashes.

This book contains the reviewed papers from CWUAAT 2016 that were invited for oral presentation. The papers that have been included were selected by extensive peer review carried out by an international panel of currently active researchers. The chapters forming the book represent an edited sample of current national and international research in the fields of inclusive and architectural design, universal access, HMI, and assistive and rehabilitative technology.

We would like to thank all those authors and researchers who have contributed to CWUAAT 2016 and to the preparation of this book. We would also like to thank the external reviewers who took part in the review process. Many thanks are also due to the reviewing members of the Programme Committee who have renewed their intention to support the workshop series. We are grateful to the staff at Fitzwilliam College for their patience and help.

Pat Langdon, and
The CWUAAT Editorial Committee
University of Cambridge
March 2016

Contents

Contributors

A. Abdolrahmani University of Maryland, Baltimore County, MD, USA

Y. Afacan Bilkent University, Ankara, Turkey

C. Amaefule University of Maryland, Baltimore County, MD, USA

A. Anåker Department of NVS Division of Occupational Therapy, Karolinska Institutet, Sweden

G. P. Bingham Department of Psychological and Brain Sciences, Indiana University, Bloomington, IN, USA

H. Boyd Designability, Bath, UK

M. D. Bradley Cambridge Engineering Design Centre, University of Cambridge, Cambridge, UK

J.-A. Bichard Helen Hamlyn Centre for Design, Royal College of Art, London, UK

E. Brulé CNRS and University Paris Saclay, Telecom ParisTech, Paris, France

J. Chakraborty Towson University, Towson, MD, USA

P. M. Chamberlain Lab4Living, Art & Design Research Centre, Sheffield Hallam University, Sheffield, UK

E. Chrysikou Bartlett School of Architecture, UCL, London, UK

P. J. Clarkson Cambridge Engineering Design Centre, University of Cambridge, Cambridge, UK

P. Cloutier Georgia Institute of Technology, Atlanta, GA, USA

R. O. Coats School of Psychology, University of Leeds, Leeds, UK

K. Coomans Department of Architecture, Research[x]Design, KU Leuven, Belgium; and D E architecten, Tervuren, Belgium

K. L. Cornish Cambridge Engineering Design Centre, University of Cambridge, Cambridge, UK

C. Craig Lab4Living, Art & Design Research Centre, Sheffield Hallam University, Sheffield, UK

M. Dexter Lab4Living, Art & Design Research Centre, Sheffield Hallam University, Sheffield, UK

H. Dong Inclusive Design Research Centre, College of Design and Innovation, Tongji University, Shanghai, China

F. Doran Helen Hamlyn Centre for Design, Royal College of Art, London, UK

B. Dubin University of Maryland, Baltimore County, MD, USA

M. Elf Division of Occupational Therapy, Karolinska Institutet, Sweden

N. Evans Designability, Bath, UK

T. Felzer Institute for Mechatronic Systems in Mechanical Engineering, Technische Universität Darmstadt, Germany

C. Galbraith University of Maryland, Baltimore County, MD, USA

T. Georgiou Centre for Research in Computing, The Open University, Milton Keynes, UK

G. A. Giannoumis Oslo and Akershus University College of Applied Sciences, Norway

E. Glazer Helen Hamlyn Centre for Design, Royal College of Art, London, UK

J.A. Goodman-Deane Cambridge Engineering Design Centre, University of Cambridge, Cambridge, UK

N. Harris Designability, Bath, UK

A. Heylighen Department of Architecture, Research[x]Design, KU Leuven, Belgium

S. Holland Centre for Research in Computing, The Open University, Milton Keynes, UK

R. J. Holt School of Mechanical Engineering, University of Leeds, Leeds, UK

A. M. Howard Georgia Institute of Technology, Atlanta, GA, USA

A. Hurst University of Maryland, Baltimore County, MD, USA

C. Jouffrais CNRS and University of Toulouse, IRIT, Toulouse, France

S. K. Kane University of Colorado Boulder, CO, USA

M. Karam Kings College London, London, UK

N. Kistamah University of Mauritius, Réduit, Mauritius

M. Kunur Cambridge Engineering Design Centre, University of Cambridge, Cambridge, UK

P. M. Langdon Cambridge Engineering Design Centre, University of Cambridge, Cambridge, UK

J. Lazar Department of Computer and Information Sciences, Towson University, Towson, MD, USA

Z. J. Liu Tongji University, Shanghai, China

J. J. Loeillet Jaguar Land Rover, Human Machine Interface, HMI Project, International Digital Lab, University of Warwick, Coventry, UK

X. Ma Inclusive Design Research Centre, College of Design and Innovation, Tongji University, Shanghai, China

J. MacCalla Zyrobotics LLC, Atlanta, GA, USA

M. P. McGuire Towson University, Towson, MD, USA

M. Mon-Williams School of Psychology, University of Leeds, Leeds, UK

J. T. Morris Rehabilitation Engineering Research Center for Wireless Technologies, Atlanta, GA, USA

J. L. Mueller Rehabilitation Engineering Research Center for Wireless Technologies, Atlanta, GA, USA

S. Naseem Department of English, Manchester Metropolitan University, Manchester, UK

F. Nickpour Inclusive Design Research Group, Brunel University London, UK

W. Ning Inclusive Design Research Centre, College of Design and Innovation, Tongji University, Shanghai, China

L. Nguyen University of Maryland, Baltimore County, MD, USA

C. O'Sullivan Cara Design Ltd., Central Research Laboratory

J. Pan College of Architectural Design and Urban Planning, Tongji University, Shanghai, China

G. Pandey Towson University, Towson, MD, USA

H. W. Park Georgia Institute of Technology, Atlanta, GA, USA

C. Phaholthep Faculty of Architecture, King Mongkut's Institute of Technology Ladkrabang (KMITL), Bangkok, Thailand

S. Ramsamy-Iranah University of Mauritius, Réduit, Mauritius

S. Rinderknecht Institute for Mechatronic Systems in Mechanical Engineering, Technische Universität Darmstadt, Germany

P. A. Rodgers Northumbria University, School of Design, UK

S. Rosunee University of Mauritius, Réduit, Mauritius

A. Sawadsri School of Interior Architecture, Faculty of Architecture, King Mongkut's Institute of Technology Ladkrabang (KMITL), Bangkok, Thailand.

H. Skates School of Environment, Griffith University, Gold Coast Australia

R. Skjerve Oslo and Akershus University College of Applied Sciences, Norway

J. van der Linden Centre for Research in Computing, The Open University, Milton Keynes, UK

I. Van Steenwinkel Department of Architecture, Research[x]Design, KU Leuven, Belgium

P.-W. Vermeersch Department of Architecture, Research[x]Design, KU Leuven, Belgium; (Full) Scale architecten, Leuven, Belgium(Full) Scale architecten, Belgium

E. Verstraeten Architectenbureau Lowette & Partners, Molenbeek-Saint-Jean, Belgium

L. Von Koch Division of Occupational Therapy, Karolinska Institutet, Sweden

S. D. Waller Cambridge Engineering Design Centre, University of Cambridge, Cambridge, UK

B. Wentz Department of Management Information Systems, Shippensburg University, PA, USA

M. A. Williams University of Maryland, Baltimore County, MD, USA

Part I
Reconciling Usability, Accessibility and Inclusive Design

Exploring the Impact of Inaccessible Redesign and Updates

B. Wentz and J. Lazar

Abstract: For many blind users, updated software versions or revised websites, apps, and operating systems can create a situation where an interface that may have been accessible is no longer accessible, more difficult to use, or confusing. Websites, apps, and cloud-based software are modified on a frequent basis, and many organizations do not have a formal process in place to ensure that those changes comply with accessibility requirements. A web-based survey was conducted to collect feedback from users who are blind to learn more about the impact that website, software, and mobile app updates can have on accessibility and use. The results of the survey illustrate the negative impact that inaccessible updates and revisions can have on users with disabilities.

1 Introduction

Websites, software, apps, and operating systems are updated so frequently that many individuals rarely pay close attention to the occurrence. A user is more likely to notice, however, when an update or newer version creates a situation in which the software or technology is no longer usable, more difficult to use, or confusing. For many of the estimated 285 million individuals worldwide who are blind or have low vision (WHO 2014), it is likely that a website, app, or software update will create significant usability challenges and frustration. Publicity frequently surrounds the creation or modification of technology that results in it becoming more inclusive, and inclusive design with a focus on the user is often touted as a positive or responsible corporate decision. A more common situation is that a website, software application, or operating system that was accessible is updated and the newer version poses accessibility barriers. The sudden dearth of accessibility and usability means that the lives, education, workplace experience, and social inclusion of many individuals are negatively affected. This exploratory study begins to investigate the impact that web, software and

B. Wentz (✉)
Shippensburg University, PA, USA
email: bwentz@ship.edu

J. Lazar
Towson University, MD, USA

P. Langdon et al. (eds.), *Designing Around People*,
DOI 10.1007/978-3-319-29498-8_1

technology changes and updates can have on blind users, based on the responses to a survey of 150 blind users.

2 Related Literature

People with disabilities often use different types of assistive technology to access computers, mobile devices, applications, and web-based information. For instance, blind users may use a screen reader, which will take what appears on the computer screen, and provide computer-synthesized speech output. Deaf or hard of hearing users may use captioning on video or transcripts instead of audio. People with motor impairments that have limited use of their hands may use a keyboard but not a pointing device (such as a mouse), or they might use an adaptive keyboard, or instead of a keyboard use speech recognition or head tracking to control their device. A set of international technical standards for making websites accessible for people with disabilities, called the Web Content Accessibility Guidelines (WCAG), has been in existence since 1999 (W3C 2012). These technical standards cover perceptual and motor impairments as well as some cognitive impairments, and are considered to be the international standard for making websites accessible. There is also a set of rules, known as WCAG2ICT, for applying the WCAG principles to all types of technologies, including operating systems and software applications. When a website, other software or OS is designed using accessibility guidelines, it meets the needs of a broad range of users. Accessible websites typically meet the needs of people with perceptual impairments (low vision or blind, deaf or hard of hearing), motor impairments (limited or no use of hands for pointing or typing), and some cognitive impairments.

A growing number of organizations are placing importance on products, applications, and web content that are designed for and usable by the widest range of users. This field of focus is often referred to as inclusive design. The basis for adhering to accessibility requirements for inclusive design is frequently derived from international standards such as WCAG, and methodologies for incorporating users directly into the development and design processes. For user experience guidelines, inclusive design research frequently points to ISO (International Organization for Standardization) standards, such as 9241 which provides guidance on usability (UsabilityNet 2006). Other ISO standards related to usability focus on things such as software development, quality standards, and ergonomics. The UXPA (User Experience Professionals Association) also maintains the Usability Body of Knowledge for the usability profession (UXPA 2010). Organizations often highlight the creation of a new product or service that adheres to inclusive design. The British Standards Institute (BSI 2005) described inclusive design as "a comprehensive framework to help all private enterprises, public sector and not-for-profit organizations ensure that disabled people's needs are considered throughout the lifecycle of a product or service." These concepts have been widely promoted through the efforts of organizations such as the EDC (Engineering Design Centre) at the University of Cambridge through their

"Inclusive Design Toolkit" project (EDC 2015). A closely related concept is that of universal design or universal usability (Shneiderman 2000).

Previous research has highlighted that blind users are more likely to avoid content if they know in advance that it will cause them accessibility problems (Bigham et al. 2007), and when there are barriers to completing their tasks due to accessibility challenges, there is a resulting loss of time (Lazar et al. 2007). Inclusive, accessible design has been an answer to these challenges, but the nature of technology is that there is often a constant stream of changes and updates. The need for revisions and new versions are not necessarily the problem. A significant problem does exist, however, when those new versions, updates, and revisions create a decrease in or lack of accessibility. Some organizations have shown an awareness of this problem by simply maintaining multiple versions of devices, software, and websites for a period of time. It has also been well-documented that this approach to the inaccessible update problem is neither equitable or inclusive (Wentz et al. 2011, Wentz and Lazar 2011). Asking users to simply use an older version, because the newer version is inaccessible, can also create the appearance that users with disabilities are not able to be at the cutting edge of technology, whereas nothing could be further from the truth. Furthermore, when users with disabilities choose not to update versions because of perceived accessibility barriers, it can lead to increased security threats (Vaniea et al. 2014).

While users can choose not to update to newer versions if they are not accessible and are aware of the barriers in advance, this scenario is becoming less prevalent due to the evolving nature of software. As more software moves from being updated every 2-3 years, with users choosing the updates, to instead being provided through the cloud, software updates become much more frequent, and users become less aware of them, since they are transparent to the user. The likelihood of having an update that causes accessibility barriers, also increases (Lazar et al. 2015). Cloud computing specifically increases the likelihood of the problem, since the user no longer is in control of version updating, and no longer "downloads an update."

3 Research Methodology

In early 2015, a web-based survey was created to collect feedback from users who are blind to learn more about the impact that website, software, and mobile app updates can have on accessibility and use. Survey data were collected during June and July 2015 from 150 respondents who were self-reported as blind and 18 years of age or older through recruitment emails sent out to organizations such as the American Council of the Blind and the National Federation of the Blind. The survey took an average of 15 minutes for respondents to complete and asked questions regarding devices used to access software and the Web as well as experiences and preferences related to software and website revisions and updates.

The survey began with an introduction to the survey and informed consent information for the respondents. Questions were adaptive, in that if a respondent did not indicate the usage of a mobile phone, no questions regarding mobile phone usage would be asked. Some survey questions required a specific answer (yes or no), a selection from a list, or a Likert-scale rating of 1 through 5. Those questions and responses will be described in section 4.1 and 4.2 below. They primarily investigated usage patterns and the existence of problems related to new versions and/or updates. Other survey questions were optional and open-ended, allowing for qualitative user feedback and responses. Those results will be described in section 4.3 below.

4 Results

4.1 Usage Patterns

The first question on the survey asked respondents to select the devices that they regularly use for software and the Web: "On a weekly basis (including both work and personal use), I use the following devices to access software and the Web (you may select more than one)." The results showed that most respondents use desktop computers (71%), laptops (68%), and mobile phones (76%) to access software and the Web. Tablet usage was reported by 18% of the respondents. This question was followed by a question asking "What is your primary desktop or laptop operating system." The majority of respondents (87%) reported that as being Microsoft Windows. For those using tablets, some version of the iPad was reported to be the dominant product (86%). For mobile phones, various iPhone models were the primary choice (84%).

4.2 Existence of Problems

The responses regarding the existence of accessibility problems after updates or newer versions was evidenced by the following survey data. When respondents were asked "Have you ever experienced a desktop or laptop operating system update that caused an accessibility problem after you installed a newer version?" 60% responded with a yes. For a question "Have you ever experienced, when you updated your desktop or laptop software to a newer version, it suddenly became inaccessible?" 55% of respondents reported this experience. For questions related to mobile devices and apps, 54% of respondents reported that a mobile device system update caused an accessibility problem, and 61% reported that they experienced an accessibility problem after updating a mobile app. A question specifically related to website revisions and updates asked "Have you ever experienced a website becoming inaccessible, when the site is completely re-designed or updated?" This resulted in an 80% response of "yes."

4.3 Tangible Impact

The survey next tried ascertain more of the impact of these problems. Respondents were asked “Has a new version or update with a website, software, or technology ever prevented you from completing a task at work?” and this resulted in a 58% response of “yes.” The majority of respondents (78%) also reported that a new version or update of a website, software or technology prevented them from using it for recreational or personal use. There was also an impact on education or training, with 51% responding that an update or new version prevented them from completing education or training.

Table 1 summarizes the responses to the question “If a new version or update of a website, software, or technology is optional, how likely are you to adopt the update or new version (on a scale of 1-5, with 1 being extremely unlikely)?”

Table 1 Responses for adopting an optional update or new version, indicating some hesitancy to adopt new versions or updates

Rating	Respondent Results
1	8%
2	14%
3	34%
4	29%
5	15%

When asked “Have you ever purchased a technology device, software, or paid web service because you knew it was more accessible than the alternatives?” 83% responded with “yes.” What a statement regarding the costs/benefits of creating accessible products! When asked “How likely are you to install security updates (on a scale of 1-5, with 1 being extremely unlikely)?” the majority of users still favored installing the security updates (with 71% of respondents selecting a 4 or 5). In a follow-up question, 58% of respondents reported no accessibility problems with security updates. When asked “How likely are you to install a screen reader update (on a scale of 1-5, with 5 being extremely likely)?” the overwhelming majority of respondents favored installing the screen reader update. The results of the screen reader update question are contained in Table 2. The majority of respondents (52%) reported no problems with screen reader updates in a subsequent question.

Table 2 Responses for screen reader update or new version, indicating few concerns with screen reader updates

Rating	Respondent Results
1	7%
2	4%
3	12%
4	18%
5	60%

4.4 User Experiences

Qualitative, open-ended questions were created to describe and provide examples of the problems experienced by users. For example, when the survey asked respondents about problems with a desktop or laptop operating system updates, responses included that they are "not accessible to a blind person, the screen reader failed to read the page, VoiceOver would [afterward] run sluggishly, OS functions were difficult to find afterward, or I had to downgrade to the previous OS." These were a sampling of the responses from the 60% of users that reported this type of accessibility problem. The question about accessibility barriers after updating desktop or laptop software to a newer version, resulted in comments such as: "I could not get into programs, buttons were not labelled, I could no longer receive email, or I couldn't navigate with the usual keystrokes." Again, this was the experience of the majority (55%) of respondents. The question related to problems when updating mobile device software to a newer version, resulted in comments such as: "my iPhone quit talking when I upgraded it, an iOS update caused the phone app to not allow the deletion of voice mails, I could no longer use certain apps efficiently, gestures that worked previously did not work after the update, or [I experienced] VoiceOver glitches."

When respondents described the problems they experienced when updating mobile apps to newer versions, they noted things such as "Facebook and Twitter would not work, certain parts of apps wouldn't work, buttons were no longer accessible, the screen reader would now lose focus on the app, many apps were no longer usable, new button labels did not make sense, and [there were] problems with apps such as Amazon, FourSquare, Pandora, Sirius XM, Dropbox, and Hulu+. Several iOS apps that used to be accessible, no longer are, including the Weather Channel (which, over the course of several updates, went from fully accessible to unusable), NFL Sunday Ticket from Directv, and Delivery.com." These comments illustrate the experience of the 61% of respondents who reported these problems.

For the question related to problems when a website is updated, there were comments such as "JAWS (screen reader) hot keys no longer worked, the website was no longer accessible with Google Chrome, there was a new CAPTCHA without audio options, dropdown menus were not accessible, new buttons were not labelled, and links and labels do not make sense." Other respondents commented that this "frequently happens with banking or finance, newspaper, sports, hotel, and shopping websites (where the shopping cart no longer works)." Other respondents noted that this "happens also with hotel and airline websites, Blackboard became less accessible with the new version, and with Amazon I frequently have to use a mobile or older version." An overwhelming 80% of respondents reported this type of experience on websites.

In an attempt to report the reactions and feelings that users experience with these occurrences, the survey asked users to "describe your initial reaction when you learn about a required new version or update with a website, software, or technology that you use." It is not a surprise that the common responses included terms such as "frustration, annoyed, apprehension, stressed, and hassle."

5 Discussion

From a compliance monitoring point of view, software, OS, and design updates pose a major challenge. The major approaches utilized for compliance monitoring related to technology accessibility often involve either expenditures as a trigger for compliance checks or the updating of content as a trigger for compliance checks. When money is spent on new technology, there are lots of procedures in place for ensuring that the money is spent properly, and among the most successful approaches for accessibility compliance has been to use procurement contracts in government, universities, and companies. For instance, the practice of utilizing procurement contracts can require that a technology be accessible, can provide an indemnification clause so that the vendor is financially responsible for accessibility barriers, and can specify the terms under which a technology will be tested for accessibility (Lazar et al. 2015). So, the financial controls can help improve accessibility. When content is updated on a public web site, there is often an office at the government, university, or company, that approves the release of information to the public (known as an office of communications, marketing, or public information). Even with large-scale content on a website, with hundreds of content contributors, those contributors can be required to sign a contract noting that they can lose their account on the content management system for posting inaccessible content (Lazar and Olalere 2011).

But software, web design, and OS updates pose a challenge to compliance because they do not go through approval channels for finance or communication.

Often, a new version arrives without users receiving any prior notification. While an internal company system may have gone through security checks on a test server before an update, if the software/OS/website is provided externally (e.g. an application provided through the cloud), often, users will just receive a new version or a slightly modified version without any warning (Lazar et al. 2015). The large web-based email providers, such as Yahoo and Google, are using this approach of multiple rounds of minute changes to the interface, with no obvious notification to users (Goel 2015). And that new version--that new modification--may have accessibility barriers. There are not yet any published best practices of how to manage compliance monitoring for versioning updates. However, two recent legal settlements in the US (one between the tax preparation provider H&R Block and the National Federation of the Blind, and one between the grocery delivery service Peapod and the US Department of Justice) have strict requirements for accessibility testing any new versions of the web site and mobile app before they are released to the public (Lazar et al. 2015).

Commercial entities should also be aware of the purchasing decisions that users with disabilities make, as was evident in the survey results. It is also noteworthy that financial and banking apps and websites were frequently mentioned by users that experienced these problems. The 80% of respondents (noted in section 4.2) that reported problems with an inaccessible new version or update to a website underscore the impact that this deterioration of inclusive design has on blind users. If an organization became aware that 80% of its customer base or employees would be impacted by an update or new version, would they take notice? One recent example is that of the Uber iOS app. In September 2015 the iOS app that was accessible for iPhone screen reader users suddenly became inaccessible because of an update, resulting in a problem that could prevent a customer base that might be likely to engage this service to be unable to request a ride. This highlights the everyday reality of versions, updates, and accessibility. As previously noted, some organizations, educational institutions and government agencies have adopted processes for ensuring that new products and content are accessible, often by leveraging a content management system to better monitor changes to the content. According to the ongoing reports of the accessibility status of web content, however (Loiacono et al. 2009, Lopez et al. 2010, Lazar et al. 2012, Lazar et al. 2013), there is a question of how well those processes are implemented.

Clearly there is a serious flaw in the longterm implementation of inclusive design. Accessible or usable for a moment in time does not mean accessible and usable forever. What is needed is some type of maintenance process as well, similar to what is endeavored for quality or change management. Future research on inclusive design should include a focus on maintaining sustainable accessibility and usability. Product roadmaps or revisions should include a plan for maintaining or improving the level of accessibility rather than merely serve as an opportunity to update or innovate at a speed that is faster than the competition. Based on the experiences of blind users, it is obvious that social inclusion and inclusive design demand results far different than the present reality.

References

Bigham J, Cavender A, Brudvik J, Wobbrock J, Ladner R (2007) WebinSitu: A comparative analysis of blind and sighted browsing behavior. In: Proceedings of the 9th International ACM SIGACCESS Conference on Computers and Accessibility, pp. 51-58, Tempe, AZ, USA

BSI (2005) New British Standard addresses the need for inclusive design. Available at: www.bsigroup.com/en-GB/about-bsi/media-centre/press-releases/2005/2/New-British-Standard-addresses-the-need-for-inclusive-design/ (Accessed in November 2015)

EDC (2015) Inclusive design toolkit. Available at: www.inclusivedesigntoolkit.com/betterdesign2 (Accessed in November 2015)

Goel V (2015) Yahoo tweaks email to make search more personal. The New York Times, 5th August 2015, available at: www.nytimes.com/2015/08/06/technology/personaltech/yahoo-tweaks-email-to-make-search-more-personal.html?_r=0 (Accessed in November 2015)

Gonçalves R, Martins J, Pereira J, Oliveira MAY, Ferreira JJP (2013) Enterprise Web accessibility levels amongst the Forbes 250: Where art thou o virtuous leader? Journal of Business Ethics 113(2): 363-375

Lazar J, Allen A, Kleinman J, Malarkey C (2007) What frustrates screen reader users on the web: A study of 100 blind users. International Journal of Human-Computer Interaction 22(3): 247-269

Lazar J, Goldstein D, Taylor A (2015) Ensuring digital accessibility through process and policy. Elsevier/Morgan Kaufmann Publishers, Amsterdam, The Netherlands

Lazar J, Olalere A (2011) Investigation of best practices for maintaining section 508 compliance in U.S. Federal Web sites. In: Proceedings of the 2011 Human Computer Interaction International Conference, pp. 498-506, Orlando, FL, USA

Lazar J, Wentz B, Akeley C, Almuhim M, Barmoy S, Beavan P et al. (2012) Equal access to information? Evaluating the accessibility of public library web sites in the State of Maryland. In: Langdon P, Clarkson J, Robinson P, Lazar J, Heylighen A (Eds.) Designing inclusive systems, pp. 185-194. Springer, London, UK

Loiacono ET, Romano Jr NC, McCoy S (2009) The state of corporate website accessibility. Communications of the ACM 52(9): 128-132

Lopes R, Gomes D, Carriço L (2010) Web not for all: A large scale study of web accessibility. In: Proceedings of the 2010 International Cross Disciplinary Conference on Web Accessibility (W4A), Article 10, ACM, New York, NY, USA

Shneiderman B (2000) Universal usability. Communications of the ACM 43(5): 84-91

UsabilityNet (2006) International standards for HCI and usability. Available at: www.usabilitynet.org/tools/r_international.htm (Accessed in November 2015)

UXPA (2010) About the usability BoK. Available at: www.usabilitybok.org/about (Accessed in November 2015)

Vaniea K, Rader E, Wash R (2014) Mental models of software updates. Paper presented at the International Communication Association, Seattle, WA, USA, in May 2014, available at: http://rickwash.com/papers/security-ica-2014.pdf (not in a proceedings, accessed in November 2015)

W3C (2012) WCAG overview. Available at: www.w3.org/WAI/intro/wcag (Accessed in November 2015)

Wentz B, Jaeger PT, Lazar J (2011) Retrofitting accessibility: The legal inequality of after-the-fact online access for persons with disabilities in the United States. First Monday 16(11): 7 November 2011

Wentz B, Lazar J (2011) Are separate interfaces inherently unequal? An evaluation with blind users of the usability of two interfaces for a social networking platform, pp. 91-97. In: Proceedings of the 2011 iConference (iConference 2011), ACM, New York, NY, USA

WHO (2014) Visual impairment and blindness. Available at: www.who.int/mediacentre/factsheets/fs282/en/ (Accessed in November 2015)

An Intersectional Perspective on Web Accessibility

R. Skjerve, G. A. Giannoumis and S. Naseem

Abstract: Socially marginalised groups experience hostility in daily life, and hostility online adds to psychological pressure. For example, hate speech, typically defined as attacks on an individual or socially marginalised group, may impact access to web content for socially marginalised groups. In addition, rendered invisibility, for example being unable to choose your gender in a web form, may act as a psychological and practical barrier to accessing web content for groups, such as genderqueer, intersex and transgender persons. Research has yet to investigate the intersectionality of web accessibility. Preliminary results from semi-structured interviews with a select group of persons that experience multiple forms of discrimination suggest that marginalized individuals expect to experience oppressive content and consider oppressive content as a part of interacting with the web. In this paper, we examine a variety of oppressive mechanisms, including ableism, racism, and transphobia, and how in combination they relate to accessing and using web content. We argue that by ensuring the accessibility of web content substantively, future researchers and practitioners can promote a more universally accessible web. By taking into consideration experiences of hostility, web developers can better support access to information and communication on the web for everyone.

1 Introduction

Research on web accessibility has typically focused on the promoting and ensuring the usability of web content for persons with disabilities as a means for achieving social inclusion. Web accessibility relates to the legal principle of equal opportunity, which, according to legal scholars, obligates service providers to take positive steps to prevent discrimination by designing web content for use by persons with disabilities. Contiguously, architects, technology developers, and disability rights advocates began to argue that information and communication technology (ICT) should be designed for the broadest possible population, i.e., for the universal design of ICT.

While research in a variety of disciplines such as cognitive and clinical psychology, anthropology and sociology have empirically examined gender

R. Skjerve (✉) · G. A. Giannoumis
Oslo and Akershus University College of Applied Sciences, Norway
email: rannveigalette@gmail.com

S. Naseem
Department of English Manchester Metropolitan University, UK

P. Langdon et al. (eds.), *Designing Around People*,
DOI 10.1007/978-3-319-29498-8_2

discrimination in a variety of contexts, this article focuses in particular on the intersectional identities of persons that experience multiple forms of discrimination based on the combination of characteristics such as disability, gender, age, or race. Thus, research has yet to examine fully the intersectionality of web accessibility or the social barriers that occur at the intersection of multiple forms of discrimination, which affect access to and use of web content. In other words, research has typically focused on the usability of web content for persons with specific impairments (e.g., the blind and partially sighted or deaf and hard of hearing) and has yet to investigate substantively the experiences of persons belonging to multiple socially marginalised groups. In this paper, we use an interdisciplinary perspective that combines computer science with disability and gender studies to examine the experiences of people that face multiple forms of discrimination online and investigate a variety of oppressive mechanisms including ableism, racism, and transphobia. This paper asks, "How, in combination, do persons experience multiple forms of discrimination, which act as barriers, in accessing and using web content?"

To illustrate the point using a hypothetical case, consider the experiences of a black gay man with a sight impairment. If information about their sexual identity could put them at risk, a gay community webpage that is designed to be compatible with screen reader would be accessible in a technological sense, but the audio broadcasting done by the reader would make the page inaccessible from a security standpoint. Considering this, one could argue that screen reader compatibility alone is not enough to make this content usable for persons experiencing multiple forms of discrimination. There would need to be a way to access the content without the risk of someone eavesdropping.

If the page has implemented alternatives to the screen reader, the audio broadcasting is no longer an issue. However, there is still the risk of someone seeing what page is being accessed. Logging out and leaving the page might not take much time, but in a situation where you have few seconds to react, it's not a viable option. Some pages have implemented a panic button that instantly logs the user out and redirects the browser to an "innocent" looking webpage, like a major newspaper. But if the person has a sight impairment, they might not be aware of the button, since the awareness of the button relies heavily on observing the visual queue. Even if the user is aware of the button, there is still the issue of navigating the page's structure fast enough to get back to the button in time.

By taking into account the context in which a person lives, we can make the web more accessible. However, security is not the only issue in the example. Assuming that the security measures are in place, there is still the question of what happens once a person is accessing the content. If you ask a gay black man what messages he receives from other users on a gay web community, you can be fairly certain that one of the types mentioned will be a messages containing one single question: "Is it true what they say about black men?"

In this example, ableism manifests in the assumption that people with disabilities are a homogenous group, homophobia manifests in the threat of physical abuse and racism manifests in its most blunt and psychologically violent way. One can see how three separate oppressive mechanisms work together and reinforce the barriers for accessing content on the web.

This article explores the experiences, such as those presented in the hypothetical case above, by analysing preliminary results from semi-structured interviews with a select group of persons that experience multiple forms of discrimination. The results suggest that individuals that are members of multiple marginalized groups expect to experience oppressive content, and consider oppressive content as a part of interacting with the web.

This article proceeds in five sections. First, this article frames the examination the intersectionality of web accessibility by reviewing previous research on web accessibility, universal design and intersectionality. Second, this article presents the methods, data and analysis used to examine the experiences of persons that experience multiple forms of discrimination in accessing and using web content. Third, this article analyses the preliminary results from semi-structured interviews with participants selected because of their experiences with the intersectionality of web accessibility. Fourth, this article discusses the results in light of previous research in web accessibility and universal design. Fifth, this article concludes by summarizing the results and providing recommendations for future research.

2 Analytic Framework

This section presents different analytical perspectives for examining the intersectionality of web accessibility and reviews research on web accessibility, universal design, and intersectionality. Research on web accessibility provides a useful framework for examining the social barriers that prevent persons with disabilities from enjoying the web on an equal basis with others. Research on universal design provides a useful framework for extending web accessibility beyond disability to include the broadest possible population, and research on intersectionality provides a framework for examining the experiences of people that are subject to multiple forms of discrimination.

2.1 Web Accessibility

With the early adoption of the web in the US and Europe in the mid-1990s, the World Wide Web Consortium (W3C) established the Web Content Accessibility Guidelines (WCAG), an international standard for web accessibility. WCAG soon spread internationally as a practical and legal solution for achieving web accessibility (Giannoumis 2015a). By the late 1990s, interest organizations had attempted to apply disability antidiscrimination legislation to ICT and the web in an effort to ensure accessibility (Giannoumis 2015b). Ensuring accessibility provides a means for promoting equality between ICT users with and without disabilities and in effect remediating the digital divide (Ellis and Kent 2015, Goggin 2015, Jaeger 2015).

Research on web accessibility has focused on the outcomes of web accessibility policies, such as WCAG. This research has examined the accessibility of web content in specific sectors, such as public libraries (Yu 2002, Stewart et al. 2005, Tatomir and

Durrance 2010, Yi 2015), education (Johnson and Ruppert 2002, Klein et al. 2003, Green and Huprich 2009), transport (Lazar et al. 2010), private enterprise (De Andrés et al. 2010), financial services (Williams and Rattray 2003) and health services (Ritchie and Blanck 2003). This research demonstrates that many private sector service providers have yet to remove barriers to accessing web content.

In addition, research has assessed web accessibility in public services including federal and regional governments in the United Kingdom (UK) and US (Jaeger 2004a-b, Jaeger 2008, Rubaii-Barrett and Wise 2008, Kuzma 2010, Olalere and Lazar 2011, Bertot et al. 2012). This research demonstrates that, although public agencies maintain a clear social responsibility for providing accessible information, service providers have yet to remove barriers that persons with disabilities experience in accessing web content.

This article emphasizes the concept web accessibility as a framework for examining the barriers experienced by persons that are subject to multiple forms of discrimination. Social barriers limit the participation of persons with disabilities on the web and this articles examines social barriers from an intersectionality perspective.

2.2 Universal Design

While web accessibility is typically associated with the removal of barriers so that persons with disabilities can use the web, recently scholars have begun to adopt a broader conceptualization of web accessibility. In a recent article, Petrie et al. (2015) posed a unified definition of web accessibility and argues that web accessibility means 'all people, particularly disabled and older people, can use websites in a range of contexts of use, including mainstream and assistive technologies; to achieve this, websites need to be designed and developed to support usability across these contexts'. Similarly Persson et al. (2014) define accessibility as 'the extent to which products, systems, services, environments and facilities are able to be used by a population with the widest range of characteristics and capabilities (e.g. physical, cognitive, financial, social and cultural, etc.), to achieve a specified goal in a specified context.'

The scope of the definitions provided by Petrie et al. (2015) and Persson et al. (2014) are similar to the definition of universal design posed in the United Nations Convention on the Rights of Persons with Disabilities (CRPD). According to the CRPD, universal design 'means the design of products, environments, programs and services to be usable by all people, to the greatest extent possible, without the need for adaptation or specialized design.'

The primary contrast between web accessibility and universally designed web content is the scope of application (Persson et al. 2014, Abascal et al. 2015, Brown and Hollier 2015). While web accessibility aims to ensure the usability of web content specifically for persons with disabilities, universally designed web content aims to ensure the usability of web content for the broadest possible populations. While the analytic distinction between web accessibility and universal design is useful point of departure for the analysis in this article, in practice the benefits of web accessibility are typically shared among a broad range of users, i.e., both people with and without disabilities. In the words of Blanck (2014), '[universal design] is well beyond a minimum standard of accessibility.'

A universal design approach, provides a broader basis for promoting and regulating the design of web content. According to the Norwegian Ministry of Children and Equality's Action Plan for universal design 'The government wants to get away from a way of thinking in which the individual is defined as the problem and in which special measures for people with disabilities are the main solution' (BLID 2009).

This article emphasizes the application of universal design principles in promoting the usability of web content for the broadest possible population. Thus, universal design, provides a useful approach for examining the experiences of persons that belong to multiple socially marginalised groups. This article explores conceptualizations of universal design by examining the barriers that persons subject to multiple forms of discrimination experience.

2.3 Intersectionality

While research has yet to fully examine web accessibility from an intersectionality perspective, scholars of intersectionality argue that race, gender, class, ability, or sexuality do not exist in isolation and therefore should not be examined separately but as part of an individual's lived experience (Crenshaw 1991, Schiek and Lawson 2011, Risam 2015). According to Schiek and Lawson (2011), intersectionality as a concept was first introduced to articulate the distinct experiences of black women, which differ from the experiences of both black men and white women. Research by Crenshaw (1991), criticized contemporary politics for neglecting the racialized experiences of black women on one hand and neglecting their gender on the other. While the concept of intersectionality has a tradition in a variety of disciplines including law, women's studies and sociology, computer scientists have yet to integrate intersectionality into examinations of web accessibility or universal design.

The UN and EU have acknowledged the relevance of intersectionality in terms of antidiscrimination – where web accessibility has its roots – and have adopted a concept similar to intersectionality, "multiple discrimination", which refers to different forms and grounds of discrimination (Schiek and Lawson 2011). Some scholars differentiate between forms of multiple discrimination where each ground of discrimination can be distinguished and intersectional discrimination where the grounds for discrimination cannot be distinguished (Schiek and Lawson 2011).

This book article adopts an intersectional approach to examining web accessibility because multiple discrimination typically suggests an 'adding up' of separate forms of disadvantage, which contrasts with the complexity of an individual's lived experience. This article aims to establish initial evidence for adopting an intersectional approach to web accessibility by examining the lived experiences of persons affected by intersectional disadvantage. This article additionally provides an opportunity for web accessibility researchers to reflect on the interdisciplinary contribution of research on intersectionality and promote a deeper and richer conceptualization of web accessibility. The focus of this article in on the disadvantage that occurs at the intersection of gender, race and disability. The experiences of those in more privileged or advantaged intersections (e.g. white, non-disabled men) is therefore not investigated here.

3 Methods

To explore the intersectionality of web accessibility, this article will analyse empirical data from semi-structured interviews with persons experiencing multiple forms of discrimination. This paper uses qualitative methods to interpret prior models of web accessibility and aims to provide new explanations to extend previous research. This article uses qualitative data and analysis to examine the experiences of individuals that experience multiple forms of discrimination to elaborate on the role of intersectionality in web accessibility as a potentially mediating factor for promoting and ensuring the universal design of web content.

It would be impossible to comprehensively account for all mediating factors associated with intersectionality and web accessibility. This article uses a purposive sample of selected participants, deliberately recruited to explain and question established relationships between web accessibility and intersectionality. The participants were selected because they belonged to multiple marginalized groups and experienced discrimination on the web. In addition, two of the authors who acted as interviewees have intersectional identities. Table 1 provides a descriptive summary of the interview participants. As all of the participants are members of more than one marginalized group, the total number of participants listed in Table 1 is larger than the number of participants interviewed.

Table 1 Descriptive summary of interview participants

Characteristic / Identity	Number of Participants
Gendered	2
Disabled	2
Racialized	2

Participants for this paper provide a locus of investigation for web accessibility within the lives and experiences of persons who are subjected to multiple forms of discrimination.

This article presents a preliminary analysis of three interviews conducted in Norway, and England. The semi-structured interviews provided data on the perspectives of persons that experience multiple forms of discrimination. Participants were recruited based on their knowledge and lived experience as members socially marginalised groups. The interview guide covered a broad range of questions related to the participants' everyday habits on the web, and their encounters with oppressive content. The interview transcripts were analysed by identifying salient themes as they pertain to conceptualizations of web accessibility and universal design.

While this paper presents the tentative findings of the study, further data collection and analysis is planned in 2015 and 2016 where additional interviews will be conducted with persons that experience multiple forms of discrimination in Norway.

4 Analysis

The results of the semi-structured interviews suggest that the social aspects of the web are important to most of the participants. Although all the participants use the web to access other kinds of information, most of the day-to-day use of the web involves social media or other kinds of social forums. Some of the participants expressed a discomfort with social media, due to the amount of information shared by others as well as themselves. However, the discomfort did not seem to be severe enough to make an impact on the way they were accessing social media.

Several of the participants talked about the freedom of non-disclosure on the web. Being able to choose what people know about you, and who knows what about you, was described as freeing by several of the participants.

> *'In the real world you might understand that my hearing isn't too good so that you take extra care of me, or don't talk to me at all. But on the web I'm just a part of the gang'*
>
> (Participant TRS)

When questioned about offensive content the participants said that they had come to expect different kind of oppressive content on the web, and because of this it did not cause any serious distress. The participants described various reactions and tactics when encountering offensive content. Strategies varied from leaving the site, to completely avoiding pages where the participant expected to encounter oppressive content.

> *'I encountered a lot of very uncomfortable articles. They were like...you know, they were using the wrong pronoun, wrong name and everything. And as a trans person myself, I felt very uncomfortable. So I just stopped accessing those kind of things, don't want to take part in the mainstream media or internet world.'*
>
> (Participant OF)

The participant expressed the opinion that it is your own responsibility to stay away from pages where you can expect to encounter oppressive content. Statements like 'I used to get upset,' implying that being upset by the oppressive content is a silly or unnecessary emotional reaction, were present in all of the interviews.

> *'In terms of content I don't, I think if I went on a webpage and the content was, if I thought "oh this is shocking" or "why have they written this" or "why is this picture there".. To be honest I'm pretty unshockable if that's a word. So I'd probably say, excuse my language but, "what the hell" and then click the back button, that's the extent to it.'*
>
> (Participant SD)

Some of participants said they would feel pressured ‘to come’ out, and relinquish the freedom of non-disclosure, due to an obligation or need to defend their communities.

> *‘What makes me “come out” as deaf? When things happen where deaf people are talked about. When I feel like it’s time to say something. Hard to say something specific, it’s something I consider on an incident to incident basis.’*
>
> (Participant TRS)

The comments sections of web pages, and avoiding them, has been a recurring issue experienced by several of the participants. The comments sections are where participants expect and experience the most outspoken oppressive content. One of the participants in particular, expressed a frustration with the ever-changing design and change in page navigation, which at times would result in involuntary encounters with the comment sections. However, most of the participants thought of these encounters more as annoyances than anything else.

The results of the semi-structured interviews suggest that barriers to access may be broader than conventionally defined in web accessibility and come closer to conceptualizations of universal design. The next section continues by summarizing and discussing the results.

5 Discussion

The results suggest that persons with intersectional identities that experience multiple forms of discrimination face barriers in accessing and using web content because of both the format and structure of web content and its substantive character. The results additionally suggest that an element of victim blaming exists in the way the participants interact with the web. The participants argue that when you access a page that you accessed before, you should know whether it can contain offensive content, and act accordingly. Emotional reactions such as anger or distress are typical and accompanied by the expectation that the experience is only one of immediate discomfort. However, in order to avoid further discomfort the participants would leave the page and limit their later access, leading to self-exclusion from parts, or most of the web.

The comment sections stands out in this aspect as a ‘house of horror’ in the world of offensive web content, and the participants stated that in general they experienced it as inconsequential and would seldom cause them to leave the page. Therefore, a tension exists between free speech and hate speech, something reflected in participants’ attitudes towards comments sections.

That the participants choose to limit what they access to avoid offensive content might not be problematic in itself. There would be little sense in accessing a white supremacy blog if one does not want to encounter racism. However, if the experience or expectancy of offensive content is limiting access to parts of the web of public interest, there is a point to be made about the page's accessibility. With this in mind, this article argues that the technological gaze of developers needs to be supplemented with a critical attitude towards possible content.

Models of web accessibility and universal design provide a useful framework for understanding the intersectional identities of the participants. This article argues that because the barriers that the interview participants encounter, particularly oppressive content is a result of marginalisation by society and sometimes cultural assumptions about who should be invited and included in considerations and approaches to web accessibility.

6 Conclusion

Considering how often the comments section of websites were mentioned by the participants, future research could usefully explore alternative ways to represent comments that prevents unintentional access, while not limiting free speech. In addition, oppressive content seems to have an effect on the participant's daily interaction with the web. The consequences vary from severe self-exclusion, to immediate but short-lived irritation. Considering this further, research on universal design should include a broader perspective, where the technological gaze is supplemented with an understanding of a person's broader context.

References

Abascal J, Barbosa SD, Nicolle C, Zaphiris P (2015) Rethinking universal accessibility: A broader approach considering the digital gap. In: Stephanidis C, Antona M (Eds.) Universal access in the information society: Aging and assistive environments. Springer

Bertot JC, Jaeger P, Hansen D (2012) The impact of polices on government social media usage: Issues, challenges, and recommendations. Government Information Quarterly 29(1): 30-40

Blanck P (2014) eQuality: The struggle for web accessibility by persons with cognitive disabilities. Cambridge University Press, New York, NY, USA

BLID (2009) Norway universally designed by 2025. The Norwegian government's action plan for universal design and increased accessibility 2009-2013, p. 9. Available at: www.regjeringen.no/globalassets/upload/bld/nedsatt-funksjonsevne/norway-universally-designed-by-2025-web.pdf (Accessed in November 2015)

Brown J, Hollier S (2015) The challenges of Web accessibility: The technical and social aspects of a truly universal Web. First Monday 20(9)

Crenshaw K (1991) Mapping the margins: Intersectionality, identity politics, and violence against women of color. Stanford Law Review 43(6): 1241-1299

De Andrés J, Lorca P, Martínez AB (2010) Factors influencing web accessibility of big listed firms: An international study. Online Information Review 34(1): 75-97

Ellis K, Kent M (2015) Disability and the Internet in 2015: Where to now? First Monday 20(9)

Giannoumis GA (2015a) Auditing Web accessibility: The role of interest organizations in promoting compliance through certification. First Monday 20(9)

Giannoumis GA (2015b) Transnational convergence of public procurement policy: A 'bottom-up' analysis of policy networks and the international harmonisation of accessibility standards for information and communication technology. International Review of Law, Computers and Technology (ahead-of-print): 1-24

Goggin G (2015) Disability and mobile Internet. First Monday 20(9)
Green RA, Huprich J (2009) Web accessibility and accessibility instruction. Journal of Access Services 6(1-2): 116-136
Jaeger P (2004a) Beyond section 508: The spectrum of legal requirements for accessible e-government web sites in the United States. Journal of Government Information 30(4): 518-533
Jaeger P (2004b) The social impact of an accessible e-democracy. Journal of Disability Policy Studies 15(1): 19-26
Jaeger P (2008) User-centered policy evaluations of section 508 of the rehabilitation act: Evaluating e-government web sites for accessibility for persons with disabilities. Journal of Disability Policy Studies 19(1): 24-33
Jaeger PT (2015) Disability, human rights, and social justice: The ongoing struggle for online accessibility and equality. First Monday 20(9)
Johnson A, Ruppert S (2002) An evaluation of accessibility in online learning management systems. Library Hi Tech 20(4): 441-451
Klein D, Myhill W, Hansen L, Asby G, Michaelson S, Blanck P (2003) Electronic doors to education: Study of high school Website accessibility in Iowa. Behavioral Sciences and the Law 21: 27-50
Kuzma JM (2010) Accessibility design issues with UK e-government sites. Government Information Quarterly 27(2): 141-146
Lazar J, Jaeger P, Adams A, Angelozzi A, Manohar J, Marciniak J et al. (2010) Up in the air: Are airlines following the new DOT rules on equal pricing for people with disabilities when websites are inaccessible? Government Information Quarterly 27(4): 329-336
Olalere A, Lazar J (2011) Accessibility of U.S. federal government home pages: Section 508 compliance and site accessibility statements. Government Information Quarterly 28(3): 303-309
Persson H, Åhman H, Yngling AA, Gulliksen J (2014) Universal design, inclusive design, accessible design, design for all: Different concepts-one goal? On the concept of accessibility-historical, methodological and philosophical aspects. Universal Access in the Information Society (4): 1-22
Petrie H, Savva A, Power C (2015) Towards a unified definition of web accessibility. In: Proceedings of the 12th Web for all Conference, pp. 35, Florence, Italy
Risam R (2015) Toxic femininity 4.0. First Monday 20(4)
Ritchie H, Blanck P (2003) The promise of the internet for disability: A study of on-line services and web site accessibility at Centers for Independent Living. Behavioral Sciences and the Law 21: 5-26
Rubaii-Barrett N, Wise LR (2008) Disability access and e-government: An empirical analysis of state practices. J. Disabil. Policy Stud. Journal of Disability Policy Studies 19(1): 52-64
Schiek D, Lawson A (Eds.) (2011) European Union non-discrimination law and intersectionality. Investigating the triangle of racial, gender and disability discrimination. Ashgate, London, UK
Stewart R, Narendra V, Schmetzke A (2005) Accessibility and usability of online library databases. Library Hi Tech 23(2): 265-286
Tatomir J, Durrance JC (2010) Overcoming the information gap: Measuring the accessibility of library databases to adaptive technology users. Library Hi Tech 28(4): 577-594
Williams R, Rattray R (2003) An assessment of web accessibility of UK accountancy firms. Managerial Auditing Journal 18(9): 710-716
Yi YJ (2015) Compliance of section 508 in public library systems with the largest percentage of underserved populations. Government Information Quarterly 32(1): 75-81
Yu H (2002) Web accessibility and the law: Recommendations for implementation. Library Hi Tech 20(4): 406-419

Representing Children Living with Visual Impairments in the Design Process: A Case Study with Personae

E. Brulé and C. Jouffrais

Abstract: Assistive technologies (ATs) must improve activities but also participations of impaired users. Thus when designing ATs, especially for children, one should consider the diversity of users and disabilities but also the educational and societal contexts, as well as subjectivities (i.e. personal experience of disability, own motivations, etc.). Co-design is a method that encompasses all those features, but it is not easy to achieve with impaired users, especially when they are children. In the context of a research project on interactive maps for visually impaired people, we first conducted a field study to better describe potential users (visually impaired people, but also parents, teachers, therapists, etc.) and their needs. Building upon this field-study, we developed a set of design cards representing users but also needs, places, goals, etc. We then designed a workshop aiming to improve the knowledge and empathy researchers had about users, ideation step of the design process. We report on how these methods facilitated the creation of inventive scenarios, interactions and prototypes, but also how they helped researchers to think about their own design and research practices.

1 Introduction

It is estimated that 19 million children live with visual impairment worldwide (WHO 2014). Ensuring their inclusion in society is critical to guarantee equal rights, and because it allows for greater independence. In particular, early inclusion in traditional school has a positive impacts on the abilities children develop (McGaha and Farra 2001, Holt et al. 2014). ATs have a role to play, as they can be highly empowering (Hurst and Tobias 2011) and reduce activity limitations. However, previous studies (Phillips and Zhao 1993, Polgar 2010, Kinoe and Noguchi 2014) show a high abandon rate of such devices, underlining the fact that they do not meet needs (usability, reliability, costs, etc.). This may relate to the fact that users are not sufficiently included in the design process (Phillips and Zhao

E. Brulé
CNRS & University Paris Saclay, Telecom ParisTech, Paris, France

C. Jouffrais (✉)
CNRS & University of Toulouse, IRIT, Toulouse, France
email: christophe.jouffrais@irit.fr

P. Langdon et al. (eds.), *Designing Around People*,
DOI 10.1007/978-3-319-29498-8_3

1993). Furthermore, the way children experience their own disability is rarely investigated (Connors and Stalker 2006). These observations show that it is necessary to understand how the adoption of technologies depends on the various aspects of disability. Numerous works have shown that having empathy for users is one approach to doing so (Wright and McCarthy 2011).

In the context of designing a collaborative interactive map for visually impaired users, we aimed at encouraging the HCI researchers of our team to better take into account users' context. The activities we proposed aimed at raising their empathy through storytelling and role playing.

In the current paper, we first describe a preliminary field-study aiming at better understanding the educational context and the experiences of visually impaired children. We then present various techniques that we used during a workshop with HCI researchers in order to improve knowledge of users' subjectivities, and to stimulate the production of speculative usage scenarios. Both were conducted as a first step of a longitudinal research project with visually impaired users and caretakers. Although the current work was specific to our context, we aim at providing insights on how personae and design cards may be used to help AT designers take into account specific needs of disability.

2 Related Work

2.1 Designing Accessible Interactive Maps and Tangible Interactions

Visual impairment has numerous consequences on cognitive development (Maurer et al. 2005), and especially on spatial cognition. Hence, there have been numerous research projects devoted to the design of assistive technologies that may improve spatial knowledge of visually impaired users (see Zeng and Weber 2011 and Brock et al. 2013 for reviews).

Tangible interaction relies on physical objects to interact with digital information. It allows simultaneous use of multiple modalities, and has been adopted in many prototypes for sighted users (Ullmer and Ishii 2000). A few research projects have aimed at designing accessible tangible devices for non-visual exploration of maps. For instance, Pielot et al. (2007) designed interactive objects in order to explore maps with audio output.

2.2 Understanding Use(r)s of Assistive Technologies

Several authors investigating Assistive Technologies (ATs) acceptance rate have underlined the importance of the stigmatization associated to such devices (Polgar 2010). Some environmental features are quite obvious (access to the care system, lack of accessibility of public places, etc.), but others are less easy to identify and may be addressed with specific methods.

The current study seeks to provide researchers with tools allowing for a better and wider description of users (including context and subjectivity) and their needs. For instance, Connors and Stalker (2006) identified that children experience disability as "impairment, difference, other people's reactions, and material barriers". When designing ATs, researchers should keep in mind that they are interfaces between: (1) the person living with impairment, including her subjective perception of herself and the world (Druin 2002); and (2) her social context. In addition, those interfaces should empower users (Hurst and Tobias 2011).

2.3 Representing Users in the Design Process

Visual impairment corresponds to a wide range of abilities, largely influenced by educational and social contexts. There are many variables to consider when describing visually impaired users. Although it would be a valuable solution to directly involve many children with diverse impairments in the design process (Druin 2002, Bailey et al. 2014), it is difficult to achieve, because of various constraints (e.g. availability, parental agreement, transportation and communication issues.).

When co-design is difficult or not possible, a method frequently used consists in the identification of representative users described as Personae (Friess 2012). Personae were proposed by Cooper (1999) as a tool for the design of interactions. They are fictitious but they embody characteristics that have been observed (e.g. professional roles, type of personality, social origins, personal history, goals, tastes, etc.). Personae are often represented with cards, and facilitate storytelling during the design process. Personae have been criticized because they represent idealized, "artificial" or stereotypical people. However, Pruitt and Grudin (2003) have pointed out that well-crafted personae are very helpful because they raise designers' sensitivity and empathy, and are an efficient communication tool within small and large teams. They may be part of a larger card deck (also including situations for example) and used in a variety of design activities, to serve as a communication tool between users and researchers (Wölfel and Merritt 2013).

3 Motivation and Objectives

A previous project on a similar topic had involved specialized teachers and visually impaired people in the design process, but not children (Brock et al. 2015). The results show that the device improved usability and satisfaction. But the designed prototype had not been implemented in the field. Furthermore, the HCI researchers involved in the project reported various design issues during work meetings. First, they lacked imagination, having difficulties coming up with new concepts of interaction techniques. Second, they were concerned by long term adoption of ATs. Many examples in the literature show that devices that have been successfully evaluated in the lab were not adopted in the field. Third, they were, in many brainstorming and evaluation sessions, working with a restricted number of users. They were afraid that this restricted population would not represent the whole targeted population. Finally, they reported that they did not manage to efficiently share notes and observations gathered in the field.

Our current research project is based on co-design. It is conducted in a research laboratory including the HCI department of a computer science research centre, and an institute for visually impaired people. It also involves a designer, a specialist in psycho-ergonomics, a start-up developing open source software, and various stakeholders of the institute who volunteered to participate (orientation and mobility instructors, specialized teachers, transcribers, and visually impaired people).

In order to understand how the existing interactive map prototype may be adapted and adopted in the classrooms, but also to provide design guidelines for the new prototypes, we decided to conduct a longitudinal field-study and to develop new design processes. Following the field-study, we proposed a two day workshop with the HCI researchers for: (1) sharing the results and recommendations provided by the field study; (2) transmitting ideation methods coming from design research; and (3) developing usage scenarios of accessible interactive prototypes. A transversal goal was to encourage HCI researchers to take into account the physical, temporal and cultural context of the users in the design process, stimulate their empathy for users, and develop an understanding of how they were considering users during the design process.

4 Preliminary Field Study

Our field study aimed to better understand the caring ecosystem of the Institute, and how caretakers (teachers, instructors, transcribers, etc.) use assistive technologies. This Institute hosts and assists hundreds of children and teenagers (up to 18 years old) living with visual impairments. It also provides rehabilitation and professional training for visually impaired adults.

4.1 Methods

The field-study consisted in twenty-seven semi-directed interviews between fifteen minutes and one hour depending on availability. Children were asked about their own experience of disability, usages of technologies, and topics of interests. Caretakers were asked about their definition of visual impairment, their roles in children's education and care practices. We also conducted four weeks of observations over six months. The results of this field-study have been reported elsewhere (Brulé et al. 2015). According to the grounded theory methodology (Charmaz 2006), they were open coded to identify concepts, and assembled by themes. In this paper, we only summarize the results that have supported the design of the workshop.

4.2 Results

About Children's experience of disability: First, the children reported *feeling impaired* when they were not able to engage in a given activity, or when they feared to failing at a task. This was especially the case for children whose impairment was late-detected, which is more likely to happen if they come from a low-income family with reduced access to the healthcare system. Second, they expressed *feeling different*, either in a positive or negative way. For instance, being able to use a smartphone without looking at it was seen as positive. But they may also feel excluded from mainstream culture, such as cinema. Third, they expressed *being concerned about other people's reactions*, such as other children telling them they are stupid. Finally the children expressed *a consciousness of material barriers* and the differences between accessibility policies and their application in everyday life.

On Caretakers' practices: First, caretakers highlighted the impact of the educational context, and especially of *inclusion in traditional schools* on children's abilities. The same impairment may have very different consequences depending on social and cultural background, as well as the specific care that children received (for instance, education in classes with sighted or in specialized schools). Second, they felt having *material barriers* in their practices, including a lack of time, finances and technical resources. Third, they reported having *strong commitments* in raising public or political awareness, but also in sharing skills with others. Fourth, most of them *engage in continuous and reflective learning*: they constantly analyse and question their methods to improve their own skills and knowledge. Fifth, they are *eager to use Do-It-Yourself or digital techniques* to design adapted tools for the children they care for. Finally, the caretakers mentioned constructive experiences with researchers or new technologies as ways to improve their practices. They would work overtime on the project.

In conclusion, it appears that children experience disability not only as activity limitations but by numerous parameters that should be considered when designing ATs. In the next section, we present the results of the ideation workshop, to see how these findings can be transmitted, understood and used.

5 Ideation Workshop

5.1 Design Cards

The design cards used in the workshop were developed by the designer, relying on the field-study results and the aims of the workshop. The set was made of personae, places and goals cards with a specific structure. The personae cards included name and surname, but also a nickname, so that participants may refer to personae informally, and not via impairment, age or gender. Furthermore, the field-study showed that context and subjectivity were important to understand usages. The cards aimed to provide personae with a social and cultural background, including date and place of birth, a general description, a list of topics of interest, as well as a personal history. An additional insert a portrait to be drawn. Finally, a field was reserved for the role(s) that personae had to play with the prototype (e.g. teaching, learning, helping, designing, etc.).

The field-study also revealed the importance of educational context (e.g. insertion in regular classes). Each place card described a location with spatial configuration and qualitative description (e.g. modern or ancient building, school, or museum).

The goal cards were initially left blank. Because each caretaker has their own objectives. It was interesting to let participants elicit caretaker practices and the associated needs. They could freely fill in the cards including needs, tasks, skills to acquire, etc. (e.g. "knowing my own size compared to the world.")

5.2 Activities

The workshop was conducted with six HCI researchers involved in the project (including one blind and one visually impaired). The workshop facilitator observed the participants, and gathered results and feedback. After each activity, the results were presented and followed by a general discussion. The organizer specifically asked participants to react to the method and the results. The workshop consisted of four activities.

Filling up persona, place, and goal cards. This activity was based on blank cards of three different types: persona, place and goal cards (Fig.1). Participants had one hour and a half to fill them, according to people, places or goals that could fit in the project. They could rely on people they had met, their office and the tasks they have to do. They also described persons that might use the intended prototype. The goal was to force participants to elicit how they were conceptualizing or stereotyping users.

There were four additional types of cards: "aesthetic" (e.g. minimalist or modern), "spatiotemporal context" (e.g. Canada 2020, India 2060, Moon 20120), "ludic mechanisms" (i.e. everyone is on the same team or against each other), and "qualitative" (i.e. the overall feeling expressed in the scenario). Ten of those cards were previously completed by the designer based on existing games.

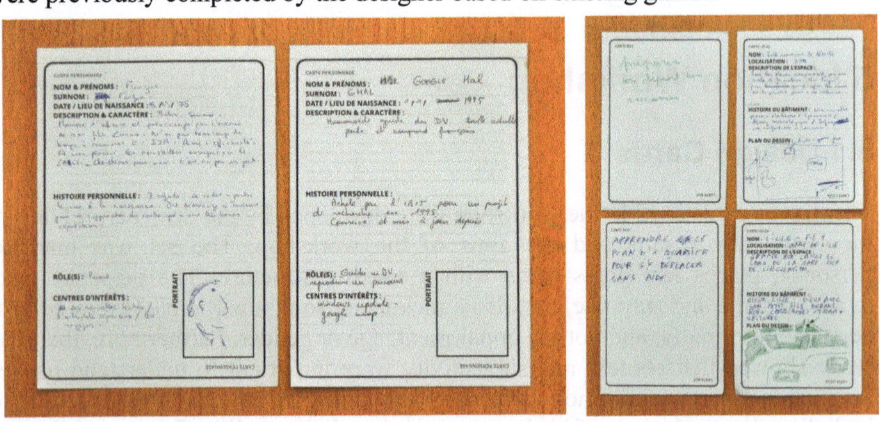

Fig. 1 From left to right: persona, goal and places cards, filled by workshop participants. We see that the personae were quite roughly described.

Imagining scenarios. Each group had to pick up three personae, one goal and one context, and imagine as many scenarios as possible with these cards.

Participants had to write down as many scenarios as possible during two hours. Finally they were asked to perform some of these scenarios (whilst blindfolded if they had to represent a visually impaired person) using everything they had at hand. The aim was for participants to better understand and describe users' subjective experiences.

Designing prototypes showing emotions. Participants were then asked to design prototypes displaying emotions. One participant selected an animal. The next participants successively picked up a temper (e.g. extrovert or nervous), and a feeling (e.g. surprised or hungry). Finally, the next participant had to describe an imaginary interactive table prototype that holds all these features (e.g. a table that looks and reacts like a surprised nervous kangaroo). Each group described two such prototypes with annotated sketches in twenty minutes. The goal was to mobilize cultural representations, i.e. a set of symbols used to communicate in a given culture.

Extended scenarios. The final activity focused on extending scenarios using the first card set (personae, places, and goals) completed with additional cards prepared by the facilitator (aesthetic, context, ludic mechanisms). The goal was to come up with completely new and speculative scenarios, as well as to extend the importance of cultural representations in scenarios.

5.3 Results

Filling up persona, place and goal cards: The participants filled 14 persona cards, 9 context cards and 12 goal cards. They wrote succinct descriptions of personae who were mainly defined by their "professional" role. The visually impaired personae were mostly described by impairment, which was not linked to a personal history. They did not contain any physical description, social background, etc. The context cards illustrated the institute classroom, various iconic buildings or speculative ones. The goal cards were mostly about acquiring new skills in geography or locomotion. There were no cards mentioning subjective, reflective or autotelic goals. The goals were highly pragmatic, thus minimizing the users' personal motivations.

Imagining scenarios: Each group came up with at least 10 to 15 scenarios. Some were pragmatic and could be immediately prototyped, such as 3D printing children figurines so that they could project themselves into a 3D model of a neighbourhood. Others were completely speculative, such as playing a game with a robotic dragon within a lunar station. They also proposed artistic settings, games or pedagogical activities. One group used many personae in scenarios, while the other group focused on goal and context cards, designing for one persona only. The participants willingly used objects found in the room (sugars, pencils, etc.) to illustrate ideas (Figure 2) but did not physically perform or play the scenarios.

Designing devices displaying emotions: The participants completed the task in less time than allocated. They all came up with rich, and annotated drawings of speculative devices. The blind participant provided verbal descriptions that were illustrated on a Dycem sheet by the facilitator. The prototypes included inventive techniques of interaction with various inputs and outputs (e.g. illumination, warming, shape changes, etc.) to express the emotional state of the device.

Extended scenarios: The participants had difficulties in imagining scenarios making actual use of aesthetic or qualitative properties. The number of generated scenarios was still high, but they had to pick up new cards frequently to get inspiration. They thought that the number of parameters was too high, and sometimes too conflicted, in order to pull something interesting out. They nevertheless came up with highly creative scenarios (e.g. large scale interaction around the prototype) and described more enthusiastically their users (e.g. clothing or motivations), which illustrates a higher degree of empathy. They also described more precisely how users interact with the device (e.g. pitch of voice, object temperature, etc.)

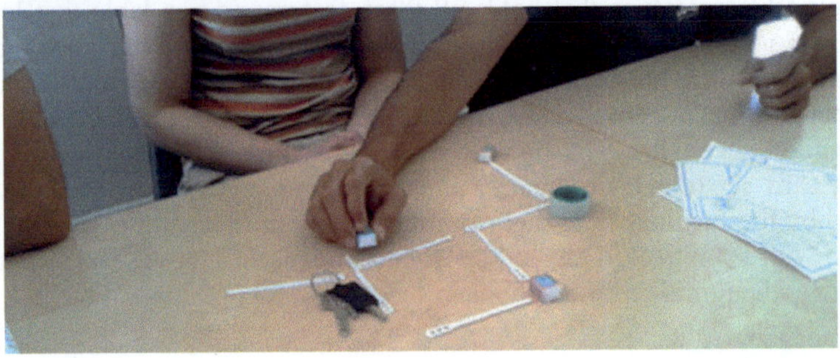

Fig. 2 Researchers prototyping scenarios with sugars, keys and other various objects

5.4 Observations

After each activity, the groups were asked to present outcomes to the others, and make comments on the activity and related aims. Although participants were used to working with scenarios, they reported having difficulties, especially in activities 3 and 4 ("Now I see that imagination is a muscle that should be flexed and trained much more"; "This is easy for you, but we are not used to it"). None of them had used similar methods before. When they were questioned about the activities and the relevance of the outcome on future research, they expressed uncertainty. They were unsure how to integrate these methods and results (e.g. the speculative scenarios) in their research activity. However, after discussion, several participants agreed that such a card set, describing potential users and goals, could be of use in the future. They emphasized that it helped them thinking outside of a task-oriented, pragmatic approach, which is often focused on impaired adults needs and experiences.

6 Discussion

The results of the field study (see Brulé et al. 2015 for extended results) were consistent with the literature on children's experience of disability. Disability encompasses many notions: feeling impaired, feeling different, a concern for others' reaction, or the existence of material barriers (Connors and Stalker 2006). The results also confirm the positive impact of inclusion (McGaha and Farra 2001, Holt et al. 2014) and the importance of rapid prototyping and new technologies (Hurst and Tobias 2011). In our case, it helped to structure the card set that was used in the workshop.

Concerning the workshop, it is interesting to note that the participants gradually proposed richer descriptions of users and interactions. Because none of them had experienced similar methods before, they were confused by the method, but also by the number of parameters. Nonetheless, it allowed them to avoid design fixations (Jansson and Smith 1991). Clearly, the workshop session led to propositions that would not have emerged from traditional brainstorming sessions. For instance, many scenarios involved interactions with rich input and output including haptics, gesture, light, temperature, etc. Some participants also described the pitch and the warmth of the prototype voice when interacting with children. On a short-term and pragmatic level, these quick ideation sessions confirmed the importance of tangible interactions, but also opened new perspectives to be prototyped and evaluated (e.g. the use of figurative objects).

However, the researchers expressed uncertainty about the "practical outcomes" of the workshop, and especially how speculative scenarios might help to design actual devices. During the discussion, the facilitator mentioned the risk of a design process mainly focused on functions and goals. They observed that it may lead to the exclusion of specific users or to failure to consider crucial aspects of interaction. They were reminded how models inherited from disability studies may help them develop other perspectives. In fact, the cards helped the researchers to think about their own practices (Schön 1983). By the end of the workshop, the participants were interested in using the design cards to better describe users, and to enable long term sharing of field observations and knowledge (the cards were preserved and may be reused). Furthermore, the card set can always be updated and may thus help framing future research projects. As co-design is not always possible, such cards may also be used by stakeholders to describe themselves and their goals.

7 Conclusion

The field-study helped us to better describe children living with visual impairment and how they interact with assistive technologies. It also showed how those interactions are shaped by a larger context (e.g. policy, culture, etc.) These observations guided the development of a set of design cards and workshop activities, which aim to improve the representation of users and increase empathy. In addition to the improvement of ideation within the team, the workshop also helped researchers to think about their knowledge of users, and highlighted how this knowledge may shape the design process. Future observations will estimate the impact it may have on the design practices within the team.

References

Brock AM, Oriola B, Truillet P, Jouffrais C, Picard D (2013) Map design for visually impaired people: Past, present, and future research. Médiation et Information, Editions L'Harmattan, Paris, France, 36 : 117-129

Brock AM, Truillet P, Oriola B, Picard D, Jouffrais C (2015) Interactivity improves usability of geographic maps for visually impaired people. Human–Computer Interaction 30(2): 156-194

Brulé E, Bailly G, Gentes A (2015) Identifier les besoins des enfants en situation de déficience visuelle : état de l'art et étude de terrain. In: Proceedings of the IHM'15

Charmaz K (2006) Constructing grounded theory: A practical guide through qualitative analysis. Sage Publications

Connors C, Stalker K (2006) Children's experiences of disability – Pointers to a social model of childhood disability. Disability and Society 22(1)

Cooper A (1999) The inmates are running the asylum. Macmillan Publishing, Indianapolis, IN, USA

Druin A (2002) The role of children in the design of new technology. Behaviour and Information Technology 21(1): 1-25

Friess E (2012) Personas and decision making in the design process: An ethnographic case study. In: Proceedings of the CHI'12, Austin, TX, USA

Holt R, Moore AM, Beckett A (2014) Together through play: Facilitating meaningful play for disabled and non-disabled children through participatory design. In: Langdon PM, Lazar J, Heylighen A, Dong H (Eds.) Inclusive designing: Joining usability, accessibility and inclusion. Springer

Hurst A, Tobias J (2011) Empowering individuals with do-it-yourself assistive technology. In: Proceedings of the 13th International ACM SIGACCESS Conference on Computers and Accessibility, pp. 11–18, New York, NY, USA

Jansson DG, Smith SM (1991) Design fixation. Design Studies (12)1

Kinoe Y, Noguchi A (2014) Qualitative study for the design of assistive technologies for improving quality of life of visually impaired. In: Yamamoto S (Ed.) HIMI 2014, Part II, LNCS 8522, pp. 602–613

Maurer D, Lewis TL, Mondloch CJ (2005) Missing sights: Consequences for visual cognitive development. Trends in Cognitive Sciences 9(3): 144-151

McGaha CG, Farran DC (2001) Interactions in an inclusive classroom: The effects of visual status and setting. Journal of visual Impairment and Blindness 95(2): 80-94

Phillips B, Zhao H (1993) Predictors of assistive technology abandonment. Assistive Technology 5(1)

Pielot M, Henze N, Heuten W, Boll S (2007) Tangible user interface for the exploration of auditory city maps. In: Oakley I, Brewster S (Eds) HAID 2007, LNCS vol. 4813: 86-97, Springer Berlin Heidelberg, Germany

Polgar JM (2010) The myth of neutral technology. In: Oishi MMK, Mitchell IM, Van der Loos HFM (Eds.) Design and use of assistive technology, Springer, New York , NY, USA

Pruitt J, Grudin J (2003) Personae: Practice and theory. In: Proceedings of the 2003 Conference on Designing for User Experience, ACM Press, San Francisco, CA, USA

Schön DA (1983) The reflective practitioner: How professionals think in action. Basic, New York, NY, USA

Ullmer B, Ishii H (2000) Emerging frameworks for tangible user interfaces. IBM Syst. J. 39: 3-4

Wright P, McCarthy J (2008) Empathy and experience in HCI. In: Proceedings of the SIGCHI Conference on Human Factors in Computing Systems, Florence, Italy

Wölfel C, Merritt T (2013) Method card design dimensions: A survey of card-based design tools. In: Kotzé P, Marsden G, Lindgaard G, Wesson J, Winckler M (Eds.) Human-computer interaction – INTERACT 2013, vol. 8117: 479-846, Springer Berlin Heidelberg, Germany

Zeng L, Weber G (2011) Accessible maps for the visually impaired. In: Proceedings of IFIP INTERACT 2011 Workshop on ADDW, CEUR

Inclusive Design and Mental Health: Policy and Legislation Challenges from the Perspective of Social Inclusion

E. Chrysikou

Abstract: Mental illness incorporates a spectrum of diseases affecting a globally increasing population. Yet, society is still accepting the institutional concept of allocating the risk associated with mental illness to closed institutions. The allocation of closed institutions as the places of treating and caring for mental illness, prevents architecture as well as the rest of the design community of seeing mental health issues as part of a community integrated design concept. On the contrary, design for mental health could form part of a more active dialogue of incorporating the needs of mentally ill people in the broader discussion of accessibility and its implications. As this is a very big and complex topic, this paper will focus on one aspect of the architectural specifications: the buildings use, and how change of legislation towards more flexibility could affect the whole deinstitutionalization prospects of a context. It also includes a case study of the Hellenic mental health facilities planning legislation and how alterations on the change of use legislation for psychiatric facilities could affect their integration outcome.

1 Background

Mental illness incorporates a spectrum of diseases affecting a globally increasing population. According to WHO, in Europe, almost 20% of the burden of disease relates to mental illness that affects one in four people at some time in life. Moreover, 9 out of 10 countries with the highest suicide rates in the world are in Europe (WHO 2013). Yet, society is still accepting the institutional concept of allocating the risk associated with mental illness to closed institutions, despite the very limited evidence on their therapeutic effectiveness, even if these are small-scale facilities (Priebe et al. 2005, Chrysikou 2014, Gilburt et al. 2014). Europe is a pioneer in the treatment and care of mental illness, but is still at the early stages of deinstitutionalization, with the majority of the mentally ill people treated in institutions rather than in the community, providing limited access to services and

E. Chrysikou (✉)
Bartlett School of Architecture UCL, London, UK
email: e.chrysikou@ucl.ac.uk

P. Langdon et al. (eds.), *Designing Around People*,
DOI 10.1007/978-3-319-29498-8_4

employment as well as a very small recognition of the contribution of carers (EIU 2014). The fact that mental illness is treated in closed and often segregated from the urban grid institutions, even if they are small in scale and considered part of what is called Community Care, is on the other hand contradictory to advancements in Social Psychiatry that happened as early as 1932, by the Soviet Government that after building small community projects, established an equivalent of what would nowadays be called a day hospital (Madianos 1980, Vostanis 1989), or even earlier by occupational therapy developments in Germany at 1929. Soon after the war, Foyer Elan Retrouve was developed by Sivadon and in the US, the Movement for Mental Health in the Community was formed, setting the ground for de-institutionalisation (Chartokolis 1989, Diebolt 1997). Since then, WHO (2001; 2005) directs that mentally ill people should be primarily treated as close to home as possible with hospitals being the last resort.

The allocation of closed institutions as the places of treating and caring for mental illness, prevents architecture and the rest of the design community from seeing mental health issues as part of a community integrated design concept. On the contrary, design for mental health could form part of a more active dialogue of incorporating the needs of mentally ill people in the broader discussion of accessibility and its implications. As this is a very big and complex topic, this paper will focus on one aspect of the architectural specifications: the buildings use, and how change of legislation towards more flexibility could affect the whole deinstitutionalization prospects of a context. It will also include a case study of national mental health facilities planning legislation and how alterations on the change of legislation for psychiatric facilities could affect their integration outcome.

2 The Need to Incorporate Mental Health in the Accessibility Discussion

Design for people with disabilities is gradually incorporated into generic architectural guidelines and briefing documentation leading to an increasingly integrated built environment. Specifications for people with disabilities start to influence broader architectural typologies, as opposed to specialised accommodation and healthcare facilities only, driven by demographic changes (Langdon et al. 2014). Moreover, design requirements for people with mobility problems, visual or other sense-related impairments have already been included in the generic building guidelines and briefs, even if there is still progress to be achieved in areas such as employment (Gomez et al. 2014). Strategies and provisions for older people appear in generic policies and architectural guidelines, incorporating those ‘designing-for-older-people’ frameworks in briefs and requirements of more generic schemes, such as social housing, shops or even entire communities with greater integrating perspectives (Glasgow 2000, Dementia Friendly Hampshire Toolkit 2012, Chrysikou et al. 2014, Care Quality Commission 2015).

This shift in architectural thinking and its effect on the built environment, eventually leads to a more integrated society. Therefore, the discussion on accessibility nowadays involves broader parts of our everyday life, such as accessible education, employment, tourism etc. (Riley 1999, Darcy and Dickson 2009, Maisel 2010). People with physical disabilities and sensory impairments as well as older people are gradually viewed from an inclusive perspective, as human capital with diverse benefits for society. There are, for instance, frequent references on the consumer power of baby-boomers and their ability to create trends and influence the market (Synchrony Financial 2014, Wu and Beyer 2015). This inclusive thinking might be occasionally so powerful that we can see an occasional shift of the argument to addressed positive aspects deriving from dealing with disability. For example, Zeisel (2010) identified the value for all of us of learning to experience life in the present tense through caring or just being involved with people with Alzheimer's.

Continuing to explore encouraging perspectives of inclusion, we will travel back at the onset of historical years. Then, Greeks perceived mental illness as a "God-sent" condition. Mentally ill people were considered to be speaking the voice of Gods. This attribute could be viewed as society introducing through mental illness an element of out of the box-thinking for its unpredictability and its disconnection from common logic and social norms. This God-sent perception of the illness stopped when St Augustin around the 4th Century AD from the theological perspective started a discussion on the relation of demons to mental illness, a relation that was confirmed by the Church two centuries late, leading to Malleus Maleficarum just before the 16th Century (Chartokolis 1989, Georgiou et al. 1993).

Since, despite some exceptions such as the Quaker movement, mental illness is still dealt as a problem that society cannot manage in an integrated way. When non-mentally ill people get to a hospital with cabs or ambulances, mentally ill people still in many parts of the western world arrive at the hospital cuffed in a police car. Similarly, for people with disabilities society tries to improve their mobility at home and at the same time make the public domain accessible for them to integrate. For the majority of people in acute mental health wards and also for all forensic patients, there is no option to visit the garden of their ward if that is not secure enough (Chrysikou 2013). The reasons could vary, from limitations of Psychiatry to provide until now successful diagnostic and treatment instruments or the reality of harm and self-harm, to the stigma or maybe, even less obvious undercurrents such as the challenging of reason and of social formation (Foucault 1972, Markus 1993).

This uncertainty related to the perception and understanding of mental illness reflects on the ways societies deal with it. Variety is very much present in the means and methods that are employed for its treatment: from a plethora of complex systems and webs of specialised facilities with varying degrees of control in Western countries to just chains on barks of trees and the absence of any form of shelter in countries such as Somalia (WHO 2010). Yet, there is a common denominator in all these attempts that on all other aspects present so many differences that direct analogies have limited value. It is what Psychiatrists call dangerousness (Chriswick 1995) and the inability of society to accept containing the risk associated with mental illness.

In short, here lies an important difference between mental illness and other disabilities regarding inclusive design. In the latter, society accepts to contain the risk, which is mainly for the individual rather than for society, explores ways for its management, with accessibility policies being one of those. This leads eventually to the facilitation of integration of vulnerable groups, such as older people, people with sensory impairments or people with mobility problems. In mental illness however, the closed mental health structures such as hospitals, hostels, community mental health wards, to name but a few and the fear of harm and self-harm still prevent society fully accepting and adopting the integrative principles of Care in the Community (Muijen 1993).

The gradual elimination of segregating lines could be enabled with the initiation of the discussion about accessibility and mental health as it shifts the perspective from clearly-defined purpose built environments to integrated places in the community. The author supports that knowledge and understanding of mental illness would promote the integration of mentally ill people in our societies. According to a service user, stigma and subsequent segregation results from a lack of knowledge and understanding (Tobias and Tobias 2015). According to scientists, mental illness is among the diseases where we have the least knowledge and understanding (Christensen et al. 2009, EIU 2014). Changing our perspective about it, and incorporating what it is already there as a theoretical model and as a recognized medical field, i.e. the principles of Care in the Community, could be a first step for the accessibility and the better integration of mentally ill people.

This paper argues that strategic planning, legislation and broader built environment interventions could play an important role towards the social integration of mentally ill people. Also, the segregative aspect that mental illness affects only a limited number of the population, compared for example to mobility or old age, needs to be addressed as a myth and it has to be reviewed as opposing to the principles of Community Psychiatry and as cultivating closed institutions in the community. The paper addresses both points. First, the importance of considering mental illness as a subject affecting society as a whole. Then, it will demonstrate new strategies that would help include mental illness in the society. The latter will be argued with the upcoming Greek legislation on the subject and how it challenges the existing broader framework of building permits.

3 A Case Study on Changing the Game

Next we will explore a very interesting case study as an example of a shift of policy from segregative to integrative, as it derived from a combination of causes that will be explored later in the paper. That is the example of Greece, the country who first accepted and protected the mentally ill as a valid part of society 3 000 years ago, for their God-sent abilities. However, modern Greece is a European Country that started its "Psychiatric Revolution" in the mid-80s and still presents a quite low placement according to the Mental Health Integration Index, being 28th out of 30 countries, followed by Romania and Bulgaria (EIU 2014). The economic crisis is amongst the reasons for this placement. Yet, despite the fact that employment, for which Greece was the 24th out of the 30 countries, is having a great influence on that Index and Greek unemployment is one of the highest in Europe, the poor access to health services, stigma and access to a stable residential environment prevent the country from achieving a better position in that ranking. As a case study, Greece sheds light in a model of de-institutionalisation that has been already applied in a European Union country with limited resources and the lessons learned could have great values to many European and European Research Area countries that start their de-institutionalisation now, such as Bulgaria, Romania and other Balkan countries or Turkey. It could also be of relevance to Israel, which is now shifting its mental health care provision from public to run by charities. However, aspects of this shift towards integration can be also relevant even in the most developed, from a psychiatric-provision perspective, countries such as the UK that is considered among the most advanced countries on the subject, as even these have a long way to go for a true integration and as several of the so called community based wards are still in hospital premises (Chrysikou 2014, Care Quality Commission 2015).

To counter the lagging of the Greek psychiatric integration, the country with the support of the European Commission, is exploring and employing a series of strategies to improve the provision of care under the Psychargos Program, i.e., a national plan that started in 2000 for the closure of the big institutions and the provision of a network of services in the community. One of the interventions of Psychargos has been the identification of problems in the licensing of all types of community mental health facilities and as a next step altering the licensing procedures, updating the building and technical equipment requirements. This attempt was based on two main objectives. The first objective constituted the design of a simpler and fairer licensing procedure. The second, that occurred as a result of the first, involved the redesign of a set of national guidelines for each facility type that would promote the support and integration of mentally ill people in the community, as European Commission indicated.

The methodology designed and used to explore the main problems that the facilities encountered constituted two main parts. The first, involved a first identification of problems regarding the issue of licenses to operate for non-for-profit mental health service providers. These are the equivalent for Greece of Mental Health Trusts, they operate in the third sector of the economy and provide the vast majority of non-hospital care. This was conducted by the Support Mechanism for the Mental Health Services and their Networking and Cooperation at a Sectoral and Peripheral level. The expertise also took into account the available reports of the Inspection Committees, of the Fire brigade and the Greek Legislation.

The second part of the methodology comprised approaching all service providers and asking their input as well as literature review on evidence and international best practice. Also, the main findings of the first part of the methodology were incorporated in order to produce a report on the situation and a set of actions that would set the basis of producing new national guidelines. The stage involved the design and administering of a questionnaire of 29 questions regarding the process of acquiring building permits and licenses to operate of the mental health facilities. This was then distributed to all 116 facilities to fill by the Support Mechanism. These comprise 53 care homes, 28 day centres, 3 mobile units, 23 protected apartments and 5 hostels. Some of these have been operating for more than 20 years, yet at the time of the research a 10% of the facilities had their operating licences still pending. There were also the psychiatric departments of the general hospitals or other types of facilities, including day centres, hostels or care homes, located inside hospital campuses, but these have been excluded. The Support Mechanism sent the completed 103 questionnaires back to the researchers for evaluation. This methodology aimed at the evaluation of the situation in Greece and would also provide an understanding on how the Trusts and in particular the facilities themselves perceive the problems they faced. It would also shed some light on what they perceive as potential solutions.

4 Findings

A key finding of the questionnaire that was sent to the facilities was that the people involved in the running of the facilities expressed the need to simplify the planning permit procedures. As building permits did not have implications for the mobile units and the apartments, here we will focus on the other three types of facilities, i.e., the care homes, the day centres and the hostels. Regarding permits 47% encountered a series of problems with strong financial and budgeting implications and an additional 8% did not specify the source of difficulties. 36% replied that the planning permit procedures affected negatively their timescale and budgeting and added to their total costs. An additional 10% mentioned that they encountered significant delays with considerable financial implications to their budget. 14% encountered problems with the site plan and the permitted uses. Additionally, 57% of the total sample proposed support measures, including the creation of a support service for the planning and the licencing or insisted on the need to reduce the time required for acquiring the licenses. This was in agreement with earlier findings of the Mechanism during the consultation period and the inspections associating complicated and time-consuming procedures to difficulties of the facilities of acquiring the necessary licences. Therefore, the expertise indicated as one of the main reasons for the lack of adequate number of community mental health facilities in Greece the complexity and the length of licensing procedures. This was either preventing trusts to expand and open new facilities or led them to operate in an obscure status, where the facilities where not fully compliant to the licensing procedures, yet the lack of alternative provisions and the lose control mechanisms enabled them to operate. As a result, the main aim of the project became the establishment of a realistic platform that would enable the facilities to operate in a legitimate way.

One of the biggest problems that was identified in the existing facilities was the change of use: it proved too lengthy and costly as a procedure or occasionally too complex to be achieved at all. Plus, there was a number of facilities who were located in areas where the change of use could not be granted at all. In that case, 67% of the facilities would have to compromise, either with expensive rents, or property outside their catchment area, often institutional looking and stigmatizing, or the fact that they did not get their license yet and until the use requirements changed, could not get it at all. As substantial pressure both from European commission that did not approve of asylums catering for mentally ill people (ECITE 1995) and also from an actual practical need, as even at this status of operation the facilities provided a necessary service and if they stopped to operate the residents would be forced to return either to asylums or to the streets, a practical solution had to be found without any further delays.

As it would be practically impossible to change overnight the dysfunctional and highly beaurocratic system of planning permissions (Economou et al. 2007,

Manolopoulos 2011) the alternative of simplifying the use requirements was examined. Thus, an initial solution was proposed by the support mechanism and was implemented with the decree of Protocol Number 107931/22-11-2013, decree with Protocol Number 107933/22-11-2013. Under these two decrees, community mental health facilities that served as accommodation, such as hostels or care homes, could be facilitated in residential areas and any property that its use was residence. Similarly, day centres did not require any more properties that were built under the healthcare use, but could be hosted in any property characterised as offices. Compared to the health or welfare uses that existed before this uses were much simpler as they allowed flexibility, increased the choice of available premises and decreased the requirements in terms of structural engineering. This of course, solved most of the problems prohibiting the opening of such facilities in Greece. Despite the change of requirements for use though, some problems remained. The most significant in terms of licensing, was the lack of the local Fire Brigade departments to recognize the adequacy of residential requirements for the function of psychiatric hostels, care homes or day centres. 33% had to make changes and 21% of the total sample found it difficult to comply, resulting in considerable delays. This was reasonable, especially if one took into account issues related to the particular function of these facilities. They accommodate more people than an ordinary family home, there is an increased dangerousness due to pathologies involved and there is a greater difficulty regarding evacuation in cases of emergencies compared to normative population.

From all the above, it became clear that there was a need to retain the simplified licensing procedure, without losing the qualitative and therapeutically necessary attributes of space, that a health related use would incorporate. The typologies of residence and office could not be fit for those purposes, as over simplistic. This was in agreement with predeceasing research findings (Chrysikou 2013) on the inadequacy of domestic typologies to fully cater for the needs of mentally ill people at acute stage or at the early stages of rehabilitation. Indeed, there were issues that rose from the co-habitation of a substantial number of people that at the same time had increased care needs. Basic needs, such as safety were compromised but the same could be said for the ability to function independently (competence) as well as users' personalisation and choice. Also, once more the oversimplifying of requirements as it were expressed in residential typologies could by no means prevent institutionalisation. The research also indicated substantial problems in evacuation plans, increased wear and tear due to tough use and inadequately tough materials and fixtures associated with residences, increased needs for security and institutional environments that provided very limited stimuli to users. Contrary to the initial aspirations, they resulted in the creation of small scale asylums in the community.

A solution to the problems deriving from oversimplification of uses and the lack of an adequate framework of guidelines for mental health facilities, was proposed the introduction of detailed guidelines referring to the specific typologies. Thus, all the problems deriving from the choice of land would be prevented allowing more choice of potential properties, saving time and costs, yet then adaptations would be necessary according to purpose. That way, the limitations that used implied could be still eliminated, but the quality would be safeguarded by fit for purpose guidelines that facilities would have to meet prior to operation. It is beyond the scope of the paper to go into more detail about the features of the guidelines, however, it is important to state that they contained all the building traits (together with all other specs) that more specific uses would mean. At the same time the flexibility of uses (residences and offices) in terms of planning permits enable a higher degree of integration of the facilities in the community as residential facilities could now be built in residential only areas and the local community could not raise legitimate NIMBYism claims for their closure. This, was not as we explained the main motive for this change of use but it was certainly an integrating element that came as a result. In that sense, even in countries where planning permits are straightforward and easy to get, the flexibility in uses relating to mental health and the ability of the facilities to be located even in purely residential areas, would be a considerable step towards their integrations as well as the accessibility of mentally ill people, as they will be enabled to access normal neighborhoods again.

Finally, another topic that rose in the legislation, was again related to the location of the facilities. According to rehabilitation theories, community mental health facilities have to be located in the community they serve. Greek legislation enabled the facilities to operate in close proximity to the community (FEK 2000). This resulted in existing facilities being located outside the population they served and sometimes segregated from the urban grid, in the fields. This was picked up and altered changing the requirement from close proximity to within the catchment area they serve, as obligatory. This aspect appears more restrictive, as it puts the proximity as inadequate and the centrality as the optimum location, yet it means a lot in terms of accessibility and breaking the barriers of NIMBYism. The new legislation might minimise the chances for out of site out of mind situations that the previous 'close to the catchment area' phrasing would enable. Mentally ill people should live and be treated within the community they belong to.

5 Conclusions

The increased numbers of mentally ill people will eventually create the pressure for facilitating the existing need of caring for these people in the community. This will mean that society will have to become able to manage dangerousness within its core. The ultimate way of this acceptance is architecture accommodating elements necessary for the universal accessibility of mental illness in generic guidelines as a result of demographics and anti-stigma campaigns, very similarly to other forms of disability and the needs of older people after the pressure of the baby-boomers. Right now, this is a future goal rather than a current reality.

Therefore, a whole range of strategies, short-, mid- and long term, as well as a range of products, from low or high-tech and from specialised to generic architectural guidelines, software applications, workplace and accommodation solutions, referring to all range of spaces, from physical to virtual, including even sectors such as gaming, entertainment or tourism to cater for the whole spectrum of a persons' needs. This means a paradigm shift for the design for mental illness as one that is happening entirely in the society, improving primarily the quality of life of the people living with the illness at some-point in their lives but also of their families and carers, who also suffer of high burnout rates as well as the effects of stigma. The broadest impact will be, however, for our entire society as it means that one of the most characteristic types of total institutions, i.e. the mental institutions (Markus 1993), will become more and more obsolete. This reality is linked to a more adaptive and a more responsible society that does not need walls of asylums (small or big) to contain its risks.

Acknowledgements

Dr Evangelia Chrysikou is Chief Investigator of the project Planning and Evaluation Methodologies for Mental Healthcare Buildings (PEMETH). Dr Chrysikou's research is funded by the European Union's Horizon 2020 research and innovation programme under the Marie Sklodowska – Curie Grant Agreement No 658244.

References

Alzheimer's Society Report (2013) Building dementia-friendly communities: A priority for everyone. Alzheimer's Society, London, UK

Care Quality Commission (2015) Right here right now: People's experiences of help, care and support during a mental health crisis. Available at: www.cqc.org.uk/sites/default/files/20150630_righthere_mhcrisiscare_full.pdf (Accessed in November 2015)

Chartokolis P (1989) Introduction in psychiatry, 2nd Ed. Themelio Publications, Athens, Greece

Christensen CM, Grossman JH, Hwang J (2009) The innovator's prescription. McGraw-Hill, New York, NY, USA

Chriswick D (1995) Dangerousness. In: Chriswick D, Cope R (Eds.) Seminars in practical forensic psychiatry. Gaskell, London, UK

Chrysikou E (2013) Accessibility for mental healthcare. Facilities 31(9/10): 418-426

Chrysikou E (2014) Architecture for psychiatric environments: Environments and therapeutic spaces. IOS Press, Amsterdam, The Netherlands

Chrysikou E, Symvoulakis E, Lionis C (2014) Home environment design and frailty: A proposal to increase impedance. In: Proceedings of the 19th WONCA EUROPE Conference, Lisbon, Portugal

Darcy S, Dickson T (2009) A whole-of-life approach to tourism: The case for accessible tourism experiences. Journal of Hospitality and Tourism Management 16(1): 32-44

Dementia Friendly Hampshire Toolkit (2012) Making Hampshire a dementia-friendly county. Finding out what a dementia friendly community means to people with dementia and carers. Available at: www3.hants.gov.uk/2012-dementia-friendly-communities-toolkit-engagement.pdf (Accessed in November 2015)

Diebolt E (1997) De la quarantaine au quarantaine: Histoire de foyer de postcure psychiatrique de l' Elan'. L' lan Retrouve, Paris, France

ECITE (1995) Parts from the report conducted on behalf of EC, on the visit in psychiatric hospitals, Autumn 1995. Tetradia Psychiatrikis (psychiatric notebooks) 54(April-June): 23-33

Economou D, Petrakos G, Psycharis Y (2007) National urban policy in Greece. In: van der Berg L, Braun E, van der Meer J (Eds.) National Policy responses to urban challenges in Europe. Ashgate, Aldershot, UK

EIU (2014) Mental health and Integration. Provision for supporting people with mental illness: A comparison of 30 European countries. The Economist Intelligence Unit

FEK (2000) 'YA No Y5v/1962/21-9-2000' FEK B' 1268/19-10-2000, article 7, paragraph 5, as it was amended and validated

Foucault M (1972) Histoire de la folie a l'age clasique'. Éditions Gallimard
Georgiou G, Vargopoulos D, Hatziioannou A (1993) The psychiatric problem analysis from prehistoric era until early Renaissance. Galen 35(6): pp 631-39
Gilburt H, Peck E, Edwards N, Naylor C, Ashton B (2014) Service transformation: Lessons from mental health. The King's Fund, London, UK
Glascow N (2000) Transportation transitions and social integration of nonmetropolitan older persons. In: Pillermer K, Glasgow N, Moen P, Wethington E (Eds.) Social integration in the second half of life, chapter 4.: The Johns Hopkins University Press, USA
Gomez JI, Langdon JA, Bichard JA, Clarkson PJ (2014) Designing accessible workplaces for visually impaired people. In: Langdon PM, Lazar J, Heylighen A, Dong H (Eds.) Inclusive designing: Joining usability, accessibility and inclusion, pp. 269-280. Springer
Langdon PM, Lazar J, Heylighen A, Dong H (2014) Inclusive designing: Joining usability, accessibility and inclusion. Springer
Madianos M (1980) Social psychiatry: Historical review, definition and ideology. Encephalos 17: 159-165
Maisel J (2010) The state of the science in universal design: Emerging research and developments. State University of Ney York at Buffalo, USA, Benthan Science Publishers
Manolopoulos J (2011) The looting of the Hellenic Republic by the Euro, the political elite and the investment community. Anthem Press, London, UK
Markus T(1993) Buildings and power: Freedom and control in the origin of modern building types. Routledge, London, UK
Muijen M (1993) Mental health services: What works? In: Weller M, Muijen M (Eds.) Dimensions of community mental health care. Saunders, London, UK
Priebe S, Badesconyi A, Fioritti A, Hansson L, Kilian R, Torres-Gonzales F et al. (2005) Reinstitutionalisation in mental health care: Comparison of data on service provision from six European countries. BMJ 330(7483): 123-6
Riley RW (1999) Schools as centres of community (Remarks as prepared for delivery to the American Institute of Architects). Department of Education, Washington, DC, USA
Synchrony Financial (2014) Balancing multi-generational retail strategies. Winning over millennials without losing boomers. Synchrony Financial
Tobias S, Tobias T (2015) In-patient bedroom design – The user perspective and the dragon café. Oral presentation on the 19th of May. Design in Mental Health Conference 2015, Birmingham, UK
Vostanis P (1989) Re-establishment of the mentally ill. Encephalos 26: 97-1984
WHO (2001) Mental health: New understanding, new hope. World Health Organization, Geneva, Switzerland
WHO (2005) Mental health: Facing the challenges, building solutions. Report from the WHO European Ministerial Conference, Helsinki, Finland. World Health Organization Regional Office for Europe, Denmark
WHO (2010) A situation analysis of mental health in Somalia. WHO Somalia Liaison Office
WHO (2013) Prevention of mental disorders and suicide. Available at: www.euro.who.int/en/what-we-do/health-topics/noncommunicable-diseases/mental-health/activities/prevention-of-mental-disorders-and-suicide (Accessed in November 2015)
Wu CF, Beyer J (2015) Making room for the baby boom: Senior living. In: Harvard Business School Case 215003. Teaching materials newsletter, Spring 2015
Zeisel J (2010) I'm still here – A breakthrough approach to understanding someone living with Alzheimer's. Piatkus Books

Part II

Designing Inclusive Assistive and Rehabilitation Systems

Designing an Innovative Walking Aid Kit; A Case Study of Design in Inclusive Healthcare Products

F. Nickpour and C. O'Sullivan

Abstract: This paper examines how products can be redesigned to allow flexibility for changes in a user's condition to give them control and ownership over their care, while offering viable, cost-effective and sustainable healthcare solutions. By focusing on the case study of the Evolvable Walking Aid Kit, we aim to investigate to what extent a modular system which has been designed to incorporate principles of affordability, evolvability and emotional durability can benefit patients. The Evolvable Walking Aid is a modular kit which can be assembled to form a walking stick, crutches, a walking frame, and variations of these aids depending on the individual's stage of their condition and fitting their anatomy. A co-design process was adopted across all stages of the project and two distinctive contexts, i.e. developing and developed regions of the world were targeted for design development. Through this case study, the rationale and potential for application of this concept to a broader context of inclusive design is suggested.

1 Walking Aids

Over 18% of the global population has moderate, severe or extreme difficulty with walking (WHO 2011). As the population continues to grow and age, this number is set to keep rising. Current walking aids and the systems for distributing them are inefficient and unsustainable so increasing attention is being given to the design of simpler and cheaper walking aids which can be adapted easily and are readily available (United Nations Enable 2007). Thus, facilitating the correct long-term support from a walking aid through adaptability, whilst making mobility affordable could be a focus.

A walking aid is an assistive device designed to facilitate walking by improving people's stability, balance and upright body posture which can provide them with the confidence and ability to live more independently (DFID 2004). A person's weight can be redistributed through a walking aid to reduce pressure, and thus

F. Nickpour (✉)
Inclusive Design Research Group, Brunel University London, UK
email: Farnaz.Nickpour@brunel.ac.uk

C. O'Sullivan
Cara Design Ltd., Central Research Laboratory

P. Langdon et al. (eds.), *Designing Around People*,
DOI 10.1007/978-3-319-29498-8_5

pain, from their lower limbs (Mac 2014). Without a walking aid the user may feel more pain, may not be able to walk, or might walk with an unstable gait (ECRI 2011). Timely access to suitable walking aids is extremely important, particularly for young people, as it can increase the likelihood of them attending school and being able to join in social activities with their peers which can change the trajectory of the rest of their lives (Consumer Focus 2010).

1.1 Increase in the Conditions Requiring Walking Aids

According to a report by the United Nations (2007), everyone is likely to experience disability at some point during their lifetime as a result of illness, accident or ageing. Disabilities are expected to continue rising globally due to population growth and medical advances (Global Health Education Consortium 2007) and consequently the demand for walking aids is predicted to continue growing (Buckingham 2013). According to a market report (Marketstrat Inc. 2013) the sales of walking aids will "soar in all regions" due to the escalating rates of chronic diseases which lead to mobility impairment. Mobility impairments can be caused by an in-born condition or congenital disorder, an accident, a disease or a condition which has been acquired over time (Colorado State University 2010). The most prevalent conditions which cause mobility impairment and typically require the use of a walking aids include: Acquired Brain Injury; Ageing; Amputations; Balance; Burns; Cerebral Palsy; Coordination; Fatigue; Hemiplegia; Infection; Multiple Sclerosis; Muscle weakness, injury, strain, sprain or brake; Muscular Dystrophy; Osteogenisis Imperfecta; Paralysis; Paraplegia; Quadraplegia; Rheumatoid arthritis; Skin irritation; Spina Bifida; Spinal Cord Injuries; Stroke; Tetraplegia; Vision loss (Active Living Alliance 2013).

1.2 Types of Support Provided by Walking Aids

Interviews with physiotherapists and observations of patients at a Neuro Rehab Centre helped provide a better understanding of why different features were required for each type of walking aid and established that most patients "get through a few different pieces of equipment" during the course of rehabilitation. Table 1 shows the three basic types of walking aid which are available with a range of variable features which enable them to facilitate walking across a broader spectrum of user requirements.

1.3 Common Components Review

The common variable features between the three main types of walking aid can be seen in Table 1. Disassembly of the three main types of walking aid revealed that many of their components were also similar to one another. This finding introduced the theory that a set of certain interchangeable components could enable a range of different walking aids to be created from the same parts.

Table 1 Basic types of walking aid

Walking aid name	**1. Walking stick/ cane**	**2. Crutch**	**3. Walking frames**
Example (image):	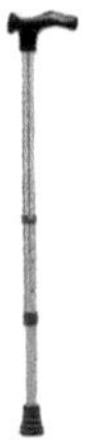 min £5	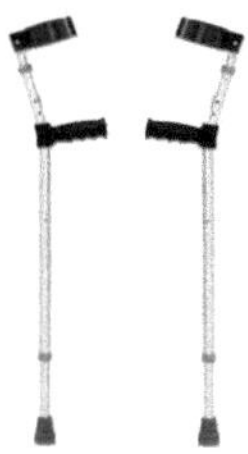 min £11	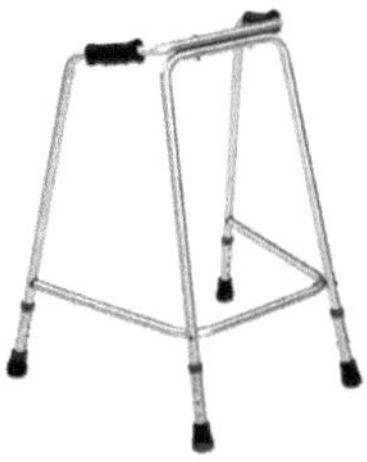 min £18
Level of support:	Low	Medium	High
Type of support:	Balance, upright posture, confidence	Weight redistribution	Stability, coordination
Variable features:	Height, handle, ferrule/ tripod/quadrupod, material	Height (axilla or forearm), handles, ferrules/foot type, elbow cuffs/underarm pads, material	Height, handles (position and shape), ferrules/front wheels, material

1.4 Importance of Correct Support and Adjustability

The conditions mentioned in section 1.1 can predominantly be improved through rehabilitation using the basic types of walking aid with the appropriate variable features listed in Table 1. The correct support can enable people to live independently and to be mobile in society and help them to reach their full potential (United Nations 2007). Changes in a person's condition are prone to take place during the course of their mobility impairment and therefore the level of support required from their walking aid, needs to change in response to the new needs (Disabled Living Foundation 2014). Using an unsuitable type of walking aid can worsen the user's condition, disrupt healing, or increase the risk of accident or injury (ECRI 2011). In the US alone, there are approximately 15 770 people hospitalised annually resulting from falls involving use of the incorrect walking aid (Stevens 2009). There is a high frequency of inappropriate walking aids being used incorrectly (Mandelstam 1997) so it is recommended that people are prescribed a walking aid after a professional health assessment of their gait, muscle strength, balance and pain rather than purchasing their own or borrowing one (Lord et al. 2001).

2 Methodology

Key insights were drawn from existing problems and opportunities identified across a broad spectrum of research sources to ensure they were valid. Both primary and secondary sources of information were included and existing literature, experts, and end users were consulted through observation, shadowing, interviews and foreign correspondence. The research was gathered through a range of qualitative data collection methods in both developed and developing regions of the world. These (developed and developing regions) were recognised as two types of contexts and explored as distinct markets for the potential solution. The co-design approach to the research helped ensure the issues and needs surrounding the product's context were accurately understood and addressed in a way which could be realistically implemented. Figure 1 provides detailed breakdown of various sources and methods used and the two contexts explored.

3 Key Findings

The most commonly highlighted issue in all contexts through various methods and sources, was the inconvenience (in terms of both access and finance) of needing different walking aids to ensure the correct support is provided. The need for adaptability in walking aid function as well as size was validated by research at rehabilitation centres, which are currently forced to have a substantial collection of walking aids that differ from one another only slightly. For example, "the different handles on the crutches cater for a range of gripping abilities" and "different types of ferrule or bases provide different levels of stability" (Mac 2014). A walking aid which is more adaptable in function as well as size would not only be safer and fit a wider range of users, but it would be financially beneficial by reducing the need for numerous different walking aids.

3.1 Transitioning between Walking Aids; Physical, Emotional and Financial Changes and Impacts

It was recognised that the process of transitioning between walking aids can have various financial, physical and emotional impacts and implications for the user. From one point of view, changing mobility aids could mean multiple purchases, thus a financial burden for the user. This could become a major barrier to access to and use of appropriate walking aid depending on the context of use (e.g. developing or developed regions of the world), provision route (e.g. private or public healthcare provision) and user's personal finance.

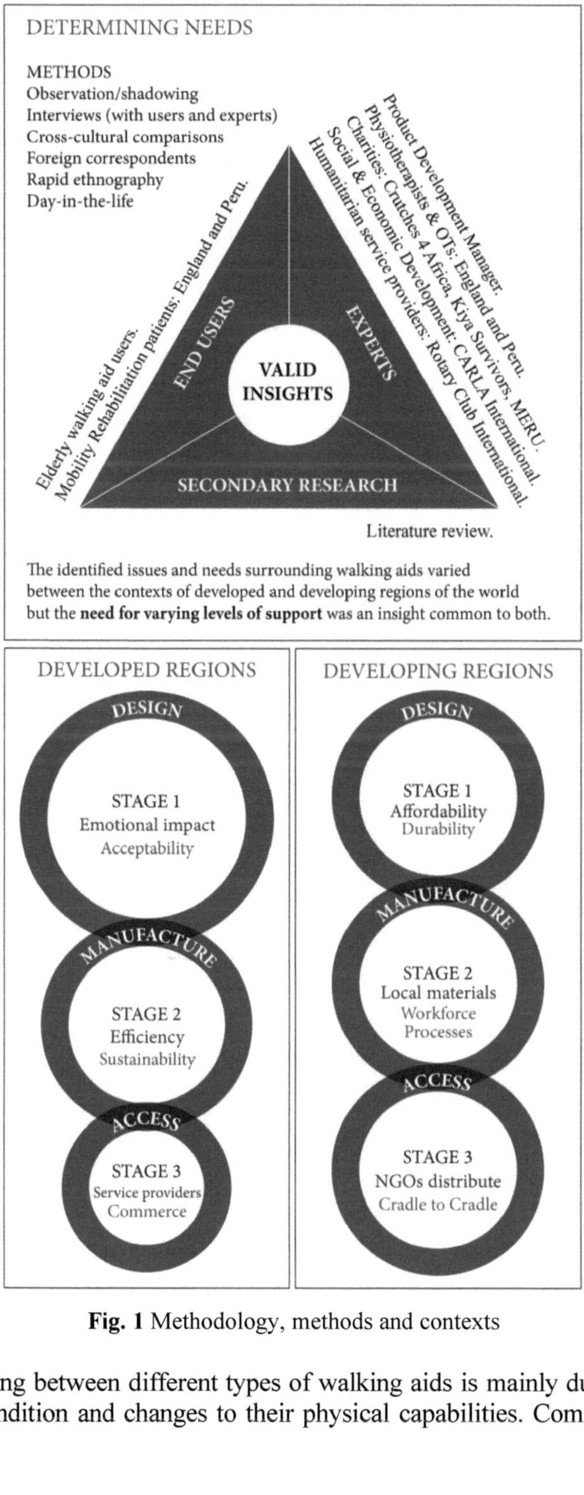

Fig. 1 Methodology, methods and contexts

Transitioning between different types of walking aids is mainly due to evolution of a user's condition and changes to their physical capabilities. Comfort and safety are key factors affected by this evolution and it is important that through this transition between walking aids, overall usability, comfort and safety of the product is well adapted to, and evolved together with the user's condition. It is also important to consider the diversity of anthropometric variables for various users and across various stages of their condition.

Shifting between various walking aids could also impact the user emotionally, most perceptibly the self-confidence, as ability to walk could have direct connection with sense of independence, overall wellbeing and perceived capability. The emotional impact of transition between walking aids could vary considerably depending on the type of transition scenario and whether the user's level of capability and therefore reliance on their walking aid was increasing or decreasing.

Two case studies of two different walking aid users (in the developed regions of the world) monitored their walking capability as their conditions changed (correlating to the level of support they required). The first user was a young female who was attending rehabilitation sessions to learn to walk. The second user was an elderly male whose mobility was deteriorating due to a problem with his health. In both cases, the progress of the condition, type of walking aid used at each stage, changes in capability and support required, and emotional impact to the changes of walking aid are illustrated in Figure 2. One key observations was the similar patterns of physical and emotional changes in both scenarios of rehabilitation and degeneration, yet in opposite directions.

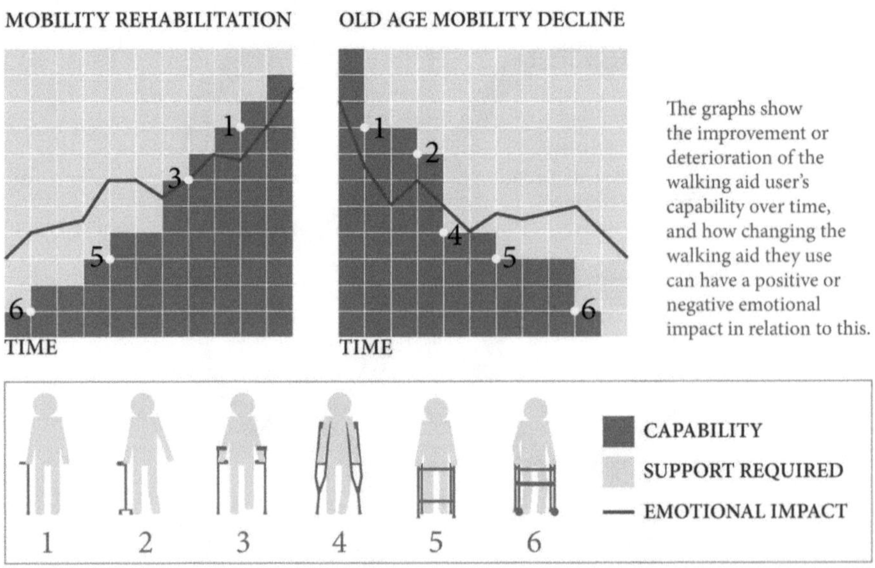

Fig. 2 Physical transitions and emotional impacts of changing walking aids - Rehabilitation and degeneration scenarios

3.2 Identifying Market Needs

The viability, feasibility and desirability of each stage of the project and product use was considered in the context of both developed and developing regions of the world. It was concluded that a solution to the identified issues would be useful and meaningful for both developed and developing regions of the world, while significantly improving different aspects in each context (see Figure 1). In the context of developing countries, the significant influence was due to the potential improvement of end users' experience on all levels (design, manufacture and access). This meant the affordability and evolvability were the key design principles. In contrast to this, developed regions already have considerable access and infrastructure for walking aid distribution, as well as manufacturing equipment and workforce availability, therefore key design principles were evolvability of the product and improving its desirability in terms of emotional needs and durability.

3.3 Existing Solutions, Standards and Regulations

No products or resources have been found in the form of a set of components which can be assembled to make various types of walking aid; however in parallel to the modularity aspect, various cutlery assessment kits have been found (Figure 3) which consist of a range of components which can be interchanged to make up different products. A patent was found for a product which attached to the handle of a mop, broom, rake or similar tool to turn it into a single arm crutch. The idea of turning existing equipment into a walking aid is something which could make sense in a low resource setting.

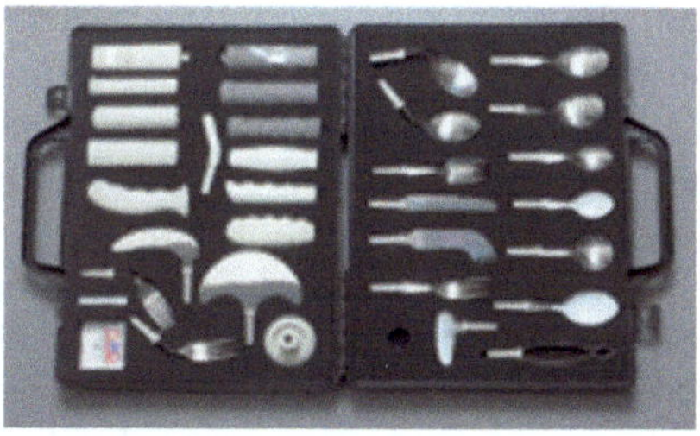

Fig. 3 Interchangeable cutlery kit (Paisley Mobility Centre 2014)

Health and safety considerations are essential in the design of a walking aid and for this reason there are several tests that the design needs to pass in order to be classed as safe to use. The main standards cover requirements and test methods for different types of walking aid but because this product intends to act as more than one type of walking aid it will need to pass the tests from all relevant standards including those for walking frames, elbow crutches, walking sticks with three or more legs, durability and friction of tips.

4 Design Principles

Through extensive user research and a collaborative approach to gaining insights, empathy for the end users was developed. In response to the validated insights and research findings, the project explored the route of designing a modular walking aid kit for use in both developing and developed regions of the world. The proposed design was to implement 'evolvability' and improve 'affordability' in the design process which would take advantage of future generational changes and reduce the long term costs of upgrading or replacing the walking aid as it could be done gradually by component rather than all at once. Longevity of such walking aid system is one major element of evolvability and it should be achieved not only on a physical but also emotional level. Emotional durability (Chapman 2005) of a walking aid system thus becomes increasingly important as the nature of transition between various walking aids has major positive or negative emotional impacts and also in the long term, it is important for the walking aid system to remain meaningful and emotionally connected to the user as their values and desires and feelings continue to change (Chapman 2005).

Thus, three main design principles were distilled from this research to be applied and referred to throughout the design process:

- design for evolvability
- design for affordability
- design for emotional durability

4.1 Concept Direction and Future Development

The concept focused on developing a walking aid kit (Figure 4) that could be tailored to the specific needs of a user in order to provide the correct support through principles of evolvability, affordability and emotional durability. The product was considered to be presented in the form of a kit, similar to Meccano®. This would require minimal technical ability to adjust, an enabling feature in the developing regions of the world. In order to define the components required in this kit, a selection of existing walking aids were disassembled and the common components and features listed. A system was then to be developed to enable them all to be connected with one another. The material selection and manufacturing process plays an important role since the product should be lightweight and robust. If focusing on developing regions of the world, simplicity to process/manufacture, with the possibility of local manufacture in the future, easy-to-transport, and cheap material are also important factors as the selection of material would take into consideration the access to resources, and the tools and energy required to process it.

The concept has received very positive feedback worldwide and is currently in the development stage in both the developing and developed regions of the world; The Evolvable Walking Aid Kit is a finalist in the Inclusive Technology Prize (Inclusive Technology Prize 2015) run by Nesta, with support from the Office for Disability Issues, Innovate UK and The Department for Business Innovation. The project has received £10,000 as well as non-financial support for the concept to be developed and prototyped for the UK market.

Also, in collaboration with Kenya High Commission in the UK, Crutches 4 Africa and local charities in Kenya, early prototypes are being developed for testing in rural areas in Kenya.

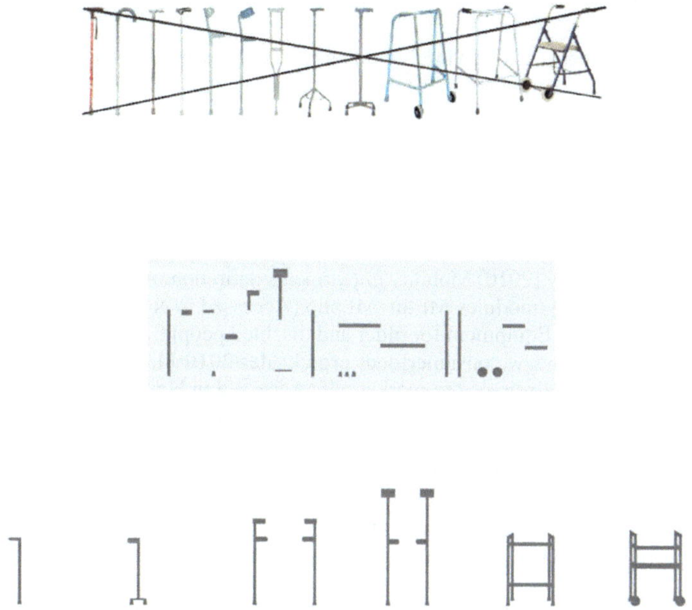

Fig. 4 Simplified concept

5 Conclusion

Through the case study of Evolvable Walking Aid Kit, this paper has explored how products can be redesigned to allow flexibility for changes in a user's condition. Thus providing comfort, control and ownership over the person's care, building meaningful, emotionally durable and connected product experiences in the long-term, while offering viable, cost-effective and sustainable healthcare solutions.

The case study of the Evolvable Walking Aid Kit, puts forward the idea of modular healthcare products that incorporate three key principles of 'evolvability', 'affordability' and 'emotional durability'. While none of these principles is new as such to inclusive design field, their combination could offer a holistic, empathic and sustainable approach to design of products, services and environments that are person-centred and evolve together with and around the person - both physically and emotionally, as their condition and context of life changes. Such rationale and potential is to be further explored, considered and applied in the wider field of inclusive design and in the design of inclusive healthcare products such as home use medical devices, hearing aids and other types of mobility products.

References

Active Living Alliance (2013) Mobility impairments general information. Available at: www.ala.ca/Content/TipSheets/Tips/mobility_impairment.asp?langid=1 (Accessed in November 2015)

Buckingham C (2013) The growth of the UK disability aids market. Available at: www.buckinghamhealthcare.co.uk/disability-aids/?s=the+growth+of&x=0&y=0 (Accessed in November 2015)

Chapman J (2005) Emotionally durable design: Objects, experiences and empathy. Earthscan, London

Colorado State University (2010) Mobility impairments definition. Available at: accessproject. colostate.edu/disability/modules/MI/tut_MI.php (Accessed in November 2015)

Consumer Focus (2010) Equipment for older and disabled people: An analysis of the market. Available at: www.consumerfocus.org.uk/files/2010/11/Equipment-for-older-and-disabled-people-an-analysis-of-the-market.pdf (Accessed in November 2015)

DFID (2004) Enhancing the mobility of disabled people: Guidelines for practitioners. Available at: r4d.dfid.gov.uk/PDF/Outputs/r8016.pdf (Accessed in November 2015)

Disabled Living Foundation (2014) Choosing walking equipment. Available at: www.dlf.org.uk/factsheets/walking (Accessed in November 2015)

ECRI (2011) Ambulation aids. Available at: www.ecri.org/Documents/PSA/February_2011/Equip1.pdf (Accessed on 30 October 2015)

Global Health Education Consortium (2007) Disability and rehabilitation in developing countries. Texas Woman's University, Dallas, TX, USA

Inclusive Technology Prize (2015) Available at: www.inclusivetechprize.org/news-blogs/ congratulations-10-finalists (Accessed in November 2015)

Mac A (2014) Physiotherapist at QEF Neuro Rehabilitation Centre. Interview on 16 September 2014

Mandelstam M (1997) Equipment for older or disabled people and the law, p. 513. Jessica Kingsley Publishers, London

Marketstrat Inc. (2013) World market for personal mobility devices (wheelchairs, scooters, walking aids). MarketStrat, Pleasanton, CA, USA

Paisley Mobility Centre (2014) Homecraft kings assessment kit 33 pieces. Available at: paisleymobilitycentre.co.uk/homecraft-kings-assessment-pieces-p-3010.html (Accessed in November 2015)

Stevens JA, Thomas K, Teh L, Greenspan AI (2009) Unintentional falls injuries associated with walkers and canes in older adults treated in U.S. emergency departments J Am Geriatr Soc. 57(8): 1464-9

United Nations Enable (2007) World programme of action concerning disabled persons. Available at: www.un.org/disabilities/default.asp?id=23 (Accessed in November 2015)

United Nations (2007) Handbook for parliamentarians on the convention on the rights of persons with disabilities. United Nations Department of Economic and Social Affairs, Geneva, Switzerland

WHO (2011) Joint position paper on the provision of mobility devices in less resourced settings. World Health Organisation Press, Geneva, Switzerland

Rhythmic Haptic Cueing for Entrainment: Assisting Post-stroke Gait Rehabilitation

T. Georgiou, S. Holland and J. van der Linden

Abstract: Restoring mobility and rehabilitation of gait are high priorities for rehabilitation from neurological conditions. Cueing using metronomic rhythmic sensory stimulation via entrainment has been shown to improve gait, but almost all previous versions of this approach have used auditory or visual cues. In contrast, we have developed and pilot-tested a prototype wearable system for rhythmic cueing based on haptics. Our initial pilot study indicated the same kinds of improvement to gait with haptics as for other cueing modalities, but haptics offer some advantages over audio and visual cues. In particular, haptics are generally more practical for use out of doors, in noisy environments, or when wishing to keep open the ability to converse freely. However, haptics also allow the precisely targeted spatial placement of cues on alternate limbs, offering the ability to manipulate attention and proprioception for therapeutic benefit. We outline the theory behind our approach and report on the iterative design of the system as part of a user-centred design evaluation process involving a wide range of stakeholders.

1 Introduction

Stroke is a sudden and devastating disease with major implications to a person's health and quality of life. In contrast to other sudden diseases, such as heart disease, stroke has a long-term disability burden. The disability impact of stroke is greater than any other chronic disease, causing a wider range of complex disabilities (including locomotion, dexterity, and communication related disabilities), making stroke a leading cause of adult disability (Adamson et al. 2004). More than half of all stroke survivors are left dependent on others for everyday activities (Intercollegiate Stroke Working Party 2012).

After acute specialist hospital care, a person's recovery can significantly improve with regular rehabilitation exercises both in the early days after a stroke and long after they return home (Galvin et al. 2009). Indeed, even rehabilitation carried out

T. Georgiou (✉) · S. Holland · J. van der Linden
Centre for Research in Computing, The Open University, Milton Keynes, UK
e-mail: Theodoros.Georgiou@open.ac.uk

P. Langdon et al. (eds.), *Designing Around People*,
DOI 10.1007/978-3-319-29498-8_6

years after a stroke can still lead to improvements. However, effective rehabilitation outside a clinical setting and without guidance can be difficult to achieve.

New wearable technologies offer the possibility of small, light inconspicuous devices, which are capable of supporting day-to-day rehabilitation exercises through appropriate guidance and monitoring. However, there are serious challenges involved in the design of such systems. Wearable healthcare systems need to take into account the physical, sensory and cognitive abilities of intended users. Addressing these problems involves user-centred design approaches, including the designing of functional prototypes that users can engage with in depth.

Prototypes help designers to understand diverse real world issues and to identify and evaluate potential improvements. They enable participants to physically explore the possibilities of new technologies, and provide a source of inspiration for future use scenarios.

In this paper we describe our approach of assisting gait rehabilitation by providing rhythmic haptic (i.e. touch-based) cues through a technology known as the *Haptic Bracelets*. The Haptic Bracelets (discussed in detail below) were originally developed (and still are used) to support the development of musical skills in learning multi-limbed rhythms (Holland et al. 2010, Bouwer et al. 2013). They were subsequently adapted for gait rehabilitation using haptic cues, drawing on the established use of rhythmic audio and visual cues for gait rehabilitation using entrainment, as outlined below.

The Haptic Bracelets are light wearable and wireless devices, designed to work in pairs, one strapped on each leg at ankle height. The devices are capable of monitoring several aspects of the wearer's gait in high resolution and provide rhythmic haptic cues through an array of vibrotactile motors. The person wearing them is instructed to feel the haptic cues and try to time their steps to that rhythm.

Before detailing the design and implementation of the Haptic Bracelets, it is useful to consider the mechanisms underlying the human ability to sense and follow a rhythm or rhythmic pattern.

2 Rhythmic Cueing for Entrainment (RCE)

The mechanisms by which an external rhythmic stimulus can affect and improve a persons gait may not be immediately obvious. The mechanism is neither stimulus response nor direct muscle stimulus, but rather biological *entrainment*.

To understand the difference, consider everyday applications of vibrotactiles, which typically focus on notifications and alerts. Applications of this kind are best understood in terms of stimulus response. When, for example, a smartphone in silent mode vibrates to give an alert, there is a necessary delay in perception while the sensory stimulus is processed, and then a further delay while any resulting human action is enacted. Broadly, this process is one of stimulus and response (though variants can involve cognitively learned responses, conditioned responses, or direct muscle responses).

Therefore, responses to notifications and alerts always involve delays. By contrast, after hearing a few initial beats, most people can generally tap along to a regular pulse in more or less exact synchronisation. This is a special case of biological entrainment.

Entrainment is a physical phenomenon whereby two rhythmic processes interact with each other until they adjust to a common (or closely related) rhythm. The phenomenon was first identified in the fields of physics and mathematics, and is characterised by the effect that one harmonic oscillator has on the motion of a second nearby powered oscillator which is oscillating at a similar frequency. More specifically, entrainment is the process where two autonomous oscillating bodies, which have different periods when they function independently, assume a common or simply related period.

Instances of entrainment must adhere to two major rules (Clayton et al. 2005):

1. **Two or more autonomous rhythmic processes or oscillators must exist.** All oscillators in the system must be able to oscillate on their own, even if they do not interact with each other. Therefore all oscillators must have an internal source of energy and not depend on the interaction for producing the oscillations. This rule distinguishes entrainment from other phenomena, such as *resonance* for example, where the oscillations stop as soon as one oscillating body (e.g. tuning fork) detaches from the other (e.g. resonance box). This in essence means that, an observation of synchronised behaviour or even a synchronous variation between two variables does not necessarily indicate entrainment.
2. **There must be a link to allow the oscillations to interact**. A link must exist between the oscillators, which is weak enough so as not cause the oscillators to lose their individuality, but is strong enough to link the interaction between the oscillators.

It was only recently (early 1990s) that biological instantiations of entrainment were identified. The human body is full of naturally occurring rhythms, with the heart beating, respiration, and various perceptual processes being just few of them. These endogenous rhythms may very easily entrain to each other within a single person (e.g. the synchronisation of respiration and heart rhythm patterns of high performance swimmers (Schäfer et al. 1998)) or with external rhythms that fit the above characterisations (e.g. singers whose heartbeats entrain to the rhythm of the music they are singing (Vickhoff et al. 2013)).

Since the early nineties, the concept of entrainment has been explicitly applied to gait rehabilitation, as detailed below.

2.1 RCE for Gait Rehabilitation

Stroke survivors commonly experience what is known as hemiparetic gait where one side of the survivor's body is physically weakened. Hemiparetic gait is characterised variously by increased step length variability (Balasubramanian et al. 2009), and temporal and spatial gait asymmetry (Chen et al. 2005). Many health problems are associated with this disorder, for example the non-paretic (stronger) limb may be exposed to higher vertical forces (Kim and Eng 2003) which can lead to joint pains (Norvell et al. 2005), degeneration (Nolan et al. 2003) and increased risk of fractures.

Entrainment can be used to help patients suffering from gait related disorders assume a more symmetrical walking rhythm (Thaut et al. 1993) via mechanisms that we will now explain.

The provision of an external rhythmic cue can assist the brain to control the movement of the leg swing in several different ways. Firstly, and most obviously the external rhythm gives a recurring reference for the period of the desired swing. Perhaps less obviously, it can also make the motion smoother, with less variability of movement trajectory and can lead to more even muscle recruitment (Thaut et al. 2015). These effects are caused by changes in muscle activation patterns, with the associated brain plasticity making it possible to re-program movement. Thus, the effect of the cue is to optimise diverse aspects of motor control via physiological period entrainment of the motor system (Thaut et al. 1999).

As already noted, different modalities can be used to deliver the rhythmic cues for entrainment: audio, visual and our proposal of haptic (summarised below).

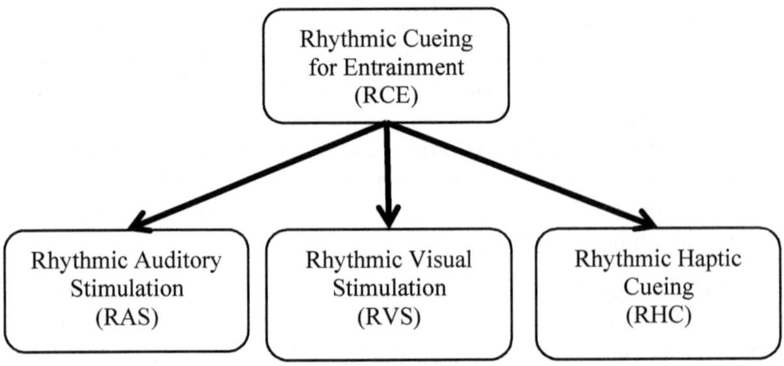

Fig. 1 Different modalities for rhythmic cueing for entrainment

2.2 Existing Applications of Entrainment to Gait Rehabilitation

The idea of using metronomic cueing to support gait rehabilitation for people suffering from various neurological conditions has been explored by researchers using a variety of sensory channels, principally auditory and visual.

Rhythmic audio cueing (RAS) delivered through headphones has been shown to lead to gait improvements with immediate effects (Thaut et al. 2007). In some cases, these improvements may last beyond the immediate application of the cues (Benoit et al. 2014).

More specifically, studies with participants suffering from post-stroke gait impairments walking on a treadmill, and RAS providing the walking rhythm, show improvements in spatial (Prassas et al. 1997) and temporal symmetry

(Roerdink et al. 2007) as well as significant improvements in step time asymmetry and the step time variability (Wright et al. 2013).

Similar encouraging results were also observed during rhythmic *visual* stimulation (RVS) where cues were projected in front of participants walking on a treadmill as stepping stones, with increase in stride length being the most prominent one (Bank et al. 2011).

Rhythmic cueing is therefore a promising approach, but the use of audio or visual cueing modes can be problematic outside the controlled environment of a lab or a clinic. When outside a clinical setting, it is generally important to keep the audio channel clear. This allows one to remain aware of the environment, or to deal with traffic or just to hold conversations while walking. Approaches involving visual cues and projections in front of a user while walking typically require extensive laboratory installations, and in any case are highly distracting.

Haptics on the other hand leave sight and hearing unobstructed. This makes haptics particularly well suited for gait rehabilitation outside controlled environments such as labs and clinics. This opens up new ways in which stroke survivors can take charge of their own rehabilitation.

Evidence suggests that rehabilitation in the home environment can be more beneficial than in a clinical setting (Hillier and Inglis-Jassiem 2010). The approach of self-managed rehabilitation has the potential to offer substantial cost savings for health services, considering that the current stroke care provision plan in the UK is estimated to cost an average of £24,855 per patient (National Audit Office 2010).

3 Rhythmic Haptic Cueing for Entrainment

In an earlier pilot study where *rhythmic haptic cueing* (RHC) was used for providing walking rhythm to a participant through RHC entrainment (Holland et al. 2014), the participant's step length was found to increase, while a range of other measures such as the paretic (affected by stroke), hip angle at toe off, peak knee flexion during swing and ankle range of motion showed significant clinical improvement indicating improved gait movement and similar walking benefits to those of audio rhythm.

This approach of using RHC for entrainment in gait rehabilitation not only helps to overcome some of the practical limitations in audio and visual cueing approaches (e.g. intrusiveness and masking of the audio and visual channel) but may also have some interesting advantages, unique to the RHC approach. RHC, for example, has the ability to target specific limbs through different spatial placement, with the potential to manipulate attention and proprioception for therapeutic benefit.

In a qualitative user-centred study aimed at investigating the views of stroke survivors and health professionals (Georgiou et al. 2015), comments from both groups both were generally positive. More specifically, all four stroke survivors agreed that the haptic cue gave them "a rhythm to walk to".

4 Technology and Prototype Development for RHC

In this section we will consider the first three iterations in the design of the Haptic Bracelets (HBI, HBII and HBIII), the prototype wearable devices we are using to assist gait rehabilitation via RHC.

Even though the earlier version (HBI) could deliver high quality rhythmic haptic cue in a precise manner, leading to clinically positive results in pilot trials, hardware limitations meant that they could only gather a limited range of gait related data, and networking limitations meant that under certain conditions data could get corrupted. This motivated us to redesign the devices from the ground up, adding sensors with higher temporal resolution for gait monitoring and better networking protocols. During this process, the devices also got smaller, lighter and gained better battery life.

HBII measured 47x34x15mm, with a custom designed and 3D printed case enclosing all the electronic components. A vibrotactile actuator of 24.9mm length and 8.8mm diameter protrudes from it on a wire of variable length. These prototype devices (designed to work in pairs of two) can be seen on Figure 2.

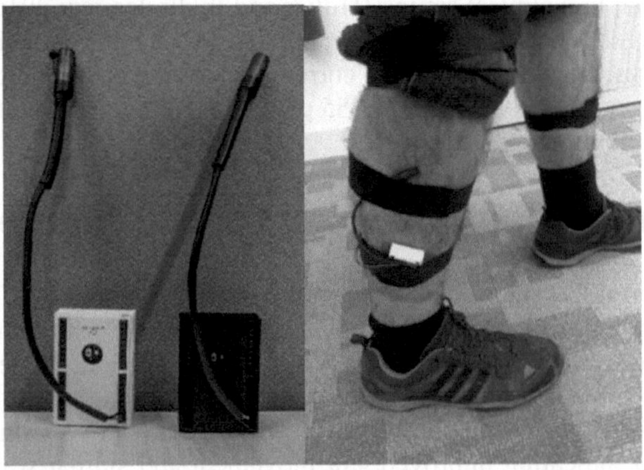

Fig. 2 Last user-tested version of the Haptic Bracelets (left). A Haptic Bracelet device strapped on a user's leg (right).

Each HBII contain a complete Inertia Monitoring Unit (IMU). The IMU is made up of a six degrees of freedom accelerometer, gyroscope and magnetometer (i.e. all sensors can measure data in three axes) and can sample data at a maximum rate of 400Hz (400 times a second) before sending them to a central control unit.

All communications between the central control unit (i.e. laptop) and the Haptic Bracelets are sent over Wi-Fi using the Open Sound Control transport control protocol. Each HBII unit is uniquely identified in the network by their IP addresses, making it easy to analyse and log data coming from specific HBII units and to send targeted instructions (e.g. when and how intensely to vibrate). All time stamping on the data received is done on the central control unit to ensure consistency, since temporal precision is important, and the local clocks on the two bracelets can drift slightly relative to each other.

The entire HBII wearable system is powered by two batteries of 3000mAh each, capable of providing a regulated 5V output. The batteries can be recharged using a standard micro-USB cable and a 5V, 1.2A charger (standard USB charger). Ease of charging is an important design goal in self-managed settings.

4.1 Participative Design Development and Evaluation

While the initial pilot study (Holland et al. 2014) raised some interesting questions regarding the design and placement of the devices from the participant's point of view, more in-depth dialogue with potential users and other major stakeholders of the system, such as physiotherapists, clinicians and health professionals was desired.

For the qualitative, more user-centred follow up study (Georgiou et al. 2015), we invited four stroke survivors (compared to one in the pilot study), three health professionals (a professor of nursing and two experienced physiotherapists) and three interaction designers. During this study, we engaged in in-depth discussions with all parties involved.

Two issues considered (Georgiou et al. 2015) were the way the devices are secured on the wearer's leg, and the control the of vibration intensity.

In the case of securing the devices, stroke survivors generally lose significant motor control on one of their hand as well as their leg (same side). That makes it difficult for them to secure a Velcro strap on their legs tightly enough. Difficulties in securing the devices on their legs without any assistance may put off users from using them, or as Mountain et al. point out: *'[...] any technological devices should be [...] usable preferably without the help of the carer, to encourage independence [...].'* (Mountain et al. 2006).

The current iteration of the HBIII system (currently under development) tries to tackle this design issue. In the new design, the Velcro straps are replaced by a tubular bandage holding all the electronic components. The user can then wear the HBIII devices as they would wear a pair of socks. The efficacy of this new strapping mechanism will have to be tested and evaluated with stroke survivors in another follow up study in the future (see Figure 3).

Stroke survivors participating in our latest study (Georgiou et al. 2015) responded positively to the haptic cueing, however a significant point was made regarding the intensity of the vibration. Due to their condition, and depending on how severe their stroke episode was, stroke survivors may have different levels of sensitivity on their limbs. For example, what may be a clearly perceptible buzz to one survivor may not be at all detectable to another.

In the first HB iteration (HBI), the intensity could be adjusted via a physical wheel on the device and through the Wi-Fi network. However, during the redesign process, that wheel was removed and the only way for adjusting the vibration intensity was through the network. This added a significant burden to the network, which interfered with the overall quality of the haptic cueing (e.g. missed and variable signal timings). In order to solve this, an Arduino Micro is used for controlling the total power received by the vibrotactiles via a technique known as Pulse Width Modulation (PWM). This allowed us to deliver haptic cues varying in intensity from a g-force of 0.5g all the way up to 10g, while retaining a well-shaped buzz via the dynamic braking of the vibrotactile motors.

In order to make the HB system more comfortable to wear, the 3D printed case protecting the electronic components for HBIII, has all edges smoothed and rounded to avoid catching on the wearers' clothes. Again, these new design features will be tested in future studies and interactive design workshops with stroke survivors and other major stakeholders (e.g. health professionals).

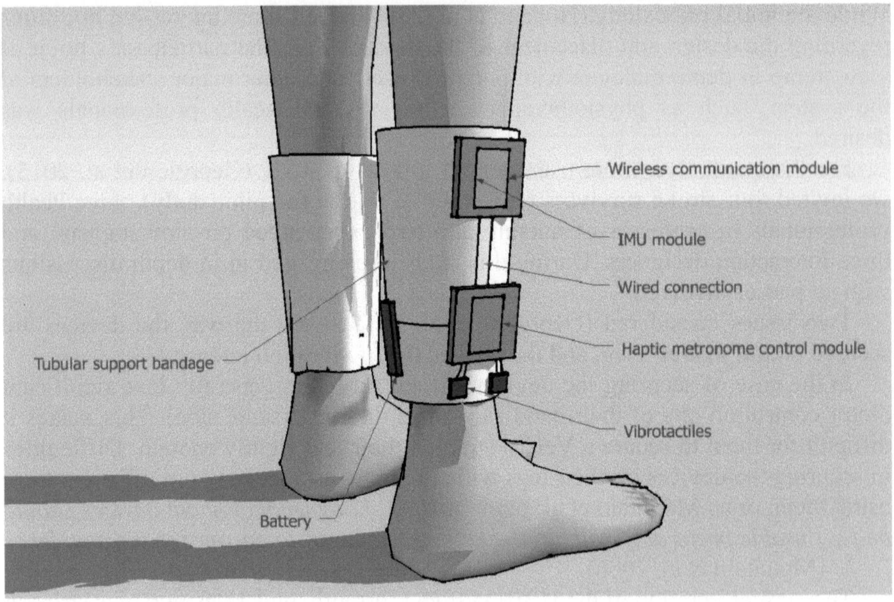

Fig. 3 Rendering of the latest Haptic Bracelet III prototype

5 Conclusion

Rhythmic cueing for entrainment is an important approach to gait rehabilitation for neurological conditions. In this paper we have outlined the theory behind this approach to rehabilitation. Walking to an audio or a visual rhythm has immediate, and sometimes lasting, gait related benefits. Haptic cueing has been shown in early pilot studies to be equally effective, and has the potential of being more suitable for use outside the controlled environment of the lab or clinic by end users. In particular, haptics leave sight and hearing unobstructed. This makes haptics particularly well suited for gait rehabilitation outside controlled environments such as labs and clinics. In this paper we have reported on three design iterations of the Haptic Bracelets, developed especially for this approach to gait rehabilitation. The designs have been guided by an on-going user-centred design evaluation process, involving a wide range of stakeholders. Rhythmic haptic cueing for entrainment promises to open up new ways in which stroke survivors can take charge of their own rehabilitation.

References

Adamson J, Beswick A, Ebrahim S (2004) Is stroke the most common cause of disability? Journal of Stroke and Cerebrovascular Diseases 13(4): 171-177

Balasubramanian CK, Neptune RR, Kautz SA (2009) Variability in spatiotemporal step characteristics and its relationship to walking performance post-stroke. Gait and Posture 29(3): 408-414

Bank PJ, Roerdink M, Peper CE (2011) Comparing the efficacy of metronome beeps and stepping stones to adjust gait: steps to follow! Experimental Brain Research 209(2): 159-169

Benoit CE, Dalla Bella S, Farrugia N, Obrig, H, Mainka S, Kotz S (2014) Musically cued gait-training improves both perceptual and motor timing in Parkinson's disease. Frontiers in Human Neuroscience 8(494)

Bouwer A, Holland S, Dalgleish M (2013) The haptic bracelets: Learning multi-limb rhythm skills from haptic stimuli while reading. In: Holland S, Wilkie K, Mulholland P, Seago A (Eds.) Music and human-computer interaction, pp. 101-122. Springer, London, UK

Chen G, Patten C, Kothari DH, Zajac FE (2005) Gait differences between individuals with post-stroke hemiparesis and non-disabled controls at matched speeds. Gait and Posture 22(1): 51-56

Clayton M, Sager R, Will U (2005) In time with the music: The concept of entrainment and its significance for ethnomusicology. European Meetings in Ethnomusicology 11(1): 1-82

Galvin R, Cusack T, Stokes E (2009) To what extent are family members and friends involved in physiotherapy and the delivery of exercises to people with stroke? Disability and Rehabilitation 31(11): 898-905

Georgiou T, Holland S, van der Linden J, Tetley J, Stockley RC, Donaldson G et al. (2015) A blended user centred design study for wearable haptic gait rehabilitation following hemiparetic stroke. In: Proceedings of the 9th International Conference on Pervasive Computing Technologies for Healthcare, Istanbul, Turkey

Hillier S, Inglis-Jassiem G (2010) Rehabilitation for community-dwelling people with stroke: Home or centre based? International Journal of Stroke 5(3): 178-186

Holland S, Bouwer AJ, Dalgelish M, Hurtig TM (2010) Feeling the beat where it counts: Fostering multi-limb rhythm skills with the haptic drum kit. In: Proceedings of the 4th International Conference on Tangible, Embedded, and Embodied Interaction, Cambridge, MA, USA

Holland S, Wright RL, Wing A, Crevoisier T, Hödl O, Canelli M (2014) A gait rehabilitation pilot study using tactile cueing following hemiparetic stroke. In: Proceedings of the 8th International Conference on Pervasive Computing Technologies for Healthcare, Oldenburg, Germany

Intercollegiate Stroke Working Party (2012) National sentinel stroke clinical audit 2010 round 7. National and local results for the clinical audit 2010. Generic report prepared on behalf of the Intercollegiate Stroke Working Party and Royal College of Physicians

Kim CM, Eng JJ (2003) The relationship of lower-extremity muscle torque to locomotor performance in people with stroke. Physical Therapy 83(1): 49-57

Mountain GA, Ware PM, Hammerton J, Mawson SJ, Zheng H, Davies R et al. (2006) The SMART project: A user led approach to developing applications for domiciliary stroke rehabilitation. In: Clarkson J, Langdon PM, Robinson P (Eds.) Designing accessible technology, pp. 135-144. Springer, London, UK

National Audit Office (2010) Progress in improving stroke care: Report on the findings from our modelling of stroke care provision. Audit Report, HMSO, London, UK

Nolan L, Wit A, Dudziñski K, Lees A, Lake M, Wychowański M (2003) Adjustments in gait symmetry with walking speed in trans-femoral and trans-tibial amputees. Gait and Posture 17 (2): 142-151

Norvell DC, Czerniecki JM, Reiber GE, Maynard C, Pecoraro JA, Weiss NS (2005) The prevalence of knee pain and symptomatic knee osteoarthritis among veteran traumatic amputees and nonamputees. Archives of Physical Medicine and Rehabilitation 86(3): 487-151

Prassas S, Thaut M, McIntosh G, Rice R (1997) Effect of auditory rhythmic cueing on gait kinematic parameters of stroke patients. Gait and Posture 6(3): 218-223

Roerdink M, Lamoth J, Kwakkel G, Wieringen C, Beek J (2007) Gait coordination after stroke: Benefits of acoustically paced treadmill walking. Physical Therapy 87(8): 1009-1022

Schäfer C, Rosenblum MG, Kurths J, Abel H (1998) Heartbeat synchronized with ventilation. Nature 392: 239-240

Thaut MH, Kenyon GP, Schauer ML, McIntosh GC (1999) The connection between rhythmicity and brain function. Engineering in Medicine and Biology Magazine 18(2): 101-108

Thaut MH, Leins AK, Rice RR, Argstatter H, Kenyon GP, McIntosh GC et al. (2007) Rhythmic auditory stimulation improves gait more than NDT/Bobath training in near-ambulatory patients early poststroke: A single-blind, randomized trial. Neurorehabil Neural Repair 21(5): 455-459

Thaut MH, McIntosh GC, Hoemberg V (2015) Neurobiological foundations of neurologic music therapy: Rhythmic entrainment and the motor system. Frontiers in Psychology 5: 1-6

Thaut MH, McIntosh GC, Prassas SG, Rice RR (1993) Effect of rhythmic auditory cuing on temporal stride parameters and EMG. Patterns in hemiparetic gait of stroke patients. Journal of Neurorehabilitation and Neural Repair 7(1): 9-16

Vickhoff B, Malmgren H, Åström R, Nyberg G, Engvall M, Snygg J (2013) Music structure determines heart rate variability of singers. Frontiers in Psychology 4 (334)

Wright RL, Masood A, MacCormac ES, Pratt D, Sackley C, Wing A (2013) Metronome-cued stepping in place after hemiparetic stroke: Comparison of a one- and two-tone beat. ISRN Rehabilitation 2013(157410): 1-5

Introducing Assistive Tactile Colour Symbols for Children with Visual Impairment: A Preliminary Research

S. Ramsamy-Iranah, S. Rosunee and N. Kistamah

Abstract: Colour has little significance for children with visual impairments, yet they use colour in their everyday life. This study explore and develop six tactile symbols to represent colour that were implemented in the learning tools of children with visual impairment. This concept was introduced to two age groups of children with low vision and totally blind by conducting learning sessions with them in their school environment. An evaluation process in terms of speed recognition of the colour symbols on the learning tools was carried out with each age group. This assessment provide an initial analysis on the response of the children to this new concept.

1 Introduction

The World Health Organisation has reported that globally about 1.4 million children are blind and/or visually impaired (WHO 2014). In Mauritius, out of a population of 1.22 million, an estimated 7800 people are visually impaired out of which about 0.07% are below the age of 20 (Government of Mauritius 2014).

Vision forms part of the learning process for children, the loss of it can interfere in their social, motor and emotional development. Important areas like communication, wakefulness, spatial concepts, balance, picture perception and language development are severely affected. The ability to perceive people and objects around are inaccurate (Rudman 2005). Therefore they have to be taught how to play and be given special attention to develop their other senses. Colour has little significance for children with visual impairments as colour is identified by using the visual sense (Eriksson 1994). However, pedagogical tools, books and daily use objects have the element of colour so this put them in a disadvantage in their daily activities. In much research conducted for children with visual impairments, the aspect of colour is conspicuously absent.

S. Ramsamy-Iranah (✉) · S. Rosunee · N. Kistamah
University of Mauritius, Réduit, Mauritius
email: s.ramsamy@uom.ac.mu

P. Langdon et al. (eds.), *Designing Around People*,
DOI 10.1007/978-3-319-29498-8_7

The aim of this study was to develop a colour system adapted for children with visual impairments in Mauritius, using simple tactile symbols that would enable them to identify colours in their pedagogical activities. The research presented in this paper was the initial part of a major scope of study involving a series of tactile symbols and their implementation. It first covers a literature review of a few concepts on colour labeling systems; a methodology comprising of the development of a first set of six tactile symbols representing the primary and secondary colours and subsequently integrated in learning tools such as ring and shaped abacus stacking and 3D geo designs, amongst others. As a result an evaluation process was carried out to analyze the children's speed of recognition in identifying the colours on each tool.

2 Literature Review

'Touch' is one of the senses that visually impaired individuals use to identify shapes and surfaces of objects. Heller and Schiff (1991) stated that many aspects of objects and space can be distinguished accurately only by touch when vision fails, such as fine textures and surface variation. The role of touch is amplified when one loses one or more major senses such as the sight. Discovering and learning new shapes can be a daunting experience for visually impaired children. They have to be guided through the shapes, and taught by taking their hands and guiding their fingers over the outline of shapes (Eriksson 1994).

Tactile symbols are classified into three types: line symbols that designate boundaries of lines, textural symbols that show areas and point symbols to indicate precise location (Kops and Gardner 1996). There are certain factors that influence tactile symbols such as the elevation height, size, shape and texture, orientation, and stimulus redundancy.

The height elevations of symbols are important when trying to identify by touch. The more pronounced the elevation height the easier to identify (Perera 2002).

There are a few systems for colour identification that have tried to relate tactile characteristics to colour for people with visual impairment. They are summarized in the following subsections.

2.1 Tactile Colour Communication

Tactile colour is a set of textured self-adhesive vinyl representing twelve colours. This system has been developed and adopted in Canada. Each texture on the vinyl is distinctive and has a particular feel which reflects a colour. Contrasting or opposite colours such as black and white are represented by contrasting textures.

The coloured textures are used to make maps, cards, and images and also for colour identification cards with embossed print and Braille, shaped identification stickers and jigsaw puzzles. Tactile colour helps visually impaired people identify colours and interpret information by touch. The textures are also used as purely tactile information for shape definition without any relation to colour. This system is not easy to implement for visually impaired children and can be confusing. It is also not standardized worldwide and so is not well known in other part of the world.

2.2 The Slade Colour System

The Slade colour system was created by Slade in 2004 with the concept of using three dimensional shapes to convey colour by touch (Vision Awareness 2014). There are sixteen different shapes, and each shape is representative of a colour. This three-dimensional concept enables blind people who have less sensitive touch to identify colour. The shapes are manufactured in plastic and applicable for playing pieces such as board games, tactile graphics, and coloured clothing buttons. Ten coloured shapes are produced as pegs specifically for board games and sixteen shapes are manufactured as colour indicating buttons for clothing and household items.

The primary range of colour indicating buttons are mostly simple geometrical shapes and they are distinguished by gripping the shapes using two fingers and thumb or by laying three fingers over the button to feel the 3D shape. Each button is about three-quarter inch width with two holes in the middle to be sewn or attached to items of clothing and objects in various ways. The shapes of the buttons can be identified at any angle. Beyond the four initial primary shapes, the identification process for the fashion range differs. According to the Royal Institute for the Blind (RNIB), these buttons are specifically appropriate for older people and for those who had lost their sight at a later stage in life and do not have a good sense of touch.

2.3 'C' System: Smart Labelling for Clothing

The 'C' system is a 'smart' labelling system for clothing designed by Coley Porter Bell using the disposable swing tag as a valuable information interface that allows independent shopping for the visually impaired (Coley Porter Bell 2002). This labelling concept consists of tactile shapes representing colour and size to be used on the swing tag and on the label of a garment. The tag also has a barcode reader that give further details of the product. There are sixteen tactile shapes with variables that enable visually impaired users to identify sixty colours. Each main shape is encased in a square with a raised outline and lined textures that represent a colour (see Figure 1). The 'C' smart labelling is complicated due to the variance in colours and patterns and the barcode reader is not user friendly for young children, so this concept is not easy to adopt in a developing country like Mauritius.

3 Designing and Creating the Tactile Symbols

The use of tactile relief symbols to communicate colours is an alternative to Braille labelling. It is simple and easier to recognize and can be learned by children with learning difficulties. As such, there is no existing system of tactile colour coding that could be compared and tested. Referring to the colour communication concept, the LEA Vision Test Systems (Repka 2002) specifically designed for children and Perera's (2002) notion of tactile perception and spatial acuity, the first version of relief symbols were developed using simplified shapes such as circle, square, line, curved line and dots. The familiarity of these shapes cut across different pedagogical tools for kindergarten and primary level and also in most research for basic understanding of tactile shapes and their interpretations (McCallum et al. 2006). The allocation of shape to specific colours was derived from initial interactions and drawing activities conducted with visually impaired children in Mauritius. The design process of the symbols was influenced by the children's prior knowledge of shapes and links to their surroundings; a small square box was associated with dark blue reflecting the blue square soap that is used for domestic laundry, circle represented red as it was associated with the red 'dot' called bindhi on the forehead of a Hindu woman. Since orange is a mixture of yellow and red, circles of smaller dimension were used to represent orange. Yellow was represented with small dots reflecting the pollens of flowers. Given that lines and curves were distinctive in the children's drawings, vertical lines represented purple and curved lines were associated with green representative of bendable grass stems.

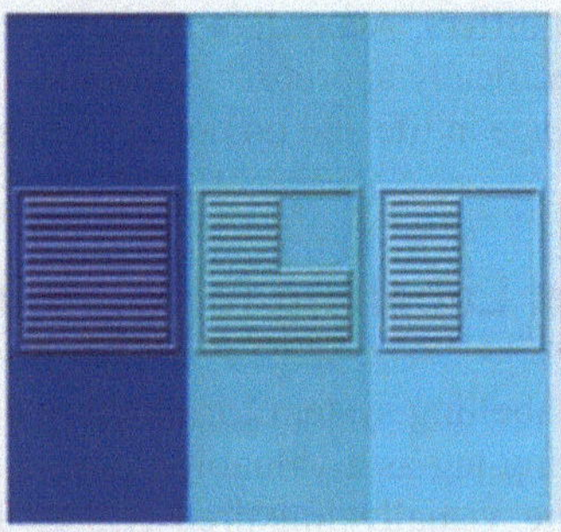

Fig. 1 Tactile Shape with raised outlines and lined textures (Bell 2002)

The set of colours started with elementary basic primary colours such as red, blue and yellow, then the secondary colours with orange, green and purple. Each colour has an associated simplistic tactile shape and size that could be easily identified and be distinctive by touch.

The symbols as shown in Table 1were designed using the CS 4.0™ Illustrator software.

The symbols were then printed with a laser printer on swell paper that was passed through a fuser. This puffed up the black ink on the paper creating a tactile relief (see Figure 2). The vertical elevation height is about 0.5 mm (Gual et al. 2014).

Table 1 Symbols representing the six primary and secondary colours

Colours	Symbols Represented
RED	
BLUE	
YELLOW	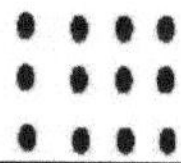
ORANGE	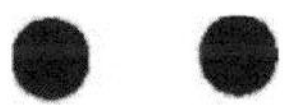
GREEN	
PURPLE	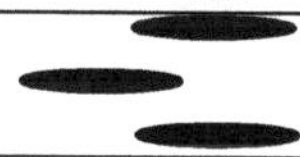

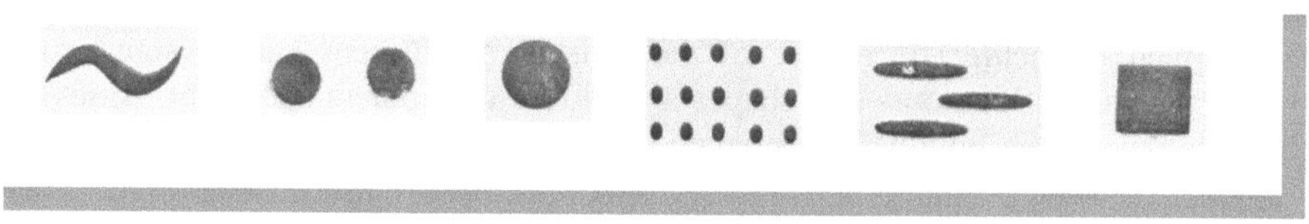

Fig. 2 Tactile relief symbols on swell paper

4 Introducing the Tactile Symbols

This part of the research began with site visits to the two local schools for the visually impaired in Mauritius. The degree of visual impairment among the children varied from partially to totally blind. The characteristics of a totally blind child were similar for both schools. Children with other apparent disabilities such as neurological disorders and brain abnormalities were not included in this study. Due to the nature of this research, informed consent and permission from parents, schools and care givers was sought, respecting all ethical procedures involving human participants.

The two schools were visited at regular intervals for a period of three months for data collection, working with the children during their pedagogical activities, studying the tools and facilities available to them and liaising with the teachers and caregivers. The tactile symbols were mounted on A4 card paper and shown to the children daily for 20 minutes for a period of 4 weeks. This enabled the children to learn the new relief symbols and associate them with the corresponding colours.

They had to be guided through the shapes, and be taught by taking their hands and guiding their fingers over the outline of shapes (Eriksson 1994).

A group of 6 boys and 8 girls with various degrees of visual impairment participated in this study. Table 2 shows the age group, category of visual impairment and gender of participants.

The participants were categorised into two age groups in either low vision (6) or totally blind (8). The sample size is small due the exclusion of all other types of physical disabilities.

Table 2 Age group, visual impairment and gender

Age group	Gender		Low vision (LV)	Totally blind (TB)
	M	F		
6-10	2	5	1	6
11-15	4	3	5	2
Total	14		6	8

The inclusion criteria required for the selected participants was their ability to communicate verbally which was essential for this study. The development level had to be in accordance with their age-level so that they can undertake the activities and tasks given to them. The degree of their visual impairment varied, some could partially distinguish colours and shapes at a close range others could not. Assessing the quantum of their blindness was beyond the scope of this research work.

4.1 Tactile Symbols on Learning Tools

Educational learning tools can help in developing a child's motor, social, intellectual and problem solving skills (Rudman 2005) as well as recognizing patterns, shapes and colours. For the purpose of this research, a few educational tools were selected for the application of the tactile symbols. The time speed per seconds of the colour symbols recognition for each participants on all learning tools was recorded. Participants with low vision were blindfolded while performing the tasks as according to Ramloll and Brewster (2002), it allows total concentration on the tasks without using their partial vision and also avoiding too strenuous effort of the eyes.

4.1.1 One to Five Ring Counter

Each tactile symbol was cut out of square labels from the swell papers and pasted onto fifteen rings representing 1 red color, 2 orange colour, 3 yellow colour, 4 green colour and 5 blue colour. The symbols were also placed at the base of each coloured rod. All the labeled rings were put in a container and the participants had to stack the coloured rings in their corresponding coloured rods (see Figure 3a).

Adopting the concept of the ManuVis test (Reimer 2008); the participants were timed in seconds for this task.

4.1.2 Shaped Abacus

In comparison to the ring counter which had rings of similar shapes and sizes, the shaped abacus had five differing shapes in different colours that needed to be stacked on five rods (Figure 3b). The tactile colour symbols were glued on the sides of all the shapes and randomly mixed in a bowl so that participants could retrieve according to colours and thread them in the coloured matching rods. The rating system was the time factor for each participant to perform the whole task.

4.1.3 Three Dimensional Geo Designs

The three dimensional geo designs were chosen for their facilitating factor for sorting, counting and identifying geometrical shapes (Figure 3c). The form constancy in geo-designs allowed visually impaired participants to interpret thin, thick, small and big shapes; however they could not recognize colour due to their disability. Out of 64 shapes of different sizes and thicknesses, only 21 shapes were chosen to apply the tactile symbols and to test with participants.

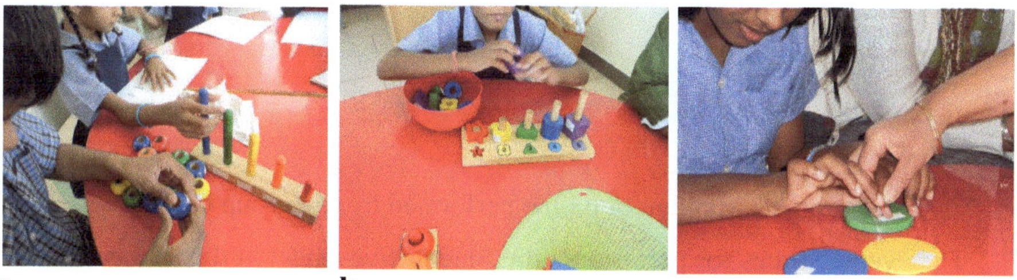

a **b** **c**

Fig. 3 Adapting symbols on learning tools: a. one to five ring b. shaped abacus c. 3D geo designs

5 Results and Analysis

The first observation after introducing the tactile relief symbols to the participants was their use of tactile scanning movement. It could be noted that the movement of the fingers was static on the symbol rather than covering all over the surface of the card paper. The application of the tactile symbols was tested on several educational tools and objects to measure the acceptability and usability of these symbols by the two groups. The evaluation methods were conducted to perceive the speed performance (per seconds) of recognizing these symbols. However only a selected few learning tools are presented in this paper.

Figure 4 shows the differences in the mean duration of participants in age group 6-10, the younger participant took longer in completing the tasks but performed significantly well in comparison to the other participants with an age gap of two to four years. The dexterity and speed performance for all participants as shown proved a good understanding of the tactile symbols.

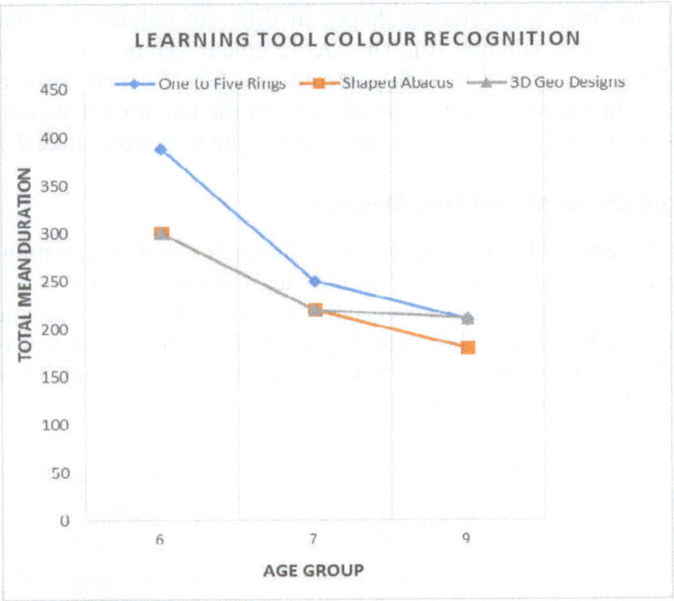

Fig. 4 Mean duration time performed by age group 6-10

The average times for performing the 'one to five rings' in this age group (M= 250 s, SD= 142.5, N=7) is higher than the 'shaped abacus' (M= 209, SD =113.8, N=7) and the 3D Geo Designs (M= 232, SD=69.4, N=7). One possible factor affecting time recognition of the 'one to five rings' task was the rounded surfaces of the rings that somehow distorted the pasted tactile symbols and made it difficult for participants to identify.

The data in Figure 5 represent the performance score of participants of age 11-15, the overall performance is good considering participants were blindfolded. However, some participants' increasing difficulty with their motor development affected their performance in the tasks.

The mean average time for 'one to five rings' (M=264, SD=106, N=7) in this age group is consistent and were reasonably well performed across all the ages. However there was a fluctuation in the performance speed of the 'shaped abacus' (M=212, SD=135, N=7) and '3D geo designs' (M=254, SD=125, N=7). In Figure 6 one can observe the differences between the age group and to what extent the younger age group surpasses the older one. The comparison seems smaller and the progress is better in the younger age group. Older children become clumsier and with adolescence in view there is certain adjustment required to cope with educational activities. Moreover their eye sight deteriorates as they grow older, affecting emotional, social and motor development.

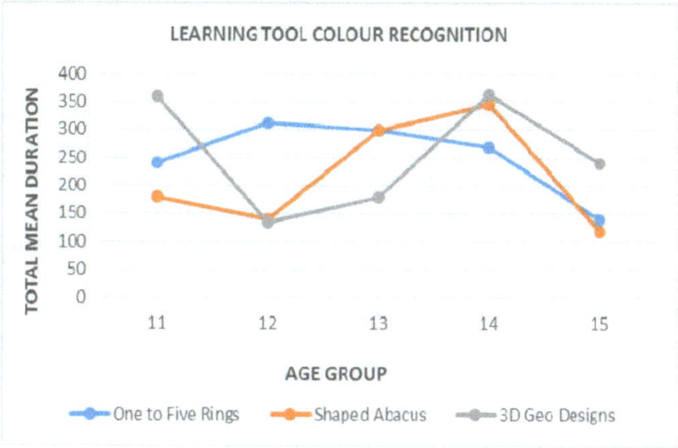

Fig. 5 Mean duration time performed by age group 11-15

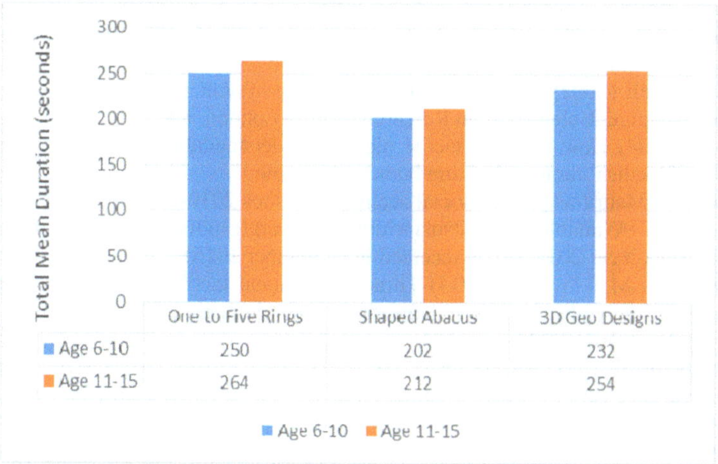

Fig. 6 Mean differences between the younger and older group

6 Conclusion and Future Work

The purpose of this study was to develop an assistive low cost tactile system to enable visually impaired children to distinguish colour. From the literature review, no appropriate system of identifying colours through touch for children with visual impairments could be found. The tactile symbols developed have proved to be effective in helping the visually impaired children recognize a mix of primary and secondary colours. The evaluation of all the tests produced a mean score for each age group and this was used to measure the ability of the participants to adopt this new methodology.

The participants were able to identify all the colours via touch after the symbols were applied. The children were very responsive to the relief symbols presented to them and they could easily associate a given shape to its corresponding colour.

The tactile colour symbols, as presented in this work, have to some extent proved to be effective and would be further tested with a much larger population.

Further experimentation will be conducted to develop and implement additional colours. The study will carry on to explore the possibility of applying these tactile symbols on clothing and accessory items. The practicality of implementing these symbols would also be investigated so that it is functional and easy to adopt.

Future work will also encompass scaling up the production of tactile colour symbols and standardize them so that it could be implemented in all products that assist the visually challenged children in Mauritius.

References

Cattaneo Z, Vecchi T, Cornoldi C, Mammarella I, Bonino D, Ricciardi E et al. (2008) Imagery and spatial processes in blindness and visual impairment. Elsevier Neuroscience and Biobehavioral Review 32: 1346-1360

Coley Porter Bell (2002) 'C'system: Smart labelling system for clothing. DBA Inclusive Design Challenge. Helen Hamlyn Research Centre, London, UK

Eriksson Y (1994) How to make tactile pictures understandable to the blind reader. PhD thesis, the Swedish library of talking books and braille

Government of Mauritius (2014) Social security statistics 2010-2014, highlights – Republic of Mauritius. Available at: statsmauritiusgovmu.org/English/StatsbySubj/Pages/Social-Security-Stats-Year-2014.aspx (Accessed in November 2015)

Gual J, Puyuelo M, Llovras J (2014) Three-dimensional tactile symbols produced by 3D printing: Improving the process of memorizing a tactile map key. British Journal of Visual Impairment 32(3): 263-278

Heller MA, Schiff W(1991) Psychology of Touch. Lawrence Erlbaum Associates, Hilldale, USA

Kops CE, Gardner EP (1996) Discrimination of simulated texture patterns on the human hand. Journal of Neurophysiology 76: 1145-1165

McCallum D, Ungar S, Jehoel S (2006) An evaluation of tactile directional symbols. British Journal of Visual impairment 24(2): 83-92

Perera S (2002) Tactile perception and design. This report is part of the Bionic Project and is funded by DTI. Tiresias Scientific Research Reports. Available at: www.tiresias.org/research/reports/tpd1.htm (Accessed in November 2015)

Ramloll R, Brewster S (2002) A generic approach for augmenting tactile diagrams with spatial non-speech sounds. In: Proceedings of CHI'02, pp. 770-771. Minneapolis, MN, USA

Reimer AM (2008) Effect of visual impairment on goal – Directional aiming movements in children. Journal of Development Medicine and Child Neurology 50: 778-783

Repka MX (2002) Use of LEA symbols in young children. British Journal of Ophthalmology 86(5): 489-490

Rudman L (2005) 143 activities, games and toys for visually impaired pre-school children (a manual for parents and teachers). South Africa

Vision Awareness (2014) Slade colour indicating buttons. www.visionawareness.co.uk/sladecolour.htm (Accessed in November 2015)

WHO (2014) Priority eye diseases: Main causes of visual impairment. World Health Organisation. Available at: www.who.int/blindness/causes/priority (Accessed in November 2015)

Virtual Reality Technology for Pain Management

Z. J. Liu and H. Dong

Abstract: Human beings have figured out numerous means to cope with pain, and virtual reality (VR) technology is a new addition to this inventory. This paper reviews relevant articles published in recent 10 years, with a focus on methods and techniques of VR application. It aims to provide a comprehensive picture of VR technology for pain management, thus aiding researchers who are interested in exploring this field further.

1 Introduction

Pain, a feeling everyone tries to avoid, may come from disease, injury, retrogression, medical treatment and other sources. Despite our dislikes, pain serves as one of the bases for numerous lives on earth. It directs beings, not only humans but also other creatures, to notice danger, to avoid threat and to seek remedy so as to survive. Therefore, human beings' strategy for coping with pain is not to eliminate it completely, but rather to relieve it and have it under control when necessary. This is what we call *pain management*.

As history progresses, humans have developed various means of pain management, e.g. chemical pharmacy, physical therapies and acupuncture. *Virtual reality* is one of the latest inventions in this field.

Virtual reality, usually abbreviated as VR, is a technology that exploits the latest advancements in computer science, in both hardware and software, to fabricate a virtual world for its users in order to create their illusion of presence in that cyberspace. Furthermore, VR has the inherent potential of being interactive because its content is generated in real time, not ahead of time, which makes the experience even more immersive. Many scholars believe that VR has a promising value in pain management mainly because it can be an effective distractor. Despite the doubts whether VR actually helps to cure a disease or physical disorder, abundant evidence has been collected showing its superiority in relieving pain and other kinds of discomfort caused by disease or the treatment procedures.

Z. J. Liu
Tongji University, Shanghai, China

H. Dong (✉)
Inclusive Design Research Centre, College of Design and Innovation, Tongji University, Shanghai, China
email: donghua@tongji.edu.cn

P. Langdon et al. (eds.), *Designing Around People*,
DOI 10.1007/978-3-319-29498-8_8

2 Methods

There are a number of studies concerning the application of VR technology in pain management. A search for articles published between 1995 and 2015 (October) from the *Web of Science* databases with the keywords "virtual reality" and "pain" gave a report as shown in Figure 1.

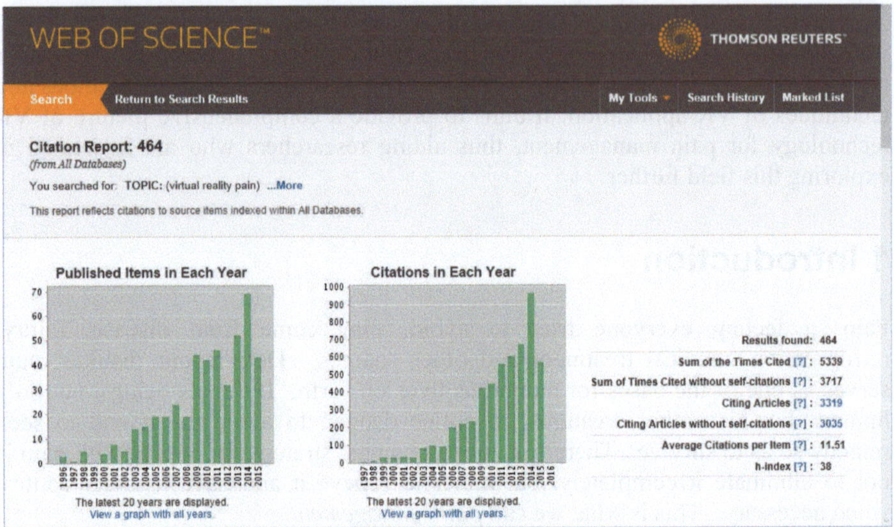

Fig. 1 A search report from Web of Science

Papers were mainly collected from *Web of Science Core Collection*, *Medline database* and *EI Compendex database*, via a search for articles published between 2006 and 2015 using key words "virtual reality" and "pain".

In total the 171 most relevant articles were read carefully and further filtered, using the following criteria:

- VR technology was used to relieve pain,
- practical data was collected from experiments and VR technology played an important role in the experiment.

Review articles were used as references but not included in the final list.

After filtering, 43 articles remained. A spreadsheet was created to compare extracted information, for example: objective of the study; demographic information of the subjects; sample size; subjects' health status; kind or source of discomfort; hardware and software used; comparative targets; research methods and procedures; measuring tools and instruments; findings and conclusion.

3 Analysis and Findings

Most of the articles were published in journals of medicine such as *Burns* (Mott et al. 2008, Konstantatos et al. 2009, Morris et al. 2010, Schmitt et al. 2011, Kipping et al. 2012), *Journal of Pain* (Hoffman et al. 2006, Rutter et al. 2009), *Pain* (Campbell et al. 2010), *Cyberpsychology & Behavior* (Gold et al. 2006, Muhlberger et al. 2007, Hoffman et al. 2009).

An encouraging trend began to emerge since 2010: Articles concerning the application of VR technology in healthcare began to appear in conferences such as *International Conference on Interactive Technologies and Games* (Czub and Piskorz 2014), *International Conference on Virtual, Augmented and Mixed Reality* (Carrino et al. 2014), *International Conference on e-Health Networking, Applications and Services* (Yeh et al. 2012) and *Systems and Information Engineering Design Symposium* (Zweighaft et al. 2012).

3.1 Objectives

It was found that 69.77% of contemporary studies are verifications of VR's analgesic effectiveness for pain caused by disease, injury or treatment, such as burn (Chan et al. 2007, Hoffman et al. 2008, Mott et al. 2008, Konstantatos et al. 2009, Morris et al. 2010, Maani et al. 2011, Schmitt et al. 2011, Kipping et al. 2012, Sil et al. 2013), cancer (Schneider and Hood 2007, Banos et al. 2013), or phantom limb pain (Carrino et al. 2014, Ortiz-Catalan et al. 2014).

Besides these, some researchers began to explore the influential factors of VR for pain management. They tried to evaluate the usefulness of head mounted display (HMD) (Dahlquist et al. 2009, Dahlquist et al. 2010a, Gordon et al. 2011), which is a signature equipment in this field. Some other studies tried to figure out whether factors like visual quality (Hoffman et al. 2006), visual content (Muhlberger et al. 2007), degree of presence (Czub and Piskorz 2014) or point of view in the virtual world (Dahlquist et al. 2010b) may affect VR's efficacy. In addition to technical factors, researchers also investigated other factors including demographic variables (Schneider et al. 2011) and psychological effects other than distraction (Loreto-Quijada et al. 2014).

Finally, some articles proposed designs of new hardware or software systems for pain management, and they usually came from computer scientists and engineers (Georgoulis et al. 2010, Villiger et al. 2011, Yeh et al. 2012, Zweighaft et al. 2012). Often these were pilot studies and tested with very small sample sizes (typically 2-3 patients).

3.2 Subjects

In most of the experiments (79.07%), sample sizes were small: usually less than 50 people participated as subjects in one experiment (Figure 2), and there were even studies based on one individual (Sil et al. 2013, Ortiz-Catalan et al. 2014). Another important finding is that children (sometimes including adolescents) were usually regarded as a special target group. 11 out of 43 articles (25.58%) explicitly claimed that they were done for children (or including adolescents). Figure 3 shows how many times children, adolescents and adults were involved.

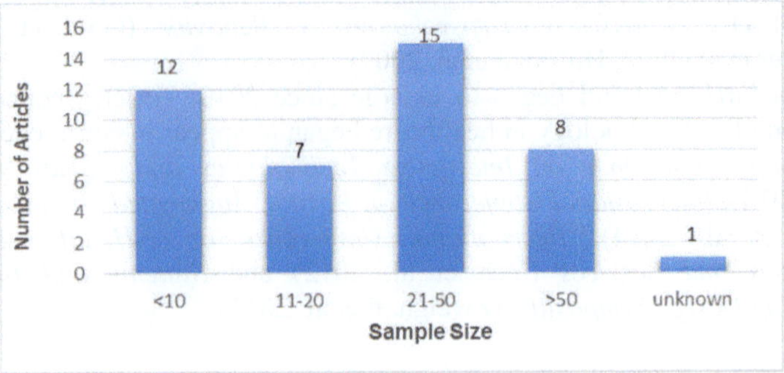

Fig. 2 Distribution of sample sizes of the 43 articles reviewed

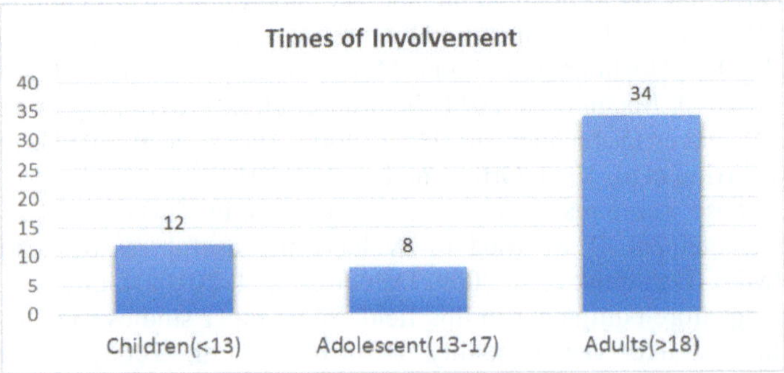

Fig. 3 Number of times when children, adolescents and adults were involved

In the 43 articles, 28 used real patients as subjects (65.12%) while 15 used healthy subjects (34.88%), usually college students, and pain was artificially created by stimuli including heat stimulus (Hoffman et al. 2006, Hoffman et al. 2007, Muhlberger et al., 2007), cold pressor (Muhlberger et al. 2007, Dahlquist et al. 2009, Rutter et al. 2009, Dahlquist et al. 2010a,b, Gutierrez-Maldonado et al. 2012, Czub and Piskorz 2014, Loreto-Quijada et al. 2014), neurometer (Gordon et al. 2011) or capsaicin cream (Campbell et al. 2010).

3.3 Technologies

Head mounted displays (HMD) were used in 26 out of 43 articles (60.47%). TVs, projections and portable game devices were also often used as output devices. On the input side, though, most of the studies still used traditional devices like keyboards, mice and gamepads. However, new technologies began to appear in a few cases in which Wii fit balance board (Kim et al. 2014), Wii remote controller (Law et al. 2011, Nilsson et al. 2013, Sil et al. 2013) and Kinect (Carrino et al. 2014) were used.

As for the software part, both linear media and interactive media were used in previous studies. Linear media were mainly videos or pre-rendered animations while interactive media could be commercial games or game-like applications. A famous application used in many studies was *SnowWorld*. There were also attempts to customize VR applications for research purposes. For instance, to compare high-quality VR with low-quality VR (Hoffman et al. 2006), or to compare hot VR environment with cold VR environment presented with heat stimulus and cold stimulus in turn (Muhlberger et al. 2007). But in general, ready-made VR applications from a third party prevailed.

3.4 Experiments

30 out of 43 studies (69.77%) included comparative experiments in which VR intervention was compared to other conditions. Standard care with no distraction usually served as the baseline (55.81%), while other distractions such as TV sets, music, books or even lollipops were also compared with VR intervention. In a few cases, VR intervention alone was compared with a compound intervention consisting of VR and other analgesia such as opioid (Hoffman et al. 2007) or hypnosis (Patterson et al. 2010).

Due to the facts that most of the studies in this field used relatively small sample sizes, within-subject design was used much more often (65.11%) than randomized control trial (between-subject design).

There were three cases in which the within-subject experiments were temporal, namely the effects were examined before and after VR intervention to determine whether pain related indicators increased or decreased (Sato et al. 2010, Banos et al. 2013, Villiger et al. 2013).

3.5 Measures

39 out of 43 studies (90.70%) measured multiple outcomes to inspect the research question from different perspectives. In a number of experiments, pain was inspected with three components: *cognitive component of pain*, *affective component of pain* and *sensory component of pain*, which were measured respectively as *time thinking about pain*, *unpleasantness* and *worst pain* with numeric or graphic scales (Gold et al. 2006, Hoffman et al. 2006, Muhlberger et al. 2007, Hoffman et al. 2008, Hoffman et al. 2009, Maani et al. 2011, Schmitt et al. 2011).

When cold pressors were used among healthy subjects, two other components were often taken into consideration, which were *pain threshold* and *pain tolerance*, measured respectively as time in seconds before subjects reported to feel painful and they withdrew their hands from the cold pressors due to unbearable pain (Rutter et al. 2009, Gutierrez-Maldonado et al. 2012, Loreto-Quijada et al. 2014). For children subjects, observation was performed by nursing staff based on FLACC (Face, Legs, Activity, Cry and Consolability) standards (Nilsson et al. 2009, Kipping et al. 2012, Nilsson et al. 2013).

Besides pain, *anxiety* and *distress* were also commonly measured. In addition to simple graphic or numeric scales, anxiety was usually measured with *State Anxiety Inventory* (Schneider and Hood 2007), *State-Trait Anxiety Inventory* (Schneider et al. 2011, Nilsson et al. 2013) and *Burn Specific Pain Anxiety Scale* (Konstantatos et al. 2009, Morris et al. 2010). Distress was usually measured with *Observation Scale of Behavioral Distress* (Windich-Biermeier et al. 2007), *Adapted Symptom Distress Scale* (Schneider and Hood 2007), *Observation Scale of Behavioral Distress* (Sil et al. 2013) and *Facial Affective Scale* (Nilsson et al. 2009, Nilsson et al. 2013). Other common outcomes are *fatigue* (Schneider and Hood 2007, Schneider et al. 2011, Botella et al. 2013), *nausea* (Gold et al. 2006, Hoffman et al. 2008, Schmitt et al. 2011, Kipping et al. 2012) and *fear* (Windich-Biermeier et al. 2007, Kim et al. 2014).

There were also attempts to obtain objective information by gathering biological data such as *pulse rate*, *respiratory rate*, *oxygen saturation* (Mott et al. 2008, Nilsson et al. 2009, Kipping et al. 2012), *brain activity* in five pain-related regions (Hoffman et al. 2007), and *body motion kinematics* (Mazzone et al. 2013). There were also inquiries about the *presence* and *fun* of the VR exposure experience (Hoffman et al. 2006, Hoffman et al. 2008, Hoffman et al. 2009, Maani et al. 2011, Schmitt et al. 2011).

3.6 Effects

35 studies suggest that VR has positive effects on pain management. Researchers believed that VR could practically help to relieve perceptible pain and other discomfort such as itching from pruritus (Magora et al. 2009). VR could not be verified to contribute to the relief of pain, anxiety or other symptoms (Schneider and Hood 2007, Konstantatos et al. 2009), or may not be eqally helpful to everyone (Morris et al. 2010, Schneider et al. 2011). There was only one study claiming that VR could increase pain level (Konstantatos et al. 2009).

4 Discussion

Most studies adopted ready-made VR products from third-party organizations. Such products might be insufficient to help explore how visual content or interaction design of a VR application might relate to analgesic efficacy. There is a lack of attention on age groups like middle-aged or elderly adults. While experiments could be performed with healthy subjects, whether such results could be applied to real patients still needs further investigation.

Comparing how a patient felt before and after a certain treatment was relatively fast and simple, but it was difficult to tell whether this was due to VR or other factors.

The authors has identifed the following research directions:

- To obtain deeper understanding of the influential factors that might affect the analgesic effect of VR intervention, such as quality, content, form and interactivity of the VR applications;
- To obtain better understanding of how VR intervention might be affected by demographic variables, like age, gender, race and health status;
- To unveil the fundamental principles of why and how VR intervention functions on a psychological and neurological level, and to discover greater potentials of it.

Acknowledgements

This study was supported by A^3 Group, an interdisciplinary research team funded by Tongji University.

References

Banos RM, Espinoza M, Garcia-Palacios A, Cervera JM, Esquerdo G, Barrajon E (2013) A positive psychological intervention using virtual reality for patients with advanced cancer in a hospital setting: A pilot study to assess feasibility. Supportive Care in Cancer 21: 263-270

Botella C, Garcia-Palacios A, Vizcaino Y, Herrero R, Banos RM, Belmonte MA (2013) Virtual reality in the treatment of fibromyalgia: A pilot study. Cyberpsychology Behavior and Social Networking 16: 215-223

Campbell CM, Witmer K, Simango M, Carteret A, Loggia ML, Campbell JN et al. (2010) Catastrophizing delays the analgesic effect of distraction. Pain 149: 202-207

Carrino F, Rizzotti D, Gheorghe C, Kabasu Bakajika P, Francescotti-Paquier F et al. (2014) Augmented reality treatment for phantom limb pain. In: Proceedings of the 6th International Conference on Virtual, Augmented and Mixed Reality, pp. 248-257, Heraklion, Crete, Greece

Chan EA, Chung JW, Wong TK, Lien AS, Yang JY (2007) Application of a virtual reality prototype for pain relief of pediatric burn in Taiwan. Journal of Clinical Nursing 16: 786-793

Czub M, Piskorz J (2014) How body movement influences virtual reality analgesia? In: Proceedings of the 7th International Conference on Interactive Technologies and Games, pp. 13-19, Nottingham, UK

Dahlquist LM, Weiss KE, Law EF, Sil S, Herbert LJ, Horn SB et al. (2010a) Effects of videogame distraction and a virtual reality type head-mounted display helmet on cold pressor pain in young elementary school-aged children. Journal of Pediatric Psychology 35: 617-625

Dahlquist LM, Herbert LJ, Weiss KE, Jimeno M (2010b) Virtual-reality distraction and cold-pressor pain tolerance: Does avatar point of view matter? Cyberpsychology Behavior and Social Networking 13: 587-591

Dahlquist LM, Weiss KE, Clendaniel LD, Law EF, Ackerman CS, McKenna KD (2009) Effects of videogame distraction using a virtual reality type head-mounted display helmet on cold pressor pain in children. Journal of Pediatric Psychology 34: 574-584

Georgoulis S, Eleftheriadis S, Tzionas D, Vrenas K, Petrantonakis P, Hadjileontiadis LJ (2010) Epione: An innovative pain management system using facial expression analysis, biofeedback and augmented reality-based distraction. In: Proceedings of the 2nd International Conference on Intelligent Networking and Collaborative Systems, pp. 259-266, Thessaloniki, Greece

Gold JI, Kim SH, Kant AJ, Joseph MH, Rizzo A (2006) Effectiveness of virtual reality for pediatric pain distraction during IV placement. Cyberpsychology & Behavior 9: 207-212

Gordon NS, Merchant J, Zanbaka C, Hodges LF, Goolkasian P (2011) Interactive gaming reduces experimental pain with or without a head mounted display. Computers in Human Behavior 27: 2123-2128

Gutierrez-Maldonado J, Gutierrez-Martinez O, Loreto-Quijada D, Nieto-Luna R (2012) The use of virtual reality for coping with pain with healthy participants. Psicothema 24: 516-522

Hoffman HG, Patterson DR, Seibel E, Soltani M, Jewett-Leahy L, Sharar SR (2008) Virtual reality pain control during burn wound debridement in the hydrotank. The Clinical Journal of Pain 24: 299-304

Hoffman HG, Patterson DR, Soltani M, Teeley A, Miller W, Sharar SR (2009) Virtual reality pain control during physical therapy range of motion exercises for a patient with multiple blunt force trauma injuries. Cyberpsychology & Behavior 12: 47-49

Hoffman HG, Richards TL, Van Oostrom T, Coda BA, Jensen MP, Blough DK et al. (2007) The analgesic effects of opioids and immersive virtual reality distraction: Evidence from subjective and functional brain imaging assessments. Anesthesia and Analgesia 105: 1776-1783

Hoffman HG, Seibel EJ, Richards TL, Furness TA, Patterson DR, Sharar SR (2006) Virtual reality helmet display quality influences the magnitude of virtual reality analgesia. Journal of Pain 7: 843-850

Kim S-S, Min W-K, Kim J-H, Lee B-H (2014) The effects of VR-based Wii Fit yoga on physical function in middle-aged female LBP patients. Journal of Physical Therapy Science 26: 549-552

Kipping B, Rodger S, Miller K, Kimble RM (2012) Virtual reality for acute pain reduction in adolescents undergoing burn wound care: A prospective randomized controlled trial. Burns 38: 650-657

Konstantatos AH, Angliss M, Costello V, Cleland H, Stafrace S (2009) Predicting the effectiveness of virtual reality relaxation on pain and anxiety when added to PCA morphine in patients having burns dressings changes. Burns 35: 491-499

Law EF, Dahlquist LM, Sil S, Weiss KE, Herbert LJ, Wohlheiter K et al. (2011) Videogame distraction using virtual reality technology for children experiencing cold pressor pain: The role of cognitive processing. Journal of Pediatric Psychology 36: 84-94

Loreto-Quijada D, Gutierrez-Maldonado J, Nieto R, Gutierrez-Martinez O, Ferrer-Garcia M, Saldana C et al. (2014) Differential effects of two virtual reality interventions: Distraction versus pain control. Cyberpsychology Behavior and Social Networking 17: 353-358

Maani CV, Hoffman HG, Morrow M, Maiers A, Gaylord K, McGhee LL et al. (2011) Virtual reality pain control during burn wound debridement of combat-related burn injuries using robot-like arm mounted VR goggles. Journal of Trauma-Injury Infection and Critical Care 71: S125-S130

Magora F, Leibovici V, Cohen S (2009) Virtual reality methodology for pruritus and pain. In: Proceedings of the 2009 Virtual Rehabilitation International Conference, pp. 202, Haifa, Israel

Mazzone B, Lighthall Haubert L, Mulroy S, Requejo P, Gotsis M, Lympouridis V et al. (2013) Intensity of shoulder muscle activation during resistive exercises performed with and without virtual reality games. In: Proceedings of the 10th International Conference on Virtual Rehabilitation, pp. 127-133, Philadelphia, PA, USA

Morris LD, Louw QA, Crous LC (2010) Feasibility and potential effect of a low-cost virtual reality system on reducing pain and anxiety in adult burn injury patients during physiotherapy in a developing country. Burns 36: 659-664

Mott J, Bucolo S, Cuttle L, Mill J, Hilder M, Miller K et al. (2008) The efficacy of an augmented virtual reality system to alleviate pain in children undergoing burns dressing changes: A randomised controlled trial. Burns 34: 803-808

Muhlberger A, Wieser MJ, Kenntner-Mabiala R, Pauli P, Wiederhold BK (2007) Pain modulation during drives through cold and hot virtual environments. Cyberpsychology & Behavior 10: 516-522

Nilsson S, Enskar K, Hallqvist C, Kokinsky E (2013) Active and passive distraction in children undergoing wound dressings. Journal of Pediatric Nursing-Nursing Care of Children & Families 28: 158-166

Nilsson S, Finnstrom B, Kokinsky E, Enskar K (2009) The use of virtual reality for needle-related procedural pain and distress in children and adolescents in a paediatric oncology unit. European Journal of Oncology Nursing 13: 102-109

Ortiz-Catalan M, Sander N, Kristoffersen MB, Hakansson B, Branemark R (2014) Treatment of phantom limb pain (PLP) based on augmented reality and gaming controlled by myoelectric pattern recognition: A case study of a chronic PLP patient. Frontiers in Neuroscience 8: 7

Patterson DR, Jensen MP, Wiechman SA, Sharar SR (2010) Virtual reality hypnosis for pain associated with recovery from physical trauma. International Journal of Clinical and Experimental Hypnosis 58: 288-300

Rutter CE, Dahlquist LM, Weiss KE (2009) Sustained efficacy of virtual reality distraction. Journal of Pain 10: 391-397

Sato K, Fukumori S, Matsusaki T, Maruo T, Ishikawa S, Nishie H et al. (2010) Nonimmersive virtual reality mirror visual feedback therapy and its application for the treatment of complex regional pain syndrome: An open-label pilot study. Pain Medicine 11: 622-629

Schmitt YS, Hoffman HG, Blough DK, Patterson DR, Jensen MP, Soltani M et al. (2011) A randomized, controlled trial of immersive virtual reality analgesia, during physical therapy for pediatric burns. Burns 37: 61-68

Schneider SM, Hood LE (2007) Virtual reality: A distraction intervention for chemotherapy. Oncology Nursing Forum 34: 39-46

Schneider SM, Kisby CK, Flint EP (2011) Effect of virtual reality on time perception in patients receiving chemotherapy. Supportive Care in Cancer 19: 555-564

Sil S, Dahlquist LM, Burns AJ (2013) Case study: Videogame distraction reduces behavioral distress in a preschool-aged child undergoing repeated burn dressing changes: A single-subject design. Journal of Pediatric Psychology 38: 330-341

Villiger M, Bohli D, Kiper D, Pyk P, Spillmann J, Meilick B et al. (2013) Virtual reality-augmented neurorehabilitation improves motor function and reduces neuropathic pain in patients with incomplete spinal cord injury. Neurorehabilitation and Neural Repair 27: 675-683

Villiger M, Hepp-Reymond M-C, Pyk P, Kiper D, Eng K, Spillman J et al. (2011) Virtual reality rehabilitation system for neuropathic pain and motor dysfunction in spinal cord injury patients. In: Proceedings of the 2011 International Conference on Virtual Rehabilitation, Zurich, Switzerland

Windich-Biermeier A, Sjoberg I, Dale JC, Eshelman D, Guzzetta CE (2007) Effects of distraction on pain, fear, and distress during venous port access and venipuncture in children andAdolescents with cancer. Journal of Pediatric Oncology Nursing 24: 8-19

Yeh S-C, Chang S-M, Chen S-Y, Hwang W-Y, Huang T-C, Tsai T-L (2012) A lower limb fracture postoperative-guided interactive rehabilitation training system and its effectiveness analysis. In: Proceedings of the 14th International Conference on E-health Networking, Applications and Services, Healthcom 2012, pp. 149-154, Beijing, China

Zweighaft AR, Slotness GL, Henderson AL, Osborne LB, Lightbody SM, Perhala LM et al. (2012) A physical workstation, body tracking interface, and immersive virtual environment for rehabilitating phantom limb pain. In: Proceedings of the 2012 IEEE Systems and Information Engineering Design Symposium, pp. 184-189, Charlottesville, VA, USA

InTacT: Insights into Telehealth and Care Technologies

P. M. Chamberlain, C. L. Craig and M. Dexter

Abstract: An ageing population, pressure on health, social care capacity and changing social roles and expectations are driving demand for innovative solutions to support independence at home for people living with long term conditions and disabilities. Digital health-technologies have been posited as one potential solution to alleviate pressures placed on existing care services, reducing overall costs and carer burden (Petersson et al. 2011). As a consequence, significant investment into telehealth and telecare has been made. However whilst advances in these technologies are moving apace, a growing body of research has suggested that significant questions still remain regarding the acceptance and ultimately adoption of these devices by end users (May et al. 2011, Greenhalgh et al. 2013).

This paper shares the findings of the initial phase of a two-year qualitative research study identifying end-users attitudes to technology in everyday life and exploring how technology might be most appropriately designed to support personal health care. Utilising a critical artefact methodology the study has focused particularly on exploring the needs of groups of individuals who are currently under-represented in this research arena including individuals from diverse ethnic communities and communities classed as being of high socio-economic need. The research has identified a number of barriers to inclusion and the need for designers to understand the broader physical and cultural contexts where health technologies are used. The paper concludes with a broader discussion of the role design in eliciting understanding and developing responses to the complex challenges facing current healthcare services.

1 The Broader Context

The World Health Organisation has described global ageing as both the 'greatest triumph and challenge of the twenty first century'. Increasing numbers of people have the opportunity to enjoy and use this extended time beyond retirement to pursue new goals, gain new skills and contribute to their families and communities. However, the extent to which individuals are able to do this will be very much

P. M. Chamberlain (✉) · C. Craig · M. Dexter
Lab4Living, Art & Design Research Centre Sheffield Hallam University, Sheffield, UK
email: P.M.Chamberlain@shu.ac.uk

P. Langdon et al. (eds.), *Designing Around People*,
DOI 10.1007/978-3-319-29498-8_9

dependent on their health. Whilst disability is not inevitable a number of common health conditions are associated with growing older including: loss of visual and hearing acuity, osteoarthritis chronic obstructive pulmonary disease and dementia. More complex health states commonly referred to as geriatric syndromes may also emerge. These are often the result of a number of underlying factors including frailty, falls, urinary incontinence and delirium (WHO 2015). Increasing frailty may occur at the same time as social networks are diminishing as a consequence of bereavement, making people increasing reliant on healthcare and placing increased pressure on existing services.

An ageing society therefore demands innovative thinking to reshape our future healthcare. Technology is considered to play a key role in changing both how and where care is delivered (Huang 2013). Most notable have been advances in telehealth and telecare technologies. Whilst terminology relating to these technologies is still evolving (RCN) it is generally accepted that telehealth refers to devices concerned with the remote monitoring of physiological data, enabling health professionals to support diagnosis and disease-management whilst Telecare comprises of systems of sensors and alarms that can detect possible problems such as smoke or gas and has the ability to alert carers or monitoring control centres should the need arise. These technologies are congruent with and support evolving paradigms of health, which place increasing responsibility on the individual to recognize and manage the symptoms of their condition (Lorig and Holman 2004).

Telehealth and telecare devices have undergone multiple iterations since their inception in the 1940s. First generation products including buzzers and pendant alarms for summoning help have been gradually augmented by second and third generations of devices which now include remote monitoring in the context of self-management approaches, with the intention of enabling individuals living with long term conditions to better manage their health. Rather than travelling to attend face-to-face appointments, placing pressure on services, telehealth can now help individuals manage their own homes and to become lay experts in their own care. At present it is estimated that 30% of the UK population have at least one chronic condition, which accounts for 70% of the total health services expenditure. The need to alleviate these costs is therefore a priority.

Given the potential of digital health technologies to increase autonomy and ease care needs significant investment in such devices has been made. Within the United Kingdom the Department of Health instigated the Whole Systems Demonstrator trial to explore the efficacy of telehealth. A similar approach was taken in North America by the Veterans Health Administration's National Home Telehealth Programme, which enrolled 50 000 patients. In Europe individual countries have developed more localized approaches. For instance in Germany the SOPHIA project has seen the widespread development and installation of multiple systems including advanced sensoring and activity monitoring through the ubiquitous television set.

However in spite of this global investment, the evidence to date supporting the use of assistive technologies such as telecare and telehealth remains mixed. Whilst initial results from the UK's whole demonstrator randomised controlled trial were extremely promising with a 45% reduction in mortality rates, a 20% reduction in emergency admissions and a 15% reduction in accidents and emergencies authors of the study have emphasized the need for caution (Steventon et al. 2012). Dixon (2012) highlighted that the trial included those with low risks, were provided with extra support and were followed up for only one year. This view was supported by subsequent studies seeking to understand the views of those who had declined to enter the trial. This research found that one of the main reasons for not participating in the study was that assistive technology was considered as a potential threat to identity and existing service use (Sanders et al. 2012, p.10). Further research is therefore required (Health Technology Strategy Board).

Low uptake of digital health technologies is not confined to high profile studies such as the Whole Systems Demonstrator Sites. In a recent article Foster et al. (2015) describe how in two linked randomized controlled trials focusing on telehealth interventions in the north of England (one for patients with depression and the other for patients raised cardiovascular disease) of the patients invited 82.9% (20,021/24,152) did not accept the study invite. The main reasons given for non-participation were telehealth related with 54.7% of decliners stating they did not have access to the skills or the use of the Internet/computers. The authors raise concerns regarding the implications of this in the context of engagement with telehealth products and services.

Much criticism has related to the patchiness of the evidence with some studies reporting positive findings whilst others do not and an overall lack of clarity exists regarding understanding of which type of technology is best suited to which condition. What is consistent however is the lack of engagement of patients and health-care professionals reflected in the low uptake of services and high-drop-out rates. A number of reasons have been proposed to account for this.

The extrinsic factors identified to account for non-adoption of telehealth include: geography, poor network coverage (Hanson et al. 2010) and affordability (Morris 2012). A meta-review and realist synthesis of existing quantitative and qualitative evidence on telehealth for chronic conditions (Salisbury et al. 2015) recognized these as contributory factors but suggested that intrinsic factors were more important, with confidence in using technology cited as the most significant construct associated with adoption. Salisbury et al. (2015) also recognized that acceptability, ease of use and integration into everyday routines were also important to patients and professionals. The meaningfulness of the technology in the broader context of the person's life was a theme explored in an earlier paper by Hanson et al. (2010), which examined factors that needed to be taken into account when designing technologies for digitally excluded older people. Although the paper does not specifically consider digital health technologies the authors highlight the need for designers to address and incorporate the values of older adults within the design process in order to ensure that the technology has meaning and currency within the person's broader habits and routines.

2 The Role of Design

The design of products is important on a number of levels. A study of community alarm services by Moray Community Health and Social Care (2009) partnership found that whilst end-users valued the service, one third of individuals only wore their alarm button some of the time or not at all because it was perceived to be too easily activated or individuals simply forgot to wear it. Bentley et al. (2014) found that non-acceptance of telehealth and telecare related to the stigmatizing aesthetics of products, which reinforced notions of vulnerability and dependency. Participants in this study reported how the look and feel of certain items such as the pendant reinforced the stereotype of telecare as being for people *'who are old and unable to cope'*. The design of interfaces raises challenging issues, as a balance must be reached between creating an interface that compensates for age related disability and promotes ease of use whilst also ensuring that potentially stigmatising designs are avoided.

Overall the literature highlights that the reason for non-acceptance of telehealth is complex. The role of design is not and should not be confined to interface development or *'traditional notions of improving usability'*. Designers need to better understand the broader physical and social environments in which these technologies will operate and how they relate to the contexts of the lives of end users. This is necessary because according to Greenhalgh et al. (2013) the things we use and make (technologies) are not neutral objects but embodiments of ourselves and our cultural values. Where a disconnect between the technology and these cultural values emerge this impacts on the individual's relationship with the world. They conclude in their study that technologies can thus be disabling as well as enabling, disempowering as well as empowering. Illness experiences and assisted living needs of older people are diverse and unique; hence do not lend themselves to simple or standardised technological solutions.

Design has much to contribute to this broader agenda and recognition of its potential to transform healthcare, drawing on a tradition of creative and divergent thinking to address these challenges has been gathering momentum. Of particular interest has been the increasing range of participatory and collaborative approaches that are being adopted to engage the end user in the design of products and services.

Within the context of telecare this is important as a number of researchers have suggested that the poor design of many devices may directly be attributed to the failure to find ways to engage end-users and to elicit understanding of their requirements. This has been difficult in telehealth and telecare since the driver for the development of the products is often from the developer and within telehealth services in hospitals '*individuals who are using the products are not usually the customer*' (Purchaser).

Hanson et al. (2010) have written extensively on the value of participatory design in the context of telehealth and telecare and the literature highlights examples of design researchers who have elicited the views of end users in order to build understanding to inform the development of telehealth and telecare products and services. The SEEDS project sought to empower older adults in developing strategies to participate in the digital economy and utilised semi-structured interviews as a way of understanding the challenges participants faced when accessing technology. Greenhalgh et al. (2013) explored what people with assisted living needs identified as being important and used ethnographic methods and cultural probes in order to elicit understanding. This study particularly highlighted the materiality of care and the value of enabling people living with chronic conditions and their carers to 'think with things'.

3 The Present Study

Insights into telehealth and care technologies (InTacT) very much draw on the value of 'thinking with things' as a method to build understanding of the factors end-users identify as being important in the design of digital health devices. The overall aim of the research is to explore the inequalities in telehealth and care technologies and identify and creatively challenge cultural (e.g. language, rituals, socio-economic) barriers to adoption.

The study explores participatory methods and approaches to engage people who are frequently under-represented in telehealth/telecare research by virtue of their age, ethnicity or socio-economic status, in meaningful ways. The focus of the first phase of the research has been to utilize a critical artefact methodology to build understanding of end-users attitudes to technology in everyday life and how it might most appropriately be adopted to support their personal healthcare.

The methodology of the present study draws on an existing body of work developed by the authors (Chamberlain and Roddis 2003, Chamberlain and Yoxall 2012, Chamberlain and Craig 2013) which uses objects and artefacts as methods to stimulate and scaffold thinking, offering valuable vehicles through which the complexities of lives can be understood. The transdisciplinary research project 'Engagingaging' exhibition provided the theatre for conversation and the medium and method for data collection and created the conduit, through which societal assumptions relating to ageing could be made visible, explored and challenged. Building on methods developed within 'Engagingaging' the principles of the traditional exhibition were distilled into a format that was more flexible, accessible and inclusive. 'Exhibition in a box' (Chamberlain and Craig 2013) took the essence of the exhibition into a suitcase, a la Duchamp that could be transported to diverse environs including the home. In doing so the home was transformed into the research arena, providing individuals with a tangible prompt to scaffold conversation.

These boxes comprised of everyday objects, photographs and textual material defined through the user-workshops undertaken in conjunction with the earlier large-scale exhibitions in 'Engagingaging'. The objects were carefully selected to code, represent and prompt further discussion on themes that had emerged from earlier research. The objects could and did combine to create objective correlatives enabling participants to express emotional responses. For example, pencil and post card prompted discussion around travel, communication, technology (analogue vs digital). The objects allowed different ways for participants to express their personal identity and creativity, prompting them to describe things they have made previously in their life and suggest new ways of doing things. The present study utilises and further tests this methodology.

The first phase of the study was undertaken in the North of England. Prior to recruitment, ethical approval was obtained, following which posters and invitations describing the research and inviting people who might be interested in taking part in a workshop/focus group exploring technology were distributed through a number of voluntary and third sector organizations. These included: Age UK, the Churches Council for Community Care and the Chinese Elders. This first phase of the research was effectively a feasibility study, focusing particularly on methods of engagement.

At this point in the research it was not a requirement for participants to be users of telehealth or telecare devices since the aim was to develop a broader understanding of participants' attitudes to digital products and devices. In total thirty-two socially and ethnically diverse community living older people were recruited. Individuals were invited to attend one of four workshops that were held in community venues and were facilitated by the research team. Each workshop lasted on average for two hours. The workshops began with a general introduction from the research team and an invitation for participants to share (verbally or through drawing) the images and associations that came to mind when they heard the word technology. Exhibition in a box was then introduced and participants were invited, in turn, to select and to respond to the objects it contained. Written consent was obtained to video and audio record the session and these were transcribed following the groups. This data was analysed using framework analysis (Ritchie and Spencer 1994). This enabled the development of a matrix of themes and related sub-topics from the data as well as identification of the links across themes, different participants and venues.

4 Findings and Discussion

The strength of the critical artefact methodology is that the objects transcend boundaries of culture, language and age and whilst the objects remain unchanging the associations they prompt and the stories they elicit are dynamic and ever changing. Across the various workshop/focus groups different objects elicited the same themes of conversation. Particularly powerful were the pencil and the post-card which participants linked to communication and the worldwide web and the key, which very much related to security. Four themes emerged during the exploration of the objects: digital beings in a digital world, navigating change, trust and control and conceptualisations of health.

4.1 Digital Beings in a Digital World

Digital technology was seen as part of everyday life and access to computers and the Internet as being necessary to undertake fundamental activities of daily living including the paying of bills and other transactions. Participants discussed the importance of e-mail and facebook as a way to engage with friends and maintain contact with family members. Lack of access was regarded as a form of social exclusion, '*This one sounds awfully melodramatic, but you just get to the point where you don't feel like a meaningful member of society*' (Workshop participant).

4.2 Navigating Change

Digital disconnectedness was a real concern and the rapid evolution of products, the speed of change as a consequence of in-built obsolescence of many digital devices were regarded as real challenges. Participants described how within the same household different generations of products existed, all of which had subtle differences requiring new learning and complex negotiation. 'Learning saturation' was a term commonly used to describe participants' experiences.

> *'As you get older your ability to retain knowledge is greater than your ability to take on new knowledge therefore to use something you already have existing knowledge of and know how it works is better than giving a new fangled object that a person could reject of find stigmatising.'*
>
> (Workshop participant)

Even when the computer products remained the same, the operating systems and interfaces were subject to constant change. Difficulties in learning how to navigate these were identified as an issue particularly given the lack of technical support. The tangibility of the critical artefacts contained within exhibition in a box and the constancy of form was contrasted with ephemerality of technological change. The pencil in particular elicited conversations regarding learning and connectivity and individuals linked this to feelings of being 'disconnected' from environments where updating of knowledge occurs such as the workplace. Others described how these challenges of mastering new technologies and products were compounded by deterioration of physical and cognitive abilities, attributing difficulties to failing memory and deterioration of skills. This was reflective of a number of people who took part in the study,

> *'We can keep on but you don't get much towards the end....I've started to lose it... it's a bit like swimming across a river, you stretch out to the bank but you can't quite reach it...'*
>
> (Workshop participant)

The metaphor of 'stretching out to the bank but not reaching it' was particularly poignant and reflected the loss of locus of control, and feelings of helplessness expressed by some participants in the research. Individuals spoke of how these feelings could lead to non-engagement with the technology. The keys contained in 'exhibition in a box' - which participants linked to security - prompted much conversation. However, whilst these keys were conceptualised as solid and unproblematic the security features associated with many of the computers were seen as tricky, particularly the need to remember multiple ever changing passwords. For a number of participants who were used to mending products the unfathomability of the digital was closely linked to issues of security and trust: '*I mean if it's a lock, someone could break in as well, but still it's something you get more – it's more understandable for me... you have a key, and a lock*' (Workshop participant).

4.3 Trust and Control

A theme emerging across all the workshops/focus groups in response to both the keys and to a series of 'what if?' cards, scenes of future technological scenarios was the importance of trust and reliability of products. This was seen as being particularly important in relation to health devices and existed on multiple levels including trusting devices not to break, trust in terms of where the information is being sent, trust in relation to accuracy. Even when there was an acknowledgement that technology could be more accurate the issue was trust '*it's just the thought isn't it? I don't trust a machine*'.

One focus group discussion centred on ways of being able to access electronic health records and how this could increase transparency and lead to increased control and involvement. One person described how her digital diabetes pen, which automatically recorded the insulin dosage, enabled her to better keep track of her medication. However, the caveat for both was that this needed to occur within the context of human relationships with medical professionals where issues and concerns could be discussed. Without this relational element it was difficult to know what to trust particularly given the number of conflicting health messages.

> *'There is no technical barrier in collecting data, it is the presentation of that data. If people are able to collect and monitor data they have to be educated to what is normal. People can get data interpretation wildly wrong either by accident of design'.*
>
> (Workshop participant)

The sensory component of many of the objects prompted conversations relating to the importance of touch, and to the relational aspects of healthcare. Fears of loneliness and loss of human contact were seen as particular concerns in relation to more remote monitoring of health: *'One of the things that frightened me to death was the idea of growing old alone, but I never thought it would happen to me'* (Workshop participant).

The sensory aspect was particularly significant for participants from the Chinese community who stressed that Chinese medicine is not predicated on 'normal ranges of data' but on the feel and pallor of the skin and on the sense of touch.

4.4 Conceptualisations of Health

Ultimately discussion across the groups regarding the qualities of products that might promote the acceptance and acceptability of digital health technologies hinged on conceptualisations of what healthcare is. The 'what if?' cards effectively embodied concepts relating to self-management and a shift in the locus of control away from medical professional to the individual and the move from care being delivered in a hospital to the home. The individuals who engaged in this present study did not see this as preferable to existing systems and struggled to come to terms with this. The efficacy of many of the current medical innovations and new paradigms of health were questioned, in particular the constant bombardment of contradictory health messages. Within this the irony that technology had contributed to people leading more sedentary lives, leading to medical problems was not lost.

Participants described the importance of seeing both evolving models of healthcare and technologies in a broader societal context. World events are constantly changing and challenging our understanding of existing technologies. Increasing publicity relating to cyber-crime, terror threats played out on a global stage all impacted on the ways participants in our study related to existing home digital technologies. The importance of this should not be underestimated, '*We talked about trust earlier on, the world has changed in ways we are still coming to terms with'* (Workshop participant).

5 Conclusion

Current literature relating to the design of telehealth and telecare has focused primarily on traditional notions of improving usability and the pursuit of stylish desirable technological solutions. An assumption has been made that designing more aesthetically appealing products will automatically increase engagement in these technologies. Early findings of this present study suggests that acceptance of digital health solutions is more complex. The present generation of health technologies are predicated on the assumption that end-users have already embraced the shift in the healthcare paradigm, which increasingly moves responsibility from the clinician and the hospital to the patient and the home. Participants in this small study raised questions regarding this and the,

> *'underpinning assumption that self-management of illness at home will occur in the same way that medical management happens in the hospital by generating, analysing and manipulating objective measures of health status'.*
>
> (Greenhalgh 2013)

Traditional qualitative research methods using structured and semi-structured interviews can preference the views of the researcher who can make assumptions about what the issues are. Exhibition in a box offered participants a space to reflect, discuss, explore and to define the real questions. The objects offered scaffolds for communication and because they were at one and the same time both concrete and abstract participants in thinking through the objects in the box were able to think outside of the box.

Acknowledgements

This article/paper/report presents independent research. This project was in receipt of funding from the Collaborations for Leadership in Applied Health Research and Care for Yorkshire and Humber (CLAHRC YH). CLAHRC YH acknowledges funding from the National Institute for Health Research (NIHR). The views and opinions expressed are those of the authors, and not necessarily those of the NHS, the NIHR or the Department of Health.

CLAHRC for YH would also like to acknowledge the participation and resources of our partner organisations. Further details can be found at clahrc-yh.nihr.ac.uk.

References

Bentley CL, Powell LA, Orell A, Mountain GA (2014) Addressing design and suitability barriers to Telecare use: Has anything changed? Technology and Disability 26: 221-235

Chamberlain P, Craig C (2013) Engagingdesign - Methods for collective creativity. In: Kurosu M (Ed.) Human-computer interaction, part I, HCII 2013, LNCS 8004. Springer
Chamberlain P, Roddis J (2003) Making sense. The Design Journal (6)1: 40-51
Chamberlain P, Yoxall Y (2012) Of mice and men. The role of interactive exhibitions as research tools for inclusive design. The Design Journal 15(1): 57-78
Dixon J (2012) Does telehealth reduce hospital costs? Six points to ponder. British Politics and Policy at LSE (09 Jul 2012), blog entry. Available at: eprints.lse.ac.uk/48410/ (Accessed in November 2015)
Foster A, Horspool KA, Edwards L, Thomas CL, Salisbury C, Montgomery AA et al. (2015) Who does not participate in telehealth trials and why? A cross sectional survey. Trials 16: 258
Greenhalgh T, Wherton J, Sugarhood P, Hinder S, Procter RN, Stones R (2013) What matters to older people with assisted living needs? A phenomenological analysis of the use and non-use of telehealth and telecare. Social Science and Medicine 93: 86-94
Hanson V, Gibson L, Coleman G, Bobrowicz A, McKay A (2010) A engaging the disengaged: How do we design technology for digitally excluded older adults? In: Proceedings of DIS 2010, Aarhus, Denmark
Huang J-C (2013) Innovative health care delivery systems: A questionnaire survey to evaluate the influence of behavioural factors on individuals' acceptance of telecare. Computers in Biology and Medicine 43(4): 281-6
Lorig KR, Holman H (2004) Self-management education: History, definition, outcomes, and mechanisms. Annals of Behavioural Medicine 26:1-7
May CR, Finch TL, Cornford J, Exley C, Gately C, Kirk S et al. (2011) Integrating telecare for chronic disease management in the community: what needs to be done? BMC Health Service Research 11:131
Morris J (2012) Integrated care for frail older people 2012: A clinical overview. Journal of Integrated Care 20(4): 257-264
Petersson I, Lilja M, Borrell L (2011) To feel safe in everyday life at home - A study of older adults after home modifications. Ageing and Society 2(5): 791-811
Ritchie J, Spencer L (1994) Qualitative data analysis for applied policy research. In: Bryman A, Burgess R (Eds.) Analysing qualitative data, pp. 173–194. Routledge, London, UK
Salisbury C, Thomas C, O'Cathain A, Pope C, Yardley L, Hollinghurst S et al. (2015) TElehealth in CHronic disease: Mixed methods study to develop the TECH conceptual model for intervention design and evaluation. BMJ Open (5)2
Sanders C, Rogers A, Bowen R, Bower P, Hirani S, Cartwright M et al. (2012) Exploring barriers to participation and adoption of telehealth and telecare within the whole system demonstrator trial: A qualitative study. BMC Health Serv Res. 12: 220
Steventon A, Bardsley M, Billings J, Dixon J, Doll H, Hirani S et al. (2012) Effect of telehealth on use of secondary care and mortality: Findings from the whole system demonstrator cluster randomized trial. British Medical Journal 2012; 344: e3874
WHO (2015) World report on ageing and health. WHO, Geneva, Switzerland. Available at: www.who.int/ageing/publications/world-report-2015/en/ (Accessed in November 2015)

Part III

Measuring Product Demand and Peoples' Capabilities

Designing the 'Perfect Day' Service Around People Living with Dementia

P. A. Rodgers

Abstract: This paper describes the author's ongoing collaborative work with Alzheimer Scotland that seeks to explore how design thinking and action might best contribute to the design and development of a range of products, services, and systems for people living with dementia. The paper focuses on one of three recently completed collaborative design projects undertaken with Alzheimer Scotland entitled 'Perfect Day'. The 'Perfect Day' project aims to better support dementia care support workers and family members who care for people living with dementia through envisioning how they describe their 'Perfect Day'. For example, David's "Perfect Day" is playing a round of golf with his friends whilst Bet's "Perfect Day" would be spent playing dominoes and poker. Overall, the key aim of this work is to better understand how design can most effectively contribute to the development of a range of products, services and systems for people living with dementia. This work, which has adopted a co-design interventionist approach, has facilitated explorations around a range of novel design contributions aimed at improving product and service innovation in a third sector context. It has also provided excellent first-hand opportunities to work with Alzheimer Scotland staff and relevant bodies, which has helped facilitate the design, development, and evaluation of a number of creative design interventions.

1 Background

With significant rises in life expectancy, the average age of Britain's population is increasing steadily. Today, the number of people living in the UK aged 65 and over outnumbers people under the age of 16. This ageing population trend is being made worse by the retirement of the so-called "baby boom generation", born during a period of rapid population growth and social change between 1946-1964. This ageing population and its subsequent impact on social services means that the National Health Service (NHS), health and social care services, public spending and the rest of UK society face dramatic changes as a result including:

P. A. Rodgers (✉)
Northumbria University, School of Design, UK
email: paul.rodgers@northumbria.ac.uk

P. Langdon et al. (eds.), *Designing Around People*,
DOI 10.1007/978-3-319-29498-8_10

- half of those born after 2007 can expect to live to over 100,
- between 2010 and 2030 the number of people aged over 65 will increase by 51%,
- the number of people aged over 85 will double during the same period.

Given these changes put enormous pressure on healthcare and social services. A key aim of government policy now is to encourage people to remain active, engage in regular exercise and refrain from behaviours that could have a detrimental effect on their health. Coupled with this the Nuffield Trust have recently predicted a 32% increase in elderly people with moderate or severe disability, and a 32% to 50% rise in over 65s with chronic diseases. Moreover, it has been claimed that unless treatment and cures are improved, the incidence of the five most common chronic conditions among the over 65s – arthritis, heart disease, stroke, diabetes and dementia – will increase by 25% by 2020 and more than 50% by 2030. This would mean that the NHS would face a £28bn to £34bn shortfall in its £110bn annual budget (Jowitt 2013).

The research, presented here, focuses on developing and implementing innovative design interventions that seek to encourage people to remain active, promote dignity, and encourage independence particulalry for people living with dementia in the post-diagnostic stage of the illness. This work focuses on reconnecting people living with dementia with their local communities, building these natural supports so that they can continue to be a source of informal support throughout the trajectory of the illness. This work has brought a dynamic approach to building the self-confidence and participation of people in the early stages of dementia and has helped counteract the social disconnection and isolation that can lead to earlier use of formal support measures.

2 The Demands of Dementia

Dementia is the umbrella term for a range of brain diseases that are progressive and chronic in their nature. Symptoms include deterioration in cognitive function, behavioural changes and functional limitations. The illness has a profound impact on society and those directly affected by the illness. Globally there are an estimated 44.4 million people with dementia, which will increase to 135 million by 2050 (Alzheimer Disease International 2013). The estimated worldwide cost of dementia is $604 billion US dollars, which equates to 1% of GDP. In the UK there are an estimated 800 000 people with dementia with the current cost of £23 billion (Alzheimer Society 2013). Amongst older people, dementia makes the largest contribution to the need for care, much more so than other types of impairment and chronic disease (Prince et al. 2013). This demand for health and social care services will continue to increase as a result of demographic changes. Responding to this challenge will require innovative ways of supporting people with dementia to live well from the early stages of the illness. Receiving a diagnosis of dementia creates a "biographical disruption", with the chronically ill "observing their former self-images crumbling away" (Bury 1982). People need support from the point of diagnosis to come to terms with this life altering event, remain connected to their community and enable them to live well with this long term illness. However, people typically do not receive support until the illness is advanced and often at the point of crisis (Alzheimer Scotland 2008). This pattern is becoming more acute as a result of pressure on health and social care budgets. Alzheimer Scotland has taken a strategic approach to counteract this failure and create systemic change through the development of the 5-Pillars Model of Post-Diagnostic Support. This led to a Scottish Government commitment for everyone newly diagnosed being entitled to one-year post diagnostic support from a named link worker (Scottish Government 2011). This Design Fellowship will be focused on this key stage in the dementia journey. Whilst there are an estimated 88,000 people with dementia in Scotland, only 50% of cases have been identified. The insidious and sporadic nature of symptoms makes it difficult to spot the early signs of dementia. People may also delay taking action fearful of having their suspicions confirmed and believing there is nothing that can be done to help in dementia (Keady and Nolan 2003). Time taken to diagnosis from the onset of symptoms may be around three years (Chrisp et al. 2011). At the point of diagnosis people will have lived with many of the difficulties dementia brings and may have become disconnected from their community. Diagnosis then brings the "sick role", challenging their identity and social position (Williams 2005).

The research, reported here, is focused on developing and implementing innovative design interventions that will promote dignity and independence for people living with dementia throughout the post-diagnostic stage of the illness. It will focus on reconnecting people to their communities, building these natural supports so that they can continue to be a source of informal support throughout the trajectory of the illness. Alzheimer Scotland works directly with over 60 link workers who provide post-diagnostic support services, which has provided an effective connection for the author (researcher) to work with people recently diagnosed and who are in the early stages of dementia. The research has brought a dynamic approach to building the self-confidence and participation of people in the early stages of dementia that has helped counteract the disconnection and social isolation that leads to earlier use of formal support and crisis intervention measures.

3 Personhood

Philosophical debates on dementia have largely focused around the fundamental nature of being and what constitutes personhood. The failure to recognise personhood and the negative impact of inappropriate care giving can result in 'malignant social psychology', which typically includes 'negative' labelling, disempowerment, infantilisation, invalidation and objectification (Kitwood 1990). One reason behind this malignance is failing to see a person and not showing the respect that properly accords a person (Kitwood 1990). Even when a person seems to have lost a significant part of what made them a unique individual, core elements of their identity will remain.

'[These] *characteristic gestures and ways of doing things are what keep alive the sense of the individual they once were, even if the more sophisticated levels of that individual have been removed.*'

(Matthews 2006)

This has important implications for any approach to providing support and services and what people require in addition to the basics of daily living. A person's sense of self and self-respect can be fostered through '*reinforcing any remaining elements of conscious self-identity*'; less conscious elements in a person's identity can be preserved through physical surroundings to retain '*physical links with their past, which help to support a sense of personhood*' (Matthews 2006). Whilst mood and behaviour may be profoundly affected, personhood is not; the individual remains the same equally valuable person throughout the course of the illness. Therefore, any potential design interventions intended to support the person with dementia should honour their personhood and right to be treated as a unique individual. In later sections of this paper, details of the 'Perfect Day' service are provided that will ensure that the individual's personhood and right to be treated as a unique individual is honoured.

4 'Perfect Day' Service

The 'Perfect Day' service has been developed predominately for Alzheimer Scotland care support workers who work with people living with dementia on a day-to-day basis. However, the 'Perfect Day' service also aims to support and inspire other stakeholders involved in the day-to-day care of individuals including family members, other Alzheimer Scotland staff, and the wider network of support personnel involved in the health and social care of people living with dementia. The service has been developed as part of the author's larger Arts and Humanities Research Council (AHRC) funded Design Research Fellowship and is built on the principles of the Scottish Dementia Working Group research sub-group's core principles for involving people with dementia in research (SDWG 2013). That is, researchers working with people with dementia must:

- Always ask people with dementia how they want to be involved in research, including at what points and in what ways they want to be updated.
- Involve people with dementia in setting research priorities (e.g. researchers asking people with dementia what a positive outcome would look like for them).
- Ensure that everyone taking part in research, especially people living with dementia, are physically and emotionally safe.
- Use language that is supportive of people with dementia and consider ways in which language can offend people living with dementia.
- Be "dementia aware" (i.e. you must be empathic not sympathetic), compassionate, knowledgeable, un-patronising, tolerant, understanding, and respectful.

- Consider "dementia time" in their expectations of research, including finding out the best time and how each individual keeps track of time.

The intention is that by following the principles outlined above will challenge researchers across all disciplines to re-consider not only how people with dementia are involved and valued in research but also how knowledge and greater understanding is constructed in dementia research (Williams 2005).

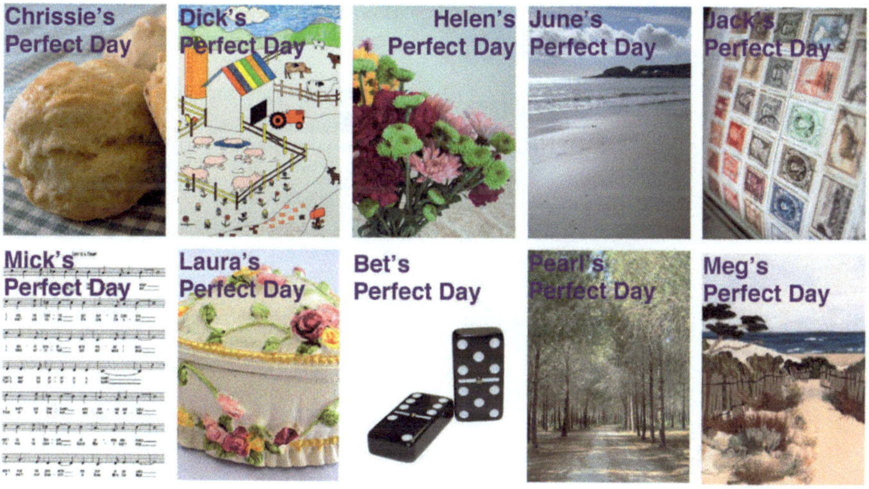

Fig. 1 Selection of "Perfect Day" cards

The "Perfect Day" service was initiated after the author visited over 20 Alzheimer Scotland day care centres across Scotland (Figure 1). During these visits the author (researcher) had first-hand opportunities to work with and communicate with people living with dementia, their family members, and the Alzheimer Scotland care support workers. From these visits, it quickly became obvious that the day-to-day work of the care support workers is very challenging and demanding. In particular, the care support workers are continually challenged to provide activities and services that are often conflicting in nature (i.e. highly personalized yet open to all, flexible yet focused, etc.) Moreover, the care support workers need to ensure that any service or activity is appropriate for a wide range of people living with dementia who may have different levels of independence, physical, cognitive and other abilities. It became abundantly clear that a service design intervention aimed at supporting Alzheimer Scotland care support workers would be very welcome.

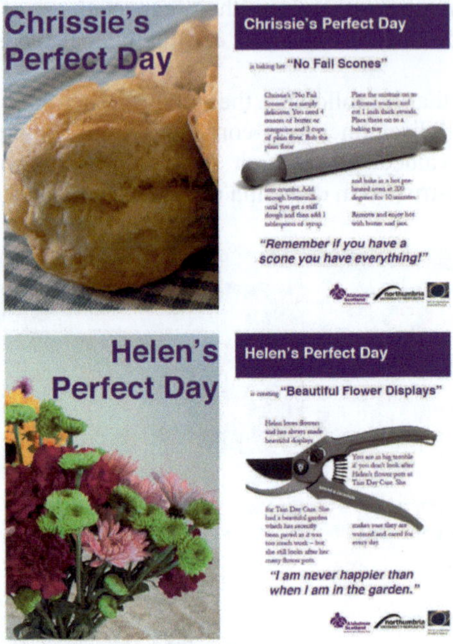
Chrissie's Perfect Day
Chrissie's Perfect Day
"No Fail Scones"
"Remember if you have a scone you have everything!"
Helen's Perfect Day
Helen's Perfect Day
"Beautiful Flower Displays"
"I am never happier than when I am in the garden."

Fig. 2 Chrissie and Helen's "Perfect Day" double-sided cards

The idea then was to explore what the 'Perfect Day' might look/feel/taste/sound like for people living with dementia. Working closely with Alzheimer Scotland Regional Managers, Deputy Regional Managers, and day care service workers a range of 'Perfect Day' examples drawn from people living with dementia all over Scotland were collected. This was undertaken in a collaborative fashion with care workers and people living with dementia. In all cases, the author would visit the day care services of Alzheimer Scotland and work closely with people living with dementia and Alzheimer Scotland support staff to create the individual's 'Perfect Day.' This was undertaken through a semi-structured interview approach, prompting the person living with dementia by asking:

- Where have you lived?
- What jobs have you done?
- What would your 'Perfect Day' look like?
- What would you do?
- Where would you do it?
- What would it involve?
- What would you need?
- Why is it perfect?

To date, the author has collected and developed a set of cards comprising over 75 double-sided 'Perfect Day' cards that day care support workers can use to help them plan and run their daily activities and sessions with people living with dementia. For example, Chrissie from Inverness has a 'Perfect Day' that is to bake her 'no fail' scones from her secret family recipe and Helen from Aberdeen has a 'Perfect Day' that is creating beautiful flower displays (Figure 2).

Senior members of Alzheimer Scotland staff believe there is much potential in exploring what people living with dementia's 'Perfect Day' might look like. Furthermore, there is potential in discovering what other people living with dementia that visit and use Alzheimer Scotland's services on a less regular basis think a 'Perfect Day' might look like? The key idea behind this service intervention is to collect over 100 'Perfect Day' stories from people living with dementia all over Scotland and then roll out the service design intervention out nationally and possibly internationally. The intention is that one person's 'Perfect Day' in Glasgow might be really enjoyable and relevant for another person's 'Perfect Day' in Orkney and vice versa. Moreover, we believe that some 'Perfect Day' ideas will be appropriate for both male and female, cover a range of abilities, and challenge care support workers to prepare and organise activities that they might never have thought of previously.

5 'Perfect Day' as Personalised Support

People with dementia and their carers require personalised and flexible support that encourages and facilitates their independence, citizenship and right to participate in society. This support needs to be delivered proactively and sensitively by skilled workers trained to a minimum of the Skilled Level of the Promoting Excellence Framework (Scottish Government 2011). Generally speaking, the vast majority of care and support for people with dementia is provided by informal carers that are usually family members (e.g. spouse, brother, sister, son, daughter). The opportunity to create best value through combining public resources with the natural supports in peoples' lives is currently not being achieved for the majority of people living with dementia. The prevalent construct of care fails to recognise community support as a resource to facilitate resilience and promote independence. Community support services can be inflexible and inappropriate, creating dependency rather than promoting independence.

A small level of consistent and high quality dementia-specialist support can complement the natural supports in people's lives. Support should utilise person-centred planning processes and be outcome-focused to enable people to live well with dementia and ensure their families enjoy as good and inclusive a life as possible. Provision of services should not be expressed in hours of care; instead, support should be designed in line with the range of approaches to self-directed support set out in the Social Care (Self-directed Support) (Scotland) Bill (Executive Bill introduced on 29th February 2012, Scottish Parliament Corporate Body, Edinburgh). Whether people wish to directly commission their own support or not, the support they are offered must allow flexibility to provide what is truly meaningful for each individual's life.

For some people, support will involve personal care and dementia-specialist day care. There may also be a need for basic home care. Personalised support goes further to enable the person and their carer to have maximum quality of life. It reinforces the right to active participation and citizenship. It provides what is meaningful and relevant for each individual in order to maintain the fabric of their life for as long as possible. Giving additional time to a person with dementia saves time in the long run; supporting a person to do things for themselves, rather than carrying out the task for them, maintains function and skills in activities of daily living. This approach to support continues to empower the person with dementia and their family to remain in control throughout the duration of the illness – thus helping to avoid crises and assisting in delaying the need for admission to institutional care.

6 Conclusions and Future Work

The 'Perfect Day' service ties in strongly with both the 'Therapeutic Interventions' pillar of Alzheimer Scotland's eight pillars model, and also the 'Personalised Support' described in the previous section (Kinnaird 2012). That is, the 'Perfect Day' service intervention will support cognitive rehabilitation and help assist the person to achieve personal goals in relation to making the most of their remaining memory and developing compensatory strategies. It is known that clinical efficacy is achieved in the use of goal-orientated cognitive rehabilitation (Clare et al. 2010, Hauer et al. 2012) and that cognitive stimulation therapy can provide mental stimulation in order to improve general functioning. There is also strong evidence of benefit to the individual's cognitive function and evidence of improvement in a person living with dementia's overall quality of life (Woods et al. 2012). To this end, the 'Perfect Day' service seeks to have an effect on promoting language, improving conversation and communication, and having fun which are all considered to have generalised benefits for people living with dementia (Spector et al. 2010).

The 'Perfect Day' activity cards proactively deliver personalised and flexible support by challenging assumptions and preconceived ideas about what is possible for people living with dementia. Current 'Perfect Day' cards include activities such as fishing, 5-a-side football, going out for a meal, hill walking, driving, painting, photography and many other challenging activities. It is acknowledged that many of the 'Perfect Day' activities and tasks are demanding and will challenge care support workers as well as people living with dementia. However, people living with dementia have created the 'Perfect Days' themselves; they are authentic accounts that will support their independence, citizenship and right to participate more fully in society.

It is envisaged that the 'Perfect Day' activities and tasks will mean giving additional time to a person with dementia. However, this will save time in the long run. By supporting a person to do things for themselves, rather than carrying out the task for them, means that the person living with dementia maintains function and skills in activities of daily living. The 'Perfect Day' approach to support will continue to empower the person living with dementia and their family to remain in control throughout the duration of the illness. Thus, helping to avoid crises and assisting in delaying the need for admission to institutional care (Oddy 2003).

The 'Perfect Day' service is viewed as a key element in Alzheimer Scotland's future 'toolkit' of interventions for people living with dementia all over Scotland. Future work on this project will include the formal roll out of the "Perfect Day" service across dementia care service centres across Scotland, using and testing them with care support workers, people living with dementia and their families. It is envisaged that the 'Perfect Day' personalised support will enable the person living with dementia and their carer network to enjoy maximum quality of life. Moreover, the service design intervention will support the rights of each person to enjoy active participation and citizenship and provide what is meaningful and relevant for each individual in order to maintain the fabric of their life for as long as possible. The next stage here is to conduct formal evaluations of the 'Perfect Day' activity cards in the near future with a range of stakeholders involved in the day-to-day care of people living with dementia. Post evaluations, the hope is that people living with dementia all over Scotland will begin to experience and enjoy their 'Perfect Days'.

Acknowledgements

The author gratefully acknowledges the financial support of the UK's Arts and Humanities Research Council (AHRC) in this work. This research project entitled 'Disrupting Dementia Care through Innovative Co-Designed Interventions' has been funded under the AHRC's Design Research Fellowship scheme (Award Ref: AH/M007677/1). The work is also generously supported by Alzheimer Scotland – the main collaborating partner. The author wishes to acknowledge the significant support of Alzheimer Scotland and the many people he has worked with over the course of the project.

References

Alzheimer Disease International (2013) Policy briefing for heads of government: The global impact of dementia 2013-2015. London, UK

Alzheimer Scotland (2008) Meeting our needs: The level and quality of dementia support services in Scotland. Edinburgh, Scotland

Alzheimer Society (2013) Defining dementia. Available at: www.alzheimers.org.uk/infographic (Accessed in November 2015)

Bury M (1982) Chronic illness as biographical disruption. Sociology of Health & Illness 4(2): 167-182

Chrisp T, Thomas B, Goddard W, Owens A (2011) Dementia timeline: Journeys, delays and decisions on the pathway to an early diagnosis. Dementia 10(4): 555-570

Clare L, Linden D, Woods RT, Whitaker R, Evans SJ, Parkinson CH et al. (2010) Goal-orientated cognitive rehabilitation for people with early stage Alzheimer's disease. American Journal of Geriatric Psychiatry 18(10): 928-939

Hauer K, Schwenk M, Zieschang T, Essig M, Becker C, Oster P (2012) Physical training improves motor performance in people with dementia. Journal of American Geriatric Society 60(1): 8-15

Jowitt J (2013) Ageing population will have huge impact on social services. The Guardian Online on 24 February 2013. Available at: www.theguardian.com/society/older-people (Accessed on 21 August 2015)

Keady J, Nolan M (2003) The dynamics of dementia: Working together, working separately, or working alone? In: Nolan M, Lundh U, Keady J, Grant G (Eds.) Partnerships in family care. Open University Press, Berkshire, UK

Kinnaird L (2012) Delivering integrated dementia care: The 8 pillars model of community support. Alzheimer Scotland, Edinburgh, Scotland

Kitwood T (1990) The dialectics of dementia: With particular reference to Alzheimer's disease. Ageing & Society 10: 177-196

Matthews E (2006) Dementia and the identity of the person. In: Hughes J, Louw S, Sabat S (Eds.) Dementia: Mind, meaning and the person. Oxford University Press, Oxford, UK

Oddy R (2003) Promoting mobility for people with dementia: A problem solving approach. Age Concern, London, UK

Prince M, Prina M, Guerchet M (2013) World Alzheimer report 2013 - Journey of caring: An analysis of long-term care for dementia. Alzheimer's Disease International, London, UK

Scottish Government (2011) Promoting excellence: A framework for all health and social services staff working with people with dementia, their families and carers. Scottish Government, Edinburgh, Scotland

SDWG (2013) Core principles for involving people with dementia in research. Scottish Dementia Working Group (Research Sub-group), University of Edinburgh, Edinburgh, Scotland

Spector A, Orrell M, Woods B (2010) Cognitive stimulation therapy: Effects on different areas of cognitive function for people with dementia. International Journal of Geriatric Psychiatry 25(12): 1253-1258

Williams S (2005) Parsons revisited: From the sick role to…? Health: An Interdisciplinary Journal for the Social Study of Health, Illness and Medicine 9(2): 123-144

Woods B, Aguirre E, Spector AE, Orrell M (2012) Cognitive stimulation to improve cognitive functioning in people with dementia. Cochrane Database Systematic Reviews 15: CD005562

Packaging Openability: A Study Involving Chinese Elders

X. Ma and H. Dong

Abstract: The aim of this study is to collect data about packaging openability from older adults in China, so as to better inform designers. It reports a survey that includes self-reporting via a questionnaire and performance tests. The study sample consists of 37 males and 33 females (from seven different regions across China), ranging from 50 to 80 years old. The study collected dexterity capability data—including the ability to pick up small objects—strength, the ability to interact with typical interfaces and visual ability. The research results will assist in the design of appropriate packaging for older people.

1 Introduction

As people get older, they become weaker, and their dexterity decreases, making it increasingly challenging to open packaging (Sudbury-Riley 2014). Lack of accessibility, understanding, perceived affordance, clarification (information) and excess packaging have all made it more difficult for older adults to access products (Winder et al. 2002, Yoxall et al. 2006, Wang and Zhao 2007, Clifford 2011, Passali et al. 2012, Dong 2013, Choi 2014). The age-related decline of capabilities has implications for design. If reduced functional capability is not taken into account in the design process, this might result in the elderly—who constitute a growing proportion of the Chinese adult population—becoming excluded from the use of many household goods. The mid-2010 sixth national census data from the Chinese National Bureau of Statistics show that members of the population aged 55 and over made up 13.26% of the total population of China (Wang 2015). Designers may have failed to keep up with demographic changes.

There are already studies about packaging openability for older adults (e.g., Yan and Yu 2005, Soininen 2011, Jégou and Liberman 2012, Wisson 2012, Brooks 2013, Clifford 2013, Khanom 2013). These studies have collected data and conducted statistical analysis by using different measurement equipment, self-reports, and performance measures (Wu et al. 2009, Bell et al. 2013, Brooks 2013, Yen et al. 2013, Yoxall et al. 2013, Rowson et al. 2014, Sudbury-Riley 2014). Packaging openability

X. Ma · H. Dong (✉)
Inclusive Design Research Centre, College of Design and Innovation, Tongji University, Shanghai, China
email: donghua@tongji.edu.cn

P. Langdon et al. (eds.), *Designing Around People*,
DOI 10.1007/978-3-319-29498-8_11

data are fundamental to the design of safe and usable packages. However, there are gaps in the ergonomics data available to designers: the majority of packaging-related work has examined issues related to the strength of consumers, particularly when opening jars. Although understanding the force required to open a jar is important, the work of Bell et al. (2013) shows that with a significant number of packaging items users struggled to open them because of issues of dexterity rather than strength. In addition, there are problems with the currently available end-user capability databases, such as the lack of data on multiple capabilities, the absence of surveys with an appropriate level of specificity in the questions, and data derived from non-representative samples of the population. Moreover, inclusive design was seldom taken into consideration when designing past experiments, and most of the research was conducted in Western countries; the database in China is very limited (Ke 2009).

This study aims to provide packaging designers with the information needed to put inclusive design into practice. The study collected information on dexterity capabilities, including strength, the ability to pick up small objects, the ability to interact with typical interfaces, the ability to access or use everyday products and visual ability.

2 Methods

This project utilized both quantitative and qualitative data collection tools. Data collection consisted of surveys as well as pictures taken from participants' daily lives. Participants were voluntary and anonymous. A total of 70 questionnaires were distributed to randomly selected adults between 50-80 years of age to ensure a sample group with an even spread of socio-economic backgrounds. Participants included 37 males and 33 females from seven cities and towns across China. All participants had the ability to live independently.

There is extensive evidence that affective states (moods or emotions) can change perceptions, thoughts and behaviours. Therefore, all tests were conducted in participants' homes, and before the start of the test, small talk with participants was used as an 'ice breaker' to reduce their discomfort with being interviewed by the researcher and help them maintain a 'normal' mood.

For the sake of fitting the national customs, a specific toolkit for Chinese ergonomics measurement has been developed through discussions and rewriting of the entire research process (Figure 1).

This toolkit was developed for inclusive design data collection based on the framework of 'Towards Better Design: An Evaluation of the Pilot Study' (Clarkson 2010). The collected data included questions about perceptions of capability and confidence in using certain products and a series of physical tests that included measures of vision, hearing, dexterity and cognition. Although the toolkit assesses many different capabilities, this paper focuses on dexterity, strength and vision because these have been identified as most relevant to package opening.

Participants who agreed to take part in this one-hour study were visited in their homes and asked for their demographic information (age, gender, any disability that may affect their ability to open packaging, colour blindness, handedness, eyesight and whether they lived alone).

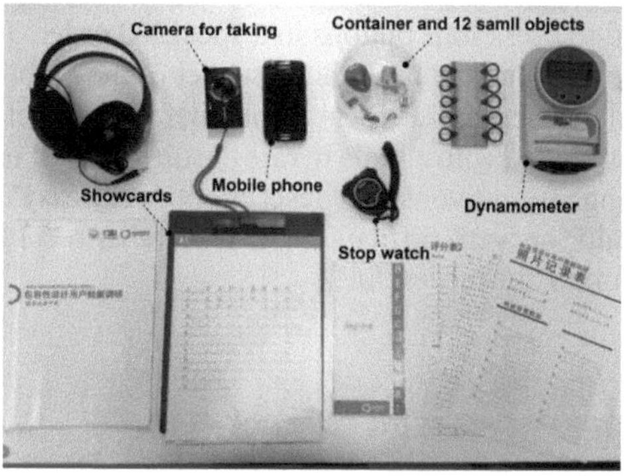

Fig. 1 The toolkit for data collection

Instruments were calibrated before the test. Before each test started, the participants were allowed to familiarize themselves with the test instruments. They adopted natural posture to ensure a true representation of the capability that can be exerted (Peebles and Norris 2002), and their posture was recorded. The following tests were conducted: the Moberg pick-up test, a grip strength test, a dexterity task and a vision test.

2.1 The Moberg Pick-up Test

The test instruments included a tape measure, a stopwatch and a container with 12 small objects inside (a ￥1 coin, a wing nut, a key, a die, a nail, a square nut, a hexagon nut, a washer, a paper clip, a cotton swab, an eraser and a pencil sharpener). These 12 small objects are widely used during everyday life in China. They were placed on a table in front of the participant, who was instructed to pick them up one at a time as quickly as possible and place them into the container. The participants did the test first with their dominant hand, then with their non-dominant hand. The time was recorded.

2.2 Grip Strength Test

A dynamometer (brand Wanqing, made in Shanghai) and a stopwatch were used for the grip strength test. When ready, the participant was asked to squeeze the dynamometer with maximum effort and to maintain maximum pressure for five seconds. After a short break, the participant was asked to squeeze the dynamometer at a comfortable level and to maintain this pressure for five seconds. The participant did the test first with their dominant hand, then with their non-dominant hand. The strength was recorded.

2.3 Dexterity Task

A mobile phone, a headphone jack and a USB cable were used for this test. The participant was asked to press four buttons in a specified order. They were then asked to insert a headphone jack into the headphone socket of the mobile phone. Finally, the participant was asked to insert the USB cable into the USB socket of the mobile phone. The participant was provided with a scale to rate the difficulty of each task. Participants could select their ratings from five verbal descriptors: 'very easy', 'easy', 'neither easy nor difficult', 'difficult', or 'very difficult'. The researcher recorded the rating and the result (i.e., 'successful' or 'unsuccessful').

2.4 Vision Test

Vision capability cards A1 and A2 were used in this test. There were twelve rows in the cards that consisted of commonly used Chinese characters (sizes for characters in each row are 9, 7.4, 6, 4.7, 4.2, 3.7, 3.3, 2.9, 2.5, 2.2, 2 and 1.8 mm). The A1 set of letters was printed in high contrast colours (i.e., black against a white background), and the A2 set of letters was printed in low contrast colours (i.e., light grey against a white background). The participant was asked to hold the cards with his or her arm outstretched at the distance they typically use when reading to look at the top set of letters (for both the high contrast and low contrast cards) and read out the letters of the smallest row that was comfortable for them to read. The participant was not initially allowed to use visual aids if they did not often wear them in their daily activities; this suggests the character size they can recognize in reading under daily conditions (coded as 'daily'), and then repeat the test with visual aids if they had in their daily life while reading; this suggest the character size they can recognize when reading under comfortable conditions (coded as 'comfort'). The researcher recorded which row the participant read and marked on the vision score sheet whether each letter in that row was identified correctly or not.

3 Results

The data received from the participants was coded by assigning a number to each scale. Numerical data were then analysed using SPSS (Version 10.0 SPSS Inc, Chicago, IL, USA). Frequencies of responses were calculated for each question. ANOVA (analysis of variance, useful for comparing three or more means for statistical significance) was used to determine the relationships between various numerical variables using SPSS. A result was considered to be significant when $p<0.05$.

Among the 70 participants (37 male, 33 female), forty-six per cent of males had achieved a high educational qualification, and 51% had achieved an intermediate education. Thirty-six per cent of females had achieved a high educational qualification, and 60% had achieved an intermediate education. Apart from one woman who lived alone, all other participants lived with their family members. Sixty per cent of males and 76% of females were unemployed (i.e., retired or unable to work).

The results of the four tests are shown in Table 1.

Table 1 Summary statistics of performance test

			Min	Max	SD	Mean	95% CI
Dexterity Test (s)	Male	DH	9.03	18.66	2.59	13.21	12.28, 14.15
		NDH	8.39	19.34	2.82	13.35	12.33, 14.37
	Female	DH	8.54	25.38	4.48	14.46	12.85, 16.08
		NDH	8.97	27.00	4.81	15.15	13.41, 16.88
Comfort Strength (kg)	Male	DH	0	26.50	6.56	6.56	6.43, 11.16
		NDH	0.50	30.20	7.03	7.03	5.86, 10.93
	Female	DH	0	25.50	7.62	7.77	5.02, 10.52
		NDH	0.70	28.50	7.25	7.77	5.16, 10.38
Max Strength (kg)	Male	DH	0	49.60	13.8	32.67	27.69, 27.64
		NDH	5.00	50.20	11.6	30.81	26.63, 34.99
	Female	DH	8.50	38.40	6.42	23.45	21.13, 25.76
		NDH	10.40	43.60	7.16	22.06	19.47, 24.64
Visual (mm)	Male	HCD	1.80	7.40	1.22	3.36	2.93, 3.79
		HCC	0	7.40	1.72	2.90	2.29, 3.51
		LCD	1.80	7.40	1.09	3.58	3.19, 3.97
		LCC	0	7.40	1.53	3.47	2.92, 4.00
	Female	HCD	0	7.40	1.45	3.51	3.00, 4.02
		HCC	0	4.70	1.48	2.55	2.02, 3.07
		LCD	0	7.40	1.59	3.98	3.41, 4.54
		LCC	0	4.70	1.19	3.02	2.60, 3.45

SD = Standard deviation; 95%CI = 95% confidence interval; DH = Dominant Hand; NDH = Non-dominant Hand; HCD = High Contrast Daily; HCC = High Contrast Comfort; LCD = Low Contrast Daily; LCC = Low Contrast Comfort

69 participants completed the study. The mean age is 62.7 years with a standard deviation of 8.86 years. 97% of the participants reported being right hand dominant; six out of 70 suffered from arthritis. The data shows that dexterity decreased with increasing age, a finding similar to those of previous research results (Frederiksen et al. 2002, Andersen-Ranberg et al. 2009, Wu et al. 2011).

The min value, max value, standard deviation, mean value and 95% confidence interval are reported according to gender. A 95% confidence interval shows the interval within which the population is likely to lie with 95% probability. Most people think daily dexterity related tasks are easy. Dexterity test time is gathered in 12.28s to 16.88s. Male participants are generally found to be significantly stronger than female participants. Most people's comfortable grip strength is under 11.16kg. On average, males have 11.40kg more maximum grip strength than females, which is 1.4kg lower than the previous research result in Qingdao, China (Wu et al. 2011).

Maximum grip strength for male is between 27.69kg and 34.99kg and for female between 21.13kg and 24.64kg.

3.1 The Moberg Pick-up Test

For the Moberg pick-up test, males took a mean time of 13.21s with their dominant hand and 13.35s with their non-dominant hand. Females took a mean time of 14.46s with their dominant hand and 15.15s with their non-dominant hand. Dexterity test times for males ranged from 11.39s to 16.99s; for females times ranged from 11.32s to 17.62s. The participants performed the test slightly faster with their dominant hand ($p=0.01$).

Age had an impact on hand dexterity in this study: participants of 50-59 years old, 60-69 years old and 70-79 years old required mean times of 13.94s, 12.96s and 17.37s, respectively. These mean times are based on the upper bound of the 95% CI (confidence interval).

A two factorial analysis of variance for dexterity performance (factors: age group and gender) shows that dexterity performance was impacted by gender ($p<0.05$) and by age ($p<0.05$). Males carried out all subsets of the Moberg pick-up test slightly faster than females. The performance of the age groups in the Moberg pick-up test was significantly different from that in the other two tests, with the 60-69 group being the fastest and the 50-59 group being the slowest to complete the test.

3.2 Grip Strength Test

The mean female grip strength was found to be only 79% of the mean male grip strength.

A pervious study showed that grip strength clearly decreases as age increases (Rowson and Yoxall 2011, Massy-Westropp et al. 2011). In this study, we found that participants 50-59 years old, 60-69 years old and 70-79 years old had a mean comfort strength of 12.91kg, 8.25kg and 8.47kg and a mean max strength of 37.05kg, 28.64kg and 25.43kg, respectively.

A two factorial analysis of variance for strength performance (factors: age group and gender) shows that strength performance was impacted by gender ($p<0.05$) and by age ($p<0.05$). One factorial analysis of variance for comfort strength performance (factors: gender) shows that comfort strength performance was not impacted significantly by gender ($p<0.05$).

3.3 Dexterity Tasks

Most of the participants found the dexterity tasks easy. For each task, the participants were asked to report how they felt when inserting a headphone cable and a USB cable into a socket. None of them found the USB task difficult.

Table 2 Dexterity task related questions (self-report) 'How difficult is it to …?'

	Very easy	Easy	Neither easy nor difficult	Difficult	Very difficult
Insert a headphone cable into socket	78.6%	18.6%	1.4%	0	1.4%
Insert a USB cable into socket	60%	18.6%	14.3%	7.1%	0

3.4 Vision Test

Presbyopia has been reported as a common visual impairment for older Chinese adults (present in 73% of males and 82% of females). On the contrary, glaucoma has been reported as a general visual impairment in Western countries. It has been suggested that economic development may have an influence on visual condition (Loh and Ogle 2004).

Males could see a mean character size of 3.36mm in a high contrast daily condition, 2.90mm in a high contrast comfort condition, 3.58mm in a low contrast daily condition and 3.47mm in a low contrast comfort condition. Women could see a mean character size of 3.51mm in a high contrast daily condition, 2.55mm in a high contrast comfort condition, 3.98mm in a low contrast daily condition and 3.02mm in a low contrast comfort condition. Participants could see the character more clearly in high contrast than in low contrast.

Visual acuity decreased with advancing age. Participants 50-59 years old, 60-69 years old and 70-79 years old required a mean character size of 3.41mm, 3.34mm and 3.61mm respectively in a high contrast daily condition; 2.35mm, 2.64mm and 3.49mm in a high contrast comfort condition; 3.46mm, 4.01mm and 4.11mm in a low contrast daily condition and 3.07mm, 3.23mm, and 3.71mm in a low contrast comfort condition. These mean sizes are based on the upper bound of the 95% CI.

A two factorial analysis of variance for visual performance (factors: age group and gender) shows that visual performance was impacted by age ($p<0.05$) and not by gender ($p>0.05$). A four factorial analysis of variance for visual performance (factors: high contrast daily condition, high contrast comfort condition, low contrast daily condition or low contrast comfort condition) shows that age significantly impacted the results of the high contrast comfort condition ($p<0.05$), with young subjects seeing much smaller characters than the older groups.

4 Discussion and Conclusions

The results of the Moberg pick-up test differ from those of earlier studies (Ng et al. 1999, Stamm et al. 2003, Amirjani et al. 2007). In this study, males carried out all subsets of the Moberg pick-up test slightly faster than females ($p<0.05$). As shown in the results, the male participants were better educated than the females. Lacking education in general, the Chinese females involved in the study did not have much of a chance to be involved in work requiring deft movement (Qu et al. 1990, Wang 2008), which may have a negative impact on female dexterity. Participants aged between 50 and 59 years needed more time to complete the dexterity test than those aged between 60 and 69. This was probably because they had not yet got used to declining dexterity and retirement, and they did not have as much experience in dealing with these situations as older participants.

In the grip strength test, the Chinese results were lower than the international ones (Laxman and Hospital 2004, Massy-Westropp et al. 2011), and similar to the results of an early study in Taiwan (Wu et al. 2009). Currently available information, such as data about physical strength, has often been collected using tests that do not actually represent how consumers use a product. For example, in past studies, tasks were carried out under ideal conditions, and participants were asked to complete tasks in a specified position (Richards et al. 1996). However, during the design process, designers have to consider how people might actually behave in the real world rather than in an ideal one. In this study, the participants were asked to perform tasks under 'normal' daily conditions.

For dexterity, the participants were asked to plug in the headphone cable. They often showed great confidence. Even if they were not successful, they thought this task was very simple and that they had successfully completed it (see Figure 2). In fact, they did not fully insert the headphones into the headphone jack.

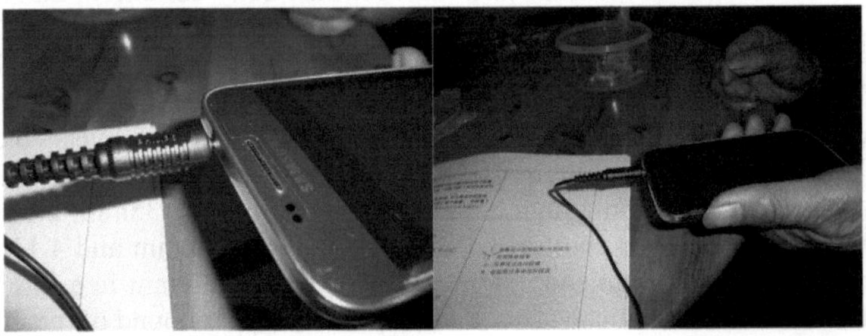

Fig. 2 The task was actually not completed successfully

Prior studies into packaging tended to concentrate on narrow and specific issues, such as brand communication, ergonomics, nutrition, consumer education or public policy implications. This study provided a multidimensional ageing framework to make sense of the packaging openability data and provided several unique insights. The data was collected from older consumers from seven different cities and towns in China; their multiple capabilities relating to packaging openability were measured.

More data relating to packaging openability are needed, such as fingertip strength, time taken to open packaging and dimension measurements of the hand. We are already working on a continuation of this research that will collect data on fingertip strength (e.g., pitch strength). It is hoped that the results from this study will motivate and inform the development of more appropriate solutions for older adults in the future through improved packaging design.

References

Amirjani N, Ashworth NL, Gordon T, Edwards DC, Chan KM (2007) Normative values and the effects of age, gender, and handedness on the Moberg pick-up test. Muscle Nerve 35: 788-792

Andersen-Ranberg K, Petersen I, Frederiksen H, Mackenbach JP, Christensen K (2009) Cross-national differences in grip strength among 50+ year-old Europeans: Results from the SHARE study. European Journal of Ageing 6: 227-236

Bell AF, Walton K, Chevis JS, Davies K, Manson C, Wypych A et al. (2013) Accessing packaged food and beverages in hospital. Exploring experiences of patients and staff. Appetite 60: 231-238

Brooks J (2013) The ageing population is pushing easy-open packaging up the agenda. Available at: www.packagingnews.co.uk/features/consumer-iq-open-questions-06-02-2013 (Accessed in November 2015)

Choi YM (2014) User capabilities versus device task demands in a tape dispenser product for persons with limited dexterity. In: Langdon PM, Lazar J, Heylighen A, Dong H (Eds.) Inclusive designing: Joining usability, accessibility and inclusion, pp.13-23. Springer International Publishing

Clarkson PJ (2010) Towards better design: An evaluation of the pilot study. Available at: discover.ukdataservice.ac.uk/catalogue?sn=6997 (Accessed in November 2015)

Clifford E (2013) Food and drink packaging trends - UK (executive summary). Mintel Group Ltd.

Clifford S (2011) Devilish packaging, tamed. Available at: www.nytimes.com/2011/06/02/business/energy-environment/02packaging.html (Accessed in November 2015)

Dong H (2013) Inaccessible packaging. Which? UK Consumer Magazine 24: 103-107

Frederiksen H, Gaist D, Petersen HC, Hjelmborg J, McGue M, Vaupel JW et al. (2002) Hand grip strength: A phenotype suitable for identifying genetic variants affecting mid- and late-life physical functioning. Genetic Epidemiology 23: 110-122

Jégou F, Liberman J (2012) Packaging research. Available at: www.education.edean.org/pdf/Case032.pdf (Accessed in November 2015)

Ke S (2009) Human factors' influence on design of packaging openability. China Packaging Industry 8: 34-36

Khanom R (2013) Soap, bath and shower products - UK (executive summary). Mintel Group Ltd.

Laxman S, Hospital O (2004) Pinch grip, power grip and wrist twisting strengths of healthy older adults. Gerontech 3: 77-87

Loh KY, Ogle J (2004) Age related visual impairment in the elderly. Medical Journal of Malaysia 59: 23-30

Massy-Westropp NM, Gill TK, Taylor AW, Bohannon RW, Hill CL (2011). Hand grip strength: Age and gender stratified normative data in a population-based study. Bmc Research Notes 4: 1-5

Ng CL, Ho DD, Chow SP (1999) The Moberg pickup test: Results of testing with a standard protocol. Journal of Hand Therapy 12: 309-312

Passali D, Gregori D, Foltran F (2012) Proper packaging for food and non-food products to avoid injuries. International Journal of Pediatric Otorhinolaryngology 76: 53-56

Peebles L, Norris B (2002) Filling 'gaps' in strength data for design. Applied Ergonomics 34: 73-88

Qu L, Zhang J, Zhou Y, Zhang J (1990) Activities of daily living (ADL) among the Chinese elderly. China Journal of Rehabilitation Medicine 7: 16-19

Richards LG, Olson B, Palmiter-Thomas P (1996) How forearm position affects grip strength. The American Journal of Occupational Therapy 50: 133-138

Rowson J, Sangrar A, Rodriguez-Falcon E, Bell AF, Walton KA, Yoxall A et al. (2014) Rating accessibility of packaging: A medical packaging example. Packaging Technology and Science 27: 577-589

Rowson J, Yoxall A (2011) Hold, grasp, clutch or grab: Consumer grip choices during food container opening. Applied Ergonomics 42: 627-633

Soininen K (2011) Dairy drinks, milk and cream - UK (executive summary). Mintel Group Ltd.

Stamm TA, Ploner A, Machold KP, Smolen J (2003) Moberg picking-up test in patients with inflammatory joint diseases: A survey of suitability in comparison with button test and measures of disease activity. Arthritis and Rheumatology 49: 626-632

Sudbury-Riley L (2014) Unwrapping senior consumers' packaging experiences. Marketing Intelligence and Planning 32: 666-686

Wang D (2008) Study on the declining physical functions and its influencing factors among the Chinese elderly aged 65 years and over. Chinese Journal of Rehabilitation Medicine 29: 1090-4

Wang X (2015) Changes in China's population structure and aging research. Journal of University of Jinan 25: 66-69

Wang X, Zhao J (2007) How to improve the packaging openability. Packaging Engineering 28: 177-178

Winder B, Ridgway K, Nelson A, Baldwin J (2002) Food and drink packaging: Who is complaining and who should be complaining. Applied Ergonomics 33: 433-438

Wisson C (2012) Crisps, salty snacks and nuts - UK (executive summary). Mintel Group Ltd.

Wu SW, Wu SF, Liang HW, Wu ZT, Huang S (2009) Measuring factors affecting grip strength in a Taiwan Chinese population and a comparison with consolidated norms. Applied Ergonomics 40: 811-815

Wu Y, Pang Z, Zhang D, Jiang W, Wang S, Li S (2011) A cross-sectional analysis of age and sex patterns in grip strength, tooth loss, near vision and hearing levels in chinese aged 50-74 years. Archives of Gerontology & Geriatrics 54: 213-220

Yan Y, Yu X (2005) Research of product packaging based on the body's comfort properties. Packaging Engineering 26: 33-36

Yen WT, Flinn SR, Sommerich CM, Lavender SA, Sanders EB (2013) Preference of lid design characteristics by older adults with limited hand function. Journal of Hand Therapy 26: 261-270

Yoxall A, Janson AR, Bradbury SR, Langley J, Wearn J, Hayes S (2006) Openability: Producing design limits for consumer packaging. Packaging Technology and Science 19: 219-225

Yoxall A, Rodriguez-Falcon EM, Luxmoore J (2013) Carpe diem, carpe ampulla: A numerical model as an aid to the design of child-resistant closures. Applied Ergonomics 44: 18-26

Walking Backwards to Quantify Visual Exclusion

S. D. Waller, J. A. Goodman-Deane, M. D. Bradley, K. L. Cornish and P. J. Clarkson

Abstract: Quantifying the proportion of the population who are unable to use a product is extremely persuasive to deliver inclusively designed solutions to market. This paper presents a new method for assessing artwork that is typically viewed at a hand-held distance, such as mobile phone icons. The assessment is performed by mounting the artwork on a wall, and then simulating reduced visual ability by viewing the artwork from further away than you normally would (i.e. walking backwards). Finally, exclusion is quantified by comparing the artwork being assessed against a vision test chart. This new method is able to capture and justify the sort of minor improvements that can really make a difference for people with age-related long sightedness, in a commercially relevant context.

1 Introduction

Inclusive design is "*the design of mainstream products and/or services that are accessible to, and usable by, as many people as reasonably possible*" (The British Standards Institute 2005). Every design decision can positively or negatively affect user exclusion. Consequently, one way of encouraging and facilitating inclusive design is through quantifying the impact of these decisions (Waller et al. 2010). This involves using survey data to estimate the number of people that would be unable to perform the task(s) required to achieve the user goals, because the demands of the tasks exceed their capabilities (Persad et al. 2007). Quantifying exclusion is intended to complement to other inclusive design methods, such as user trials (Aldersey-Williams et al. 1999), standards (W3C World Wide Web Consortium 2008) and expert opinion (Poulson et al. 1996). In particular, these other methods are excellent at uncovering user issues, but quantifying the corresponding exclusion is important to encourage businesses to actually do something about these issues (Waller et al. 2010).

The focus of this paper is on quantifying exclusion for artwork that is intended to be viewed from a hand-held position. This covers many products that people rely on on a daily basis, such as mobile phones, medicine labels, food packaging and

S. D. Waller (✉) · J. A. Goodman-Deane · M. D. Bradley · K. L. Cornish · P. J. Clarkson
Cambridge Engineering Design Centre, University of Cambridge, Cambridge, UK
email: sam.waller@eng.cam.ac.uk

P. Langdon et al. (eds.), *Designing Around People*,
DOI 10.1007/978-3-319-29498-8_12

medical devices. Use of these products is significantly affected by age-related long sightedness, which is by far the most common vision condition, affecting around 83% of people aged over 45 (Holden et al. 2008). The impact of this issue is increasing, 31% of the population were aged 60+ in 2014, and this is predicted to increase to 41% by 2034 (ONS 2015).

However, many designers are young, so age-related long sightedness is easily overlooked (Zitkus et al. 2013). Furthermore, when assessing the visual demand of handheld products, typical design practice relies heavily on experience and personal judgement, typified by the phrase "*I can see it, I think it is fine*". This is known to be a misconception in the design industry (Pheasant 1996, Cornish et al. 2015).

Existing methods for quantifying exclusion include comparing against standardised tasks, comparing against data-driven personas, or assessing the degree of simulated acuity loss through which the task remains possible (Porter et al. 2004, Cardoso 2005, Persad et al. 2007, Waller et al. 2010, Helen Hamlyn Centre for Design 2012, Goodman-Deane et al. 2014). Quantifying visual exclusion by simulating acuity loss is particularly advantageous as it is more objective than judging against standardised tasks or data-driven personas, and much faster and more economical than user trials (with enough users to meaningfully estimate population exclusion).

There are many visual impairment simulation tools available, including the 'Cambridge Simulation Glasses' and 'Impairment Simulator Software' available within the 'Inclusive Design Toolkit' (Clarkson et al. 2015); and the VINE (2015) SimSpecs. However, most of these tools rely on the designer having access to special hardware, such as blurry glasses, or specialist simulation software.

This paper presents a novel method for simulating visual acuity loss by mounting the artwork on a wall, and then viewing the artwork from further away than you normally would (i.e. walking backwards). For example, if the artwork is typically viewed at 70 cm, and the assessor has Snellen VA 6/6 (Beech and Singleton 1997), then if the assessor instead views the artwork at 140 cm, this is equivalent to simulating VA 6/12.

Simulating reduced visual ability in this manner eliminates the need for any specialist hardware or software, and also enables the designer to quickly and easily vary the level of simulated loss on a continuous scale. In particular, this continuous scale operates all the way from best corrected vision to severe visual impairment. Walking forwards and backwards allows for very fine adjustment of the simulated acuity loss, much more so than any commercially available simulation glasses.

Modifying the viewing distance is often used in ad-hoc ways in design practice, and was noted during designer interviews conducted as part of Cornish et al. (2015)'s research. However, to the authors knowledge, nothing has yet been published on calibrating a modified viewing distance with particular levels of visual acuity loss, or the corresponding population exclusion.

However, it is important to note that modifying the viewing distance is only practical when dealing with flat artwork that is typically hand-held. There are many viable and important design scenarios that match this scope, such as those discussed earlier. However, simulation glasses remain the authors' recommended approach for quantifying exclusion associated with graphical details that are intended to be perceived at a distance, or for understanding and assessing an interaction involving hand-eye coordination, such as opening packaging or interacting with a mobile phone interface.

This paper first examines the use of survey data to quantify visual exclusion, then formally describes the assessment method, and then presents some worked examples.

2 Using Survey Data to Quantify Visual Exclusion

Ocular accommodation is the ability of the eye to change focus between near and far. As people get older, the accommodative ability of the eye inevitably decreases (Vassilieff and Dain 1986). As a result, the performance for near vision tasks becomes heavily dependent on the availability and actual use of appropriate reading glasses.

In real-world near-vision tasks, the user will choose a viewing distance that is comfortable for them. If the user has uncorrected age-related long sightedness, they may choose to view things at 'arms length'. If the user has uncorrected myopia, they may choose to view things 'close to the nose'.

Therefore, in order to quantify exclusion for real-world near vision tasks, it is important to use near-vision survey data which tests people's ability to distinguish visual stimuli that has been printed on card, and given to the participants to hold in their hands and choose their own viewing distance. The method presented here could be combined with any survey data that meets this condition, although this paper focuses on data from the 2010 Better Design Survey (Clarkson et al. 2012, Tenneti et al. 2013), which was designed by the authors (and others). The details of this survey, the visual stimuli used, and the full survey data are available in the public domain (Clarkson et al. 2012).

Test chart letter characters, as used in the Better Design Survey, are considered a better visual stimuli than reading words in paragraphs, because reading words involves considerably more complex processes than does recognising letters, and is therefore more affected by the cognitive ability of the survey participant (Kitchin and Bailey 1981).

The Better Design Survey covered the full range of ability evident within the population, without pre-screening or focusing on disability and impairment. The survey took place inside people's own homes, in real-world lighting conditions. The sample size was relatively small at 362 people, but this is considered sufficient for the purposes here to demonstrate proof of concept.

This survey measured peoples' near-vision ability while they were wearing any visual aids that they wear 'for the majority of the day'. Participants were given a near vision test chart that is approximately reproduced in Figure 1, and asked 'please identify the smallest row of letters that is **comfortable** for you to read'. The percentage of sample who chose each of the different rows is provided in Table 1.

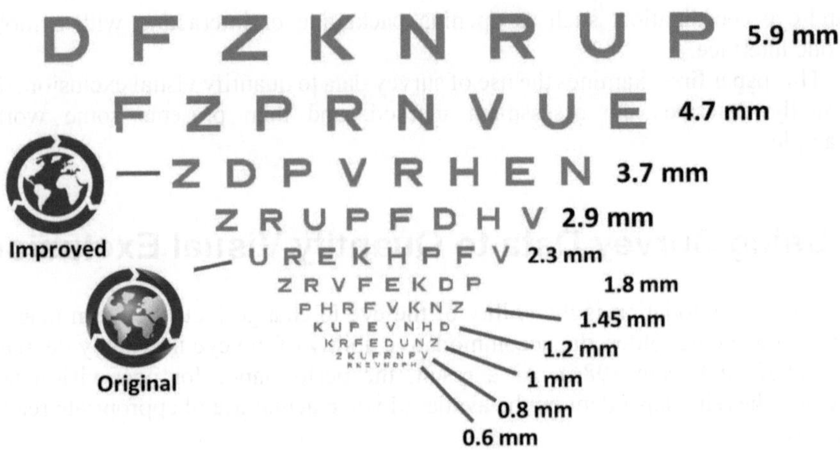

Fig. 1 A reproduction of the near vision test chart used within the Better Design Survey. The 7.4mm row is not shown as it had zero frequency count. Efforts have been made for these letters to appear at the actual size used in the survey, however some scaling and loss of printed clarity may have been inevitable in publication. The assessed positions of the logos in the worked example in Section 4 are also shown.

Table 1 Frequency counts for the Better Design Survey data, based on the near vision test chart shown in Figure 1.

Letter size (mm) of the comfort row	% Sample
0.60 (or better)	12.3
0.80	25.8
1.00	14.0
1.20	15.2
1.45	8.2
1.80	8.6
2.30	5.1
2.90	5.4
3.70	2.9
4.70	1.3
5.90	1.1
7.40	0.0
Cannot read chart	0.0

The survey also collected many other measures of near-vision ability, with and without specialist reading aids, including the threshold size of letters that participants were able to read, in addition to the row they considered comfortable. The method presented herein could be used to quantify exclusion based on these other survey measures, but this is not considered here. The chosen measure of 'perceived comfort', while using any visual aids that they wear for the majority of the day, was considered the most widely applicable to real-world design scenarios.

3 Assessment Method

This assessment method quantifies exclusion by:

- Firstly, identifying the size of test chart characters that are of equivalent visual clarity to the design being assessed;
- Secondly, using a cumulative version of the frequency counts from the survey data to estimate the visual exclusion for the design.

The procedure is intended for an assessor with good vision, who does not experience refractive error at any of the viewing distances involved in the design assessment. The authors designed the vision module within the Better Design Survey, so had easy access to the actual test charts that were used in the survey. The procedure described below assumes that the assessor is also able to obtain one of these test chart cards, and the section on 'further work' describes how this might be possible. The full procedure is as follows:

- Mount the design to be assessed, and the Better Design Survey test chart card, next to each other on a wall, in a position with good lighting;
- Choose which feature of the design you are assessing;
- Walk forwards and backwards to find the maximum distance at which you can comfortably see the feature being assessed;
- At this distance, now look at the vision chart. Identify the row of letters that best matches the feature you are assessing, in terms of visual clarity. Note the height of the capital letters for this row, which is provided on the test chart, as shown in Figure 1;
- The visual exclusion can now be quantified by looking up this letter size in Table 2, or using the graph in Figure 2;
- Repeat the procedure with at least 1 other assessor. Preferably someone who has not seen the design before;
- Discuss the assessment, considering the following prompts:
    - **What** do 'users' really need to 'see' in order to interpret the design?
    - **Why** is the 'feature' difficult to interpret (e.g. size, contrast, spacing)?
    - **How** can the design be improved?
- Improve the design to make it visually clearer, based on the insights gained from this discussion.

Table 2 and Figure 2 were created by calculating a cumulative version of the frequency counts from the survey (shown in Table 1). It is assumed that the percentage of survey sample who could not comfortably see the design being assessed is identical to the percentage of the survey sample who could not comfortably see the equivalent row on the test chart, which is determined by the above procedure.

By comparing the design side-by-side against the test chart letter characters, the procedure should mostly eliminate variability arising from:

- the ambient lighting in which the test is performed;
- the assessors' choice of how hard they struggle before deciding something cannot be 'seen';
- the eyesight ability of the assessors.

The procedure presented herein cannot directly quantify visual exclusion due to colourblindness, or other visual issues beyond visual acuity. However the procedure can be performed with either a full-colour or greyscale version of the artwork. Assessing a greyscale version is the easiest way to ensure the design is colour redundant, which is considered best practice. Greyscale versions of artwork are assessed in the example considered in this paper.

Table 2 The percentage of survey sample who cannot comfortably see the design being assessed, for use in the procedure described in Section 3

x-height of test-chart letter that has similar visual clarity to the design being assessed (mm)	Percentage of survey sample who cannot comfortably see the design being assessed
0.60	87.7%
0.80	61.9%
1.00	47.9%
1.20	32.7%
1.45	24.5%
1.80	15.8%
2.30	10.8%
2.90	5.4%
3.70	2.5%
4.70	1.1%
5.90	0.0%

One difficulty in using the method is determining what the users will really need to be able to 'see' in order to successfully interpret the artwork, which depends on both the usage context and the users' past experience. This issue is inevitable in any kind of 'expert appraisal' but can partly be mitigated by repeating the assessment with a variety of assessors, including at least one who has never seen the design before, and one who has observed actual user behaviour. The assessments should also be repeated by role-playing different scenarios, one based on a novice user and one based on an expert user.

Different assessors and different scenario assumptions will inevitably lead to different predictions of exclusion. The authors recommend using multiple assessors to deliberately expose these differences, in order to provoke a discussion that can further improve the design.

4 Examples

4.1 Designing Our Tomorrow Website

The assessment process described above was used to examine the Designing Our Tomorrow logo that was produced by a professional design agency, which is shown in Figure 1 (labelled 'original'). The process found that the visual clarity of the original logo was roughly equivalent to 2.3 mm size test chart characters, corresponding to visual exclusion of 10.8 % (see Figure 2)

The authors studied the logo from the distance at which they could just perceive the country shapes. In doing so, they realised that the gap between Africa and South America is the most recognisable feature that communicates the logo is a picture of the world.

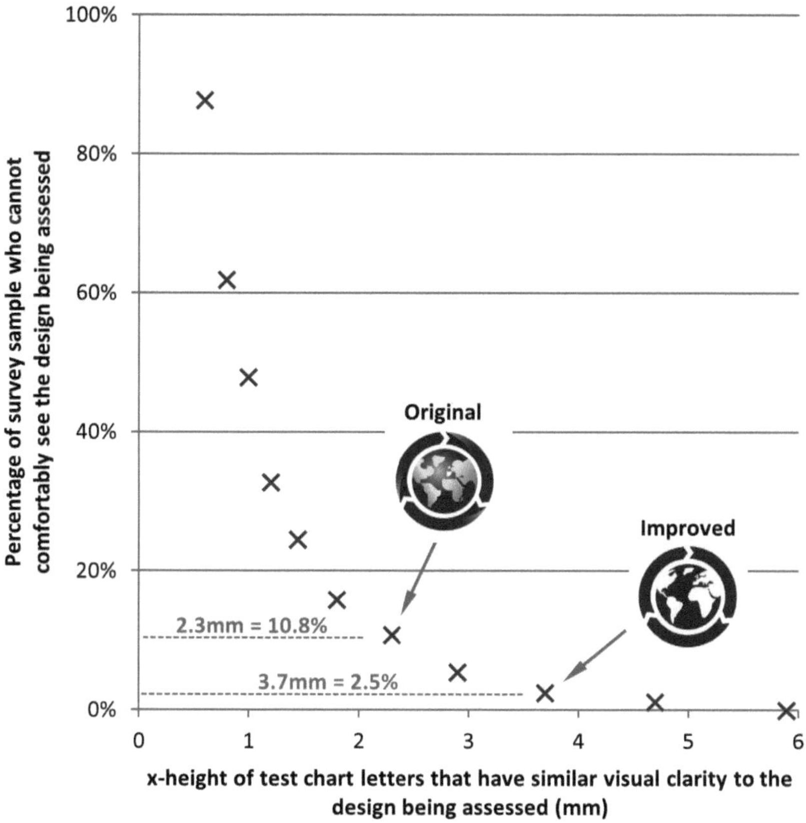

Fig. 2 Graph plotting the results shown in Table 2, together with the assessed positions of the worked example

Having realised this, the authors identified improvements that could be made to make this key feature more distinctive. In particular, they removed lighting effects and colour gradients, increased the contrast, increased the separation between the countries and zoomed and cropped the globe to focus more directly on this feature.

The assessment process was repeated with the new version of the logo, which is also shown in Figure 1 (labelled 'improved'). The improved version was found to be roughly equivalent to 3.7 mm size test chart characters, corresponding to a visual exclusion of 2.5% (see Figure 2). These quantified exclusion figures helped to justify modifying the design agency's work, and the improved version is now live on www.designingourtomorrow.com (accessed in November 2015).

4.2 Usage in Consulting

Versions of the method presented here have also been used by the authors in consulting contexts, for several years, to provide recommendations and justifications for Unilever to optimise its images for e-commerce. One such example was informing decisions made in the early stage design and development of an e-commerce image for Dove Beauty Cream bars, and the original and improved versions of this image are shown in Figure 3. The improved version was live at the time of writing on Tesco's, Asda and other UK grocery websites.

The client provided this quote to describe the benefit of the method presented herein:

> *'This assessment worked extremely well to communicate how easy to use our images were for our customers, to both internal and external stakeholders, as the percentage exclusion is a relatively easy concept to explain and understand. The speed of application of the method also allowed us to iterate design solutions with the knowledge of how inclusive they were. In the business of designing user experiences for customers using visually challenging environments, such as those found on mobile screens, this has proved to be extremely powerful.'*
>
> (Unilever global e-commerce director)

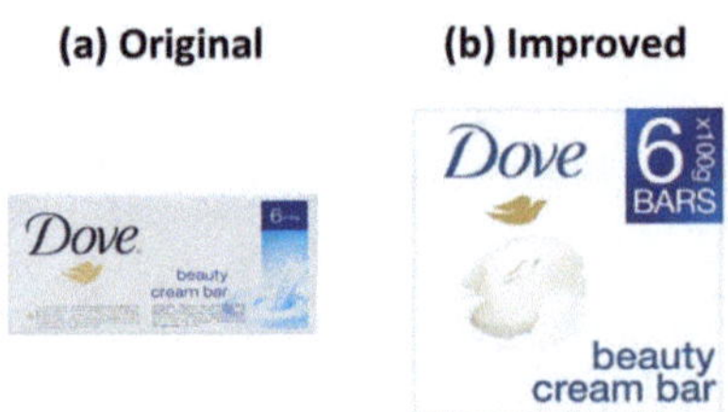

Fig. 3 Original and improved images for Dove Beauty Cream bars

5 Conclusions and Further Work

The authors have used this method in consulting contexts and found it to be quick, repeatable, able to capture minor improvements, and objective. The method is experiential, which helps the assessor to generate and quantify improvements in the graphic artwork.

By comparing physical sizes directly in a like-for-like manner, this procedure should eliminate much of the variability arising from different eyesight abilities of different assessors. Comparatively, the equivalent procedure that uses simulation glasses first requires an assessor eyesight calibration step.

Further work intends to investigate how to make this method more suitable for use in industry. In particular, the method is most effective when the actual test charts from the survey are used. However the authors are currently considering a variety of methods that use visual prompts that are more readily available and distributable, an early version of a mobile website is currently available at www.inclusivedesigntoolkit.com/seeit.

Further work is needed to test the usability of the method by its target user group, namely clients and designers involved in the commission and production of graphical artwork that is flat and handheld. Further work could also customise the method to directly assist target setting and benchmarking in business contexts, directly considering the client-designer relationship.

Any method for quantifying exclusion uses a simplified and extremely approximate model. However, the Unilever case study demonstrates that this inclusive design method was agile enough to inform design decisions in real time and justify them commercially. The subsequent sales feedback suggests the project successfully improved the user experience for millions of people.

References

Aldersey-Williams H, Bound J, Coleman R (Eds.) (1999) The methods lab: User research for design. Design for Ageing Network, London, UK

Beech J, Singleton C (1997) The psychological assessment of reading. Psychology Press

British Standards Institute (2005) BS 7000-6:2005, design management systems, managing inclusive design. Guide

Cardoso C (2005) Design for inclusivity: Assessing the accessibility of everyday products. PhD thesis, University of Cambridge, Cambridge, UK

Clarkson PJ, Coleman R, Hosking I, Waller S (2015) Inclusive design toolkit. Cambridge Engineering Design Centre, Cambridge, UK. Available at www.inclusivedesigntoolkit.com (Accessed in November 2015)

Clarkson PJ, Huppert FA,Tenneti R,Waller S, Goodman-Deane J, Langdon PM et al. (2012) Towards better design, 2010. [data collection]. UK Data Service, SN: 6997. Available at: dx.doi.org/10.5255/UKDA-SN-6997-1 (Accessed in November 2015)

Cornish K, Goodman-Deane J, Clarkson PJ (2015) Visual accessibility misconceptions held by graphic designers and their clients. In: Sharples S, Shorrock S, Waterson P (Eds.) Contemporary ergonomics and human factors 2015, pp. 72-79. Taylor and Francis

Goodman-Deane, J, Waller S, Cornish K, Clarkson PJ (2014) A simple procedure for using vision impairment simulators to assess the visual clarity of product features. In: Universal access in human-computer interaction. Design and development methods for universal access, pp. 43-53. Springer International Publishing

Helen Hamlyn Centre for Design (2012) Designing with people website: designingwithpeople.rca.ac.uk/people (accessed in November 2015)

Holden BA, Fricke TR, Ho SM, Wong R, Schlenther G, Cronjé S et al. (2008) Global vision impairment due to uncorrected presbyopia. Archives of Ophthalmology 126(12): 1731-9

Kitchin JE, Bailey I (1981) Task complexity and visual acuity in senile macular degeneration. Australian Journal of Optometry 63: 235-242

ONS (2015) National population projections, 2014-based statistical bulletin. Available at: www.ons.gov.uk/ons/rel/npp/national-population-projections/2014-based-projections/stb-npp-2014-based-projections.html (Accessed in November 2015)

Persad U, Langdon P, Clarkson J (2007) Characterising user capabilities to support inclusive design evaluation. Universal Access in the Information Society 6(2): 119-135

Pheasant S (1996) Bodyspace: Anthropometry, ergonomics and the design of work. Taylor and Francis, London, UK

Porter JM, Case K, Marshall R, Gyi D, Oliver RSn (2004) Beyond Jack and Jill: Designing for individuals using HADRIAN. Int. J. Indus. Ergon. 33 (3): 249-264

Poulson D, Ashby M, Richardson S (1996) USERfit: A practical handbook on user-centred design for rehabilitation and assistive technology. HUSAT Research Institute for the European Commission

Tenneti R, Goodman-Deane J, Langdon P, Waller S, Ruggeri K, Clarkson PJ et al. (2013) Design and delivery of a national pilot survey of capabilities. International Journal of Human Factors and Ergonomics 2(4): 281-305

Vassilieff A, Dain S (1986) Bifocal wearing and VDU operation: A review and graphical analysis. Applied Ergonomics 17(2): 82-86

VINE (2005) Visual impairment North-East, website. Available at: www.vine-simspecs.org.uk/html/index.html (Accessed in November 2015)

Waller SD, Langdon PM, Clarkson PJ (2010) Using disability data to estimate design exclusion. Universal Access in the Information Society 9(3): 195-207

W3C World Wide Web Consortium (2008) Web content accessibility guidelines 2.0 (WCAG 2.0). Available at: www.w3.org/TR/WCAG20/ (Accessed in November 2015)

Zitkus E, Langdon P, Clarkson PJ (2013) Inclusive design advisor: Understanding the design practice before developing inclusivity tools. Journal of Usability Studies 8(4): 127-143

How and Why Do People Adopt ICT Products? A Preliminary Model Based on Literature Review

J. Pan and H. Dong

Abstract: Technology is developing at an unprecedented rate, but the adoption of it, especially among older population, is relatively slow. While information communication technology (ICT) provides great opportunities to improve older people's quality of life, it is known that many older people are excluded from ICT. The reason can be at least two fold: 1) the usability barrier of technology, 2) the lack of motivation of the users. This paper focuses on the latter through exploring how and why people adopt ICT products. It reviews theories of technology acceptance, innovation diffusion, and motivation, and proposes a preliminary model to explain the factors and theories influencing the adoption of ICT products.

1 Background

In the 21st century, from transportation to communication, Information and Communication Technology (ICT) products can be found in all the domains of our life. They have brought great benefits to people.

However, it has been found that ICT products sometimes put off people, especially the older population. On one hand, numerous studies suggest that people experience difficulty, frustration, or exclusion when using technology products (e.g. Philips report, www.inclusivedesigntoolkit.com); on the other hand, many older people prefer to be left behind instead of learning the foreign technology that they have never encountered before (Mieczakowski and Clarkson 2013). Much of inclusive design research focuses on the usability of technology, while very few studies focus on motivating people to adopt technology.

In order to motivate people, we first need to understand how and why people adopt ICT products. Relevant psychology theories are reviewed and synthesized, based on which a preliminary model was developed to explain the process and the influencing factors of people's adoption of ICT products. This will form a theoretical foundation for further studying on motivating older people to adopt ICT.

J. Pan
College of Architectural Design and Urban Planning, Tongji University, Shanghai, China

H. Dong (✉)
Inclusive Design Research Centre, College of Design and Innovation, Tongji University, Shanghai, China
e-mail: donghua@tongji.edu.cn

P. Langdon et al. (eds.), *Designing Around People*,
DOI 10.1007/978-3-319-29498-8_13

2 Methods

This paper focuses on three main theories:

- technology acceptance theories,
- innovation diffusion theory,
- motivation theories.

A variety of technology acceptance models were analysised to form the basis of the preliminary theoretical model. Then, the innovation diffusion theory was used to reorganize the constructs in the model. Finally, motivation theories were referenced to explain the links and show theory foundations of the preliminary model.

3 Building the Preliminary Model Based on Technology Acceptance Theories

After reviewing many technology acceptance theories and models, the authors summarized the mostly used models (see Table 1): the Theory of Reasoned Action (Fishbein and Ajzen 1975), the Theory of Planned Behavior (Ajzen 1991), the Technology Acceptance Model (TAM) (Davis 1989) and extended Technology Acceptance Model (TAM2) (Venkatesh and Davis 2000), and the Decomposed Theory of Planned Behavior (Taylor and Todd 1995).

Theories of technology adoption can be traced back to the Theory of Reasoned Action (TRA) developed by Fishbein and Ajzen in 1975. TRA is based on the assumption that individuals are rational decision makers who constantly calculate and evaluate the relevant behavior beliefs in the process of forming their attitude toward the behavior.

Based on the TRA, Davis (1989) develops the Technology Acceptance Model (TAM) to find out what factors cause people to accept or reject an information technology. He suggestes that perceived usefulness and perceived ease of use are the two most important individual beliefs about using an information technology. In the Information Systems field, TAM has arguably become the most influential theory. From then on, “Perceived usefulness” and “Perceived ease of use” can be seen in all the models and theories of technology acceptance.

Table 1 Technology acceptance models

Model	Constructs
TRA (Fishbein et al. 1975)	• Belief and evaluations; • Attitude towards behavior; • Normative beliefs and motivation to comply; • Subjective norms; • Behavior intention; • Actual behavior.
TAM (Davis 1989)	• Perceived usefulness; • Perceived ease of use; • Attitude towards usage; • Intention to use; • Actual Usage.
TAM2 (Venkatesh and Davis 2000)	• Perceived usefulness; • Perceived ease of use; • Intention to use; • Usage Behavior; • Subjective norm; • Image; • Job relevance; • Output Quality; • Result Demonstrability; • Experience; • Voluntariness.
TPB (Ajzen 1991)	• Belief and evaluations; • Attitude towards behavior; • Normative beliefs and motivation to comply; • Subjective norms; • Behavior intention; • Actual behavior; • Control Beliefs and perceived facilitation; • Perceived behavior control.
DTPB (Taylor and Todd 1995)	• Perceived usefulness; • Ease of use; • Attitude towards usage; • Behavior intention; • Actual Behavior; • Perceived behavior control; • Compatibility; • Peer influence; • Superior's influence; • Subjective norm; • Self-efficacy; • Resource facilitating conditions; • Technology facilitation conditions.

More factors such as external variables have been introduced by other researchers. A widely known extended TAM is called TAM2 (Venkatesh and Davis 2000). Social influences (e.g. subjective norm, voluntariness, and image) and cognitive instrumental processes (e.g. job relevance, output quality, result demonstrability, and perceived ease of use) have been added to predict the adoption of an information technology.

Ajzen (1991) develops the Theory of Planned Behavior (TPB) to extend TRA. TRA is used to predict an individual's behavior only in a voluntary situation while TPB also takes mandatory situations into consideration. He adds a new construct of perceived behavioral control, which originates from the self-efficacy theory.

Taylor and Todd (1995) decompose the three main constructs of TPB (i.e. Attitude towards behavior, Subjective norm, and Perceived behavior control) in detail, and develops the model Decomposed Theory of Planned Behavior (DTPB)

The relation between these models is summarized in Figure 1. All these models intend to investigate factors that influence people's actual behavior including technology acceptance. The "+" in the figure means a new factor being introduced while "-" means the existing factor being removed.

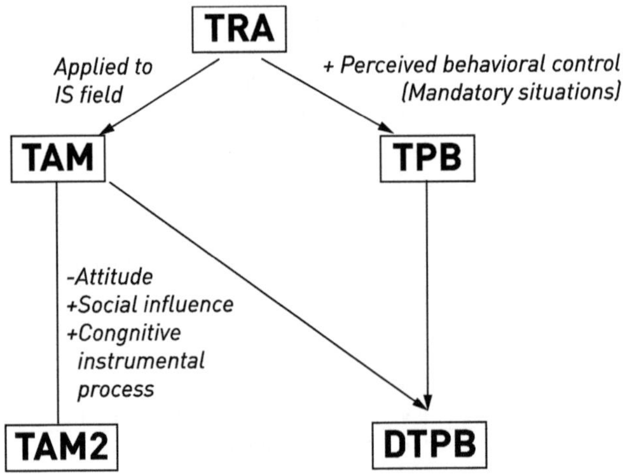

Fig. 1 Relation between different models

From these models, six main constructs that influence people's adoption of ICT products can be extracted: i.e. Perceived Usefulness; Perceived Ease of Use; Attitudes; Social Influence; Intention to Use; and Actual Usage. the relations between each of these constructs cannot be incorporated by one single model that exits, but they are all measured in at least one model, as shown in Figure 2.

Because "Perceived Usefulness" and "Perceived Ease of Use" of ICT products are formulated by the interaction between the user and products, the characteristics of the user and the characteristics of ICT products should be taken into consideration to understand how the new product will be received by potential users (Figure 3).

The "Characteristics of the user" include demographic information (age, gender, education, income etc.), user competence (physical and cognitive) and users' needs. The 'Characteristics of ICT products' include price, quality, function, appearance and complexity. Lots of characteristics have been mentioned by different researchers (Rogers 1995, González et al. 2012, Mitzner et al. 2014, Wang 2014). Some of them are difficult to measure. The constructs listed in this paper are mainly based on design experience, which are relatively more visible and measurable. The relations between these constructs are based on subjective analysis and need validation in specific contexts.

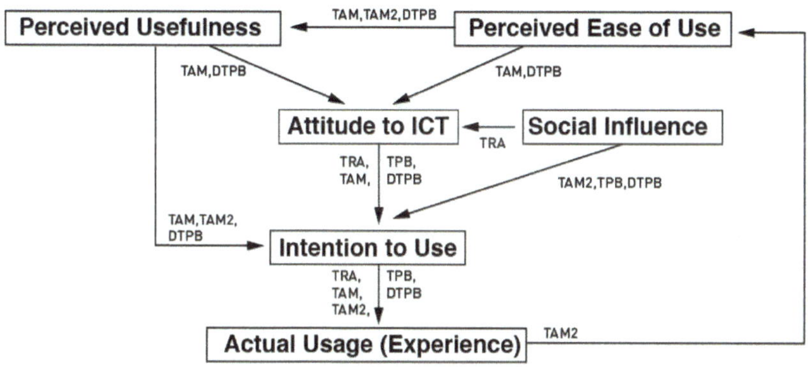

Fig. 2 Main constructs of existing models and their relations

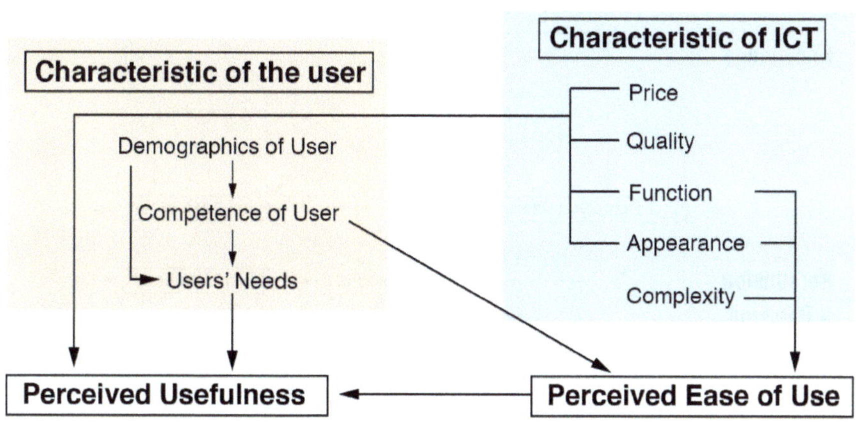

Fig. 3 How the characteristic of the user and the ICT product affect 'Perceived Usefulness' and 'Perceived Ease of Use' (ICT in the figure is short for ICT products)

4 Applying the Innovation Diffusion Theory to Technology Acceptance Models

Diffusion of Innovation (DOI) Theory, developed by E. M. Rogers in 1962 has been used to study a variety of innovations. It explains how an idea, practice or object diffuse and be accepted by people. ICT products are not new in the world, but for new adopters they can still be seen as innovations. Therefore this theory can also be applied to this study.

The Innovation-Decision Process Model (Rogers 2010) helps to answer how people adopt ICT products. There are five stages:

- Knowledge: know how the ICT product functions;
- Persuasion: formulate the intention of adopting ICT products based on intrinsic and extrinsic motivations;
- Decision: decide whether to adopt or reject these ICT products;
- Implementation: actually begin using the ICT products;
- Confirmation: get reinforcement or reverse previous decision after using the ICT products adopted.

Based on these stages, the authors reorganized the existing constructs of the preliminary model and added three new items, i.e. 'Perceived Usefulness', 'Perceived Ease of Use' and 'Behavior Outcome', to show how and why people adopt ICT products (Figure 4).

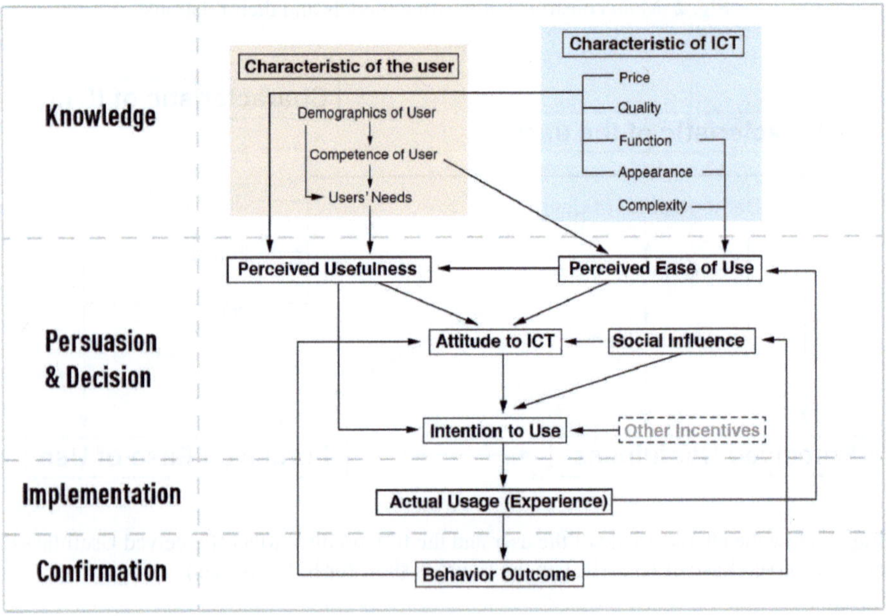

Fig. 4 Relations between different models

Table 2 Relevant motivation theories

1	**Drive Need Desire**	Three Needs Theory	Mcdougall 1908
		Needs as Personality	Murray 1938
		Maslow's Hierarchy of Needs	Maslow 1970
		Drive (Reduction) Theory	Hull 1943
2	**Expectancy -Value Theory**	Valence-Instrumentality-Expectancy Theory	Vroom 1964
		Achievement Motivation Theory	Atkinson 1964
			Covington 1992
			Wigfield and Eccles 2000
		Field Theory	Lewin 1943
		Social Learning Theory	Rotter 1954
3	**Attribution Theory**	Common sense psychology	Heider 1958
		Correspondent inference theory	Jones and Davis 1965
		Co-variation model	Kelley 1967
		Three-dimensional Model	Weiner 1980
4	**Incentive Theory**	Intrinsic and Extrinsic Motivation	Deci and Ryan 1985
		Operant conditioning	Skinner 1938
5	**Self -Efficacy**	Triadic Reciprocal Determinism	Bandura and Walters 1963
		Social Cognitive Theory	Bandura 1986
6	**Goal setting Theory**	Goal Setting and Performance	Locker and Lathem 1990
		Goal commitment	Locker et al. 1988

5 Providing Evidence Using Motivation Theories

Motivation theories explain human behavior: the choice of a particular action, persistence with it, and effort expended on it (Dörnyei 2000). The relation of different constructs in the impact model can be partly explained and evidenced by motivation theories.

The numbers of theories listed in Table 2 were added to the newly built model to show where motivational evidence can be found in this model.

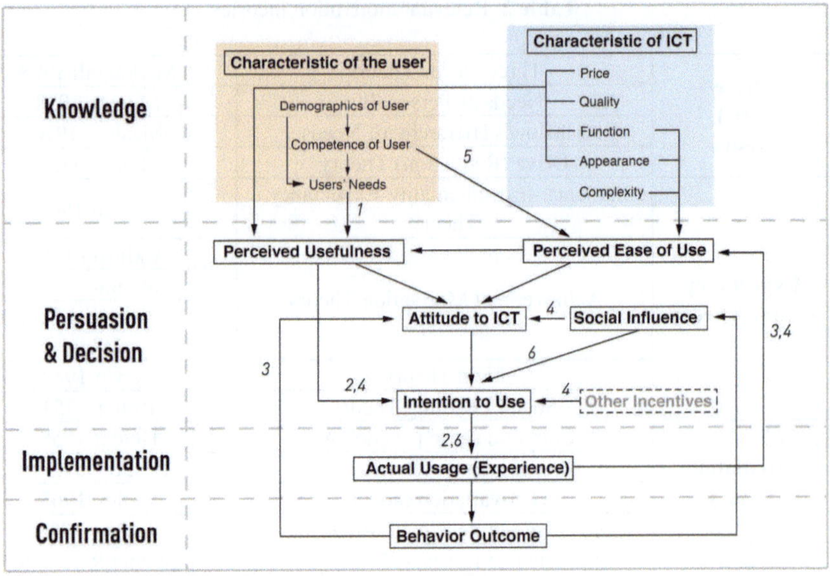

Fig. 5 Impact model of ICT product adoption with motivational evidence (ICT in the figure is short for ICT products)

6 Conclusion

The preliminary model shows how and why people adopt ICT products. It extends the traditional Technology Acceptance Model and is organized using the framework of Innovation Diffusion stages. It provides some answers to the question how and why people adopt ICT products. Such an understanding can help designers think about what they may do to motivate people to use ICT products.

However, although some of the relations between different constructs in the model can be evidenced by motivation theories and existing models of technology acceptance, more practical evidence is needed.

Further studies will focus on how the added constructs impact on the whole technology adoption process, especially regarding age-related factors.

References

Ajzen I (1991) The theory of planned behavior. Organizational Behavior and Human Decision Processes 50(2): 179-211
Atkinson JW (1964) An introduction to motivation. Van Nostrand, Princeton, NJ, USA

Bandura A (1986) Social foundations of thought and action: A social cognitive theory. Prentice Hall, Upper Saddle River, NJ, USA
Bandura A, Walters RH (1963) Social learning and personality development. Holt, Rinehart & Winston, New York, NY, USA
Covington MV (1992) Making the grade: A self-worth perspective on motivation and school reform. Cambridge University Press, New York, NY, USA
Davis FD (1989) Perceived usefulness, perceived ease of use, and user acceptance of information technology. MIS Quarterly 13(3): 319-340
Deci EL, Ryan RM (1985) Intrinsic motivation and self-determination in human behavior. Plenum, New York, NY, USA
Dörnyei Z (2000) Motivation in action: Towards a process oriented conceptualization of student motivation. British Journal of Educational Psychology 70(4): 519-538
Fishbein M, Ajzen I (1975) Belief, attitude, intention and behavior: An introduction to theory and research, pp. 561-562. Addison- Wesley, Reading, UK
González A, Paz Ramírez M, Viadel V (2012) Attitudes of the elderly toward information and communications technologies. Educational Gerontology 38(9): 585-594
Heider F (1958) The psychology of interpersonal relations. Wiley, New York, NY, USA
Hull CL (1943) Principles of behavior. Appleton-Century-Crofts, New York, NY, USA
Jones EE, Davis KE (1965) A theory of correspondent inferences: From acts to dispositions. Advances in Experimental Social Psychology 2(1): 219-266
Kelley HH (1967) Attribution theory in social psychology. In: Levine D (Ed.), Nebraska Symposium on Motivation, pp. 192-238. University of Nebraska Press, Lincoln, NE, USA
Lewin K (1943) Defining the field at a given time. Psychological Review 50: 292-310
Locke EA, Latham GP (1990) A theory of goal setting and task performance. Prentice-Hall, Upper Saddle River, NJ, USA
Locke EA, Latham GP, Erez M (1988) The determinants of goal commitment. Academy of Management Review 13(1): 23-39
Maslow AH (1970) Motivation and personality, 3rd Ed. Harper & Row, New York, NY, USA
McDougall W (1908) An introduction to social psychology. Methuen, London, UK
Mieczakowski A, Clarkson PJ (2013) Ageing, adaption and accessibility: Time for the inclusive revolution! Cambridge Engineering Design Centre, UK
Murray HA (1938) Explorations in personality. Oxford University Press, New York, NY, USA
Rogers EM (2010) Diffusion of innovations, pp.163-210. Simon and Schuster, New York, NY, USA
Rotter JB (1954) Social learning and clinical psychology. Prentice Hall, Englewood Cliffs, NJ, USA
Skinner BF (1938) The behavior of organisms: An experimental approach. Appleton-Century, New York, NY, USA
Taylor S, Todd P (1995) Decomposition and crossover effects in the theory of planned behavior: A study of consumer adoption intentions. International Journal of Research in Marketing 12(2): 137-155
Venkatesh V, Davis FD (2000) A theoretical extension of the technology acceptance model: Four longitudinal field studies. Management Science 46(2): 186-204
Vroom VH (1964) Work and motivation. Wiley, New York, NY, USA
Weiner B (1980) A cognitive (attribution) – emotion – action model of motivated behavior: An analysis of judgments of help-giving. Journal of Personality and Social Psychology, 39: 186-200
Wigfield A, Eccles JS (2000) Expectancy–value theory of achievement motivation. Contemporary Educational Psychology 25(1): 68-81

Wang Z (2014) Difference analysis of the influence of personal characteristics on technology acceptance – The mainland and Chinese Taiwan. Science and Technology Management Research (in Chinese)

A Clock That Does Not Tell the Time: How the Day Clock Meets the Needs of People Living with Dementia

H. Boyd, N. Evans and N. Harris

Abstract: Time disorientation is common in dementia, and can cause difficulty in knowing what day or time it is, or whether it is day or night. Some time orientation products exist to mitigate this, but the need for a simpler product was highlighted by relatives of people with dementia. The Day Clock was developed to meet this need, displaying only the day of the week and part of the day, by working in consultation with people with dementia, carers and healthcare professionals. Questionnaires and user trials were used to fully understand the product requirements. The design was further developed with a commercial partner and supplied as a market product. The Day Clock was evaluated with 123 people with dementia or memory problems as part of a local memory technology lending library, and the majority of goals set using Goal Attainment Scaling by people with dementia and their carers were met as a result of using the Day Clock. There was good acceptability and evidence of efficacy of the Day Clock, in what was one of the largest formal evaluations to date of assistive technology for people with dementia. Understanding the requirements of people living with dementia and their carers, and carrying out iterative design, has underpinned the development of this product and justifies the final design of the Day Clock which gives the day of the week and part of the day but does not tell the time.

1 Background

Disorientation in time is frequently experienced by people with dementia, who may have difficulty knowing what time it is and distinguishing between day and night, and so are unable to follow a daily routine. This often causes confusion, anxiety and distress. Orientation is reliant on the connection of disparate neural systems such as those of memory, attention and sense of time. Dementia affects the structure and chemistry of the brain and progressively impairs a person's ability to remember, understand, communicate and reason. A qualitative study by Nygård

H. Boyd · N. Evans (✉) · N. Harris
Designability, Bath, UK
email: ninaevans@designability.org.uk

P. Langdon et al. (eds.), *Designing Around People*,
DOI 10.1007/978-3-319-29498-8_14

and Johansson describes how the skills of knowing when something is happening and judging lengths of time can become impaired and be challenging for people living with dementia and their primary carers. Environmental compensation with time aids offers potential for support (Nygård and Johansson 2001, Topo et al. 2007).

Large, clear-faced clocks or calendar clocks that show analogue time with the date or digital displays that offer time, day and date information are commercially available. However, few are specifically designed for dementia; the exception being the Forget Me Not calendar. This is a picture frame design and shows the day, date and time of day developed by Inger Hagen and evaluated as part of the Enabling Technologies for People with dementia (Enable Project 2001), (http://enableproject.org). This European project highlighted the lack of motivation for people with dementia to use assistive technology and the pivotal role of the carer in facilitating the selection and use of assistive technology. It also underlined the need for further development and evaluation of assistive technology and positively concluded that people with dementia and their carers could actively contribute to the design process.

2 Identifying the Need

The unmet need for a different type of orientation aid came about through persistent telephone enquiries to the Occupational Therapist at Designability (a research and development charity) from relatives looking for a display solution to help with time of day orientation for people with dementia. At the time of the project, the existing commercial products typically showed information about the date, time and day, and while these suited some people with time orientation problems, there was clearly a group of potential users whose needs were not being met. Carers described requests for frequent reassurance of the day of the week and the part of the day, and there was a suggestion that the exact date and time were unnecessary and potentially confusing for some users. We therefore embarked upon a user centred design project to understand the user requirements and develop and evaluate concepts. This paper describes the design and development of an alternative time orientation product for people with dementia and its subsequent evaluation as part of a local technology lending library.

3 User Requirements

We conducted an informal survey of nine participants composed of carers and Occupational Therapists to inform the user requirements of a simple time orientation product. The carers each had detailed experience of an individual with dementia whereas the Occupational Therapists had a broad professional understanding of a wider population with dementia. At this stage we were keen to develop a concept which was likely to be appropriate for evaluation by people with dementia. They identified requirements as the ability to tell what part of the day it was, to distinguish between day and night, to be able to link time to routine and a need to reduce anxiety about time. When asked to rank the priority of information displayed, the day of the week and part of day (e.g. morning or afternoon) were ranked as most important.

4 Development of a Design Concept

We proposed a simple display concept which only indicated the day of the week and part of the day (morning, afternoon, evening or night). This was more detailed than the "day/night" clocks available for children and adults, and it was felt that this would be more orientating for users, since events in people's lives tend to occur in these terms, e.g. on a Monday afternoon or on a Wednesday evening. The distinction between evening and night was considered a helpful one, since night time is usually associated with sleeping and evening is associated with being a later stage of the day when one would usually be awake, and the blurring of sleep/wake cycles is one of the key problem areas in time disorientation. The words "Now it's" were added in order to make any display seem live or current, in case the words "Monday morning" were considered to be a static statement.

In order to create a display using these words, with the aim of creating a product, the resulting output had to be as low cost as possible and mechanical means and custom-built electronic set ups were therefore discounted. Some text displays used commercially in showrooms or marketing displays were considered but were also cost-prohibitive, not flexible enough or not available in suitable sizes and formats to meet the needs of a consumer design. The proposed route in the first instance was to use low-cost, commercially available digital photo frames which allowed content to be displayed as a series of images in a timed fashion, and could be set to a real time.

The concept was reviewed by nine Carers and Occupational Therapists, who volunteered to complete a postal questionnaire on the detailed concept design. This asked about the exact wording used, the time of day periods, the appearance of the screen and where it would be displayed. Overall the concept was rated positively. A dementia carers' group liked the simplicity and acknowledged that, *"most people know days"* but added caution about whether a display would be believed.

Prototype day clocks were then produced by generating a series of jpeg images which displayed the required content (e.g. "Now it's Monday Morning"). The chosen format was white text on a black background to give maximum contrast, and in lower case to enable easy reading of the shapes of the words. The chosen font was a sans serif font (Arial) in bold and the words were made as large as possible on the screen for ease of reading. The text was centred to give a balanced feel.

These images were given ordered alphanumeric filenames which ensured that they were displayed in the correct sequence, and duplicated so that one image was displayed each hour, set using a one-hour interval setting on the digital photo frame. This series could then be played repeatedly by many commercially available digital photo frames by copying the images onto a memory card or USB stick. The one-hour interval was needed because the four parts of the day, morning, afternoon evening and night, were not of equal lengths, so a simple, "change every six hours" approach was not appropriate, and a six-hour time interval was rarely available on digital photo frames; a one-hour setting was more common. The chosen timings for parts of the day, based on the feedback from the review panel, were:

- morning: 7am - 12 noon,
- afternoon: 12 noon - 5pm,
- evening: 5pm - 10pm,
- night: 10pm - 7am.

Some critics suggested that morning should begin at midnight, but those familiar with the issues of time disorientation readily understood that "night" in this context is strongly associated with "time in bed (possibly asleep)", given that the aim here is to encourage good sleep/wake cycles in order to try to improve overall time orientation. Describing 1am as "morning" to someone with time disorientation was considered to be counterproductive.

A brief set of clear instructions was generated to enable the users to set up the day clocks themselves using supplied pre-loaded memory cards containing the series of generated images.

5 User Trial of Prototype

Four prototypes were then supplied to four pairs of volunteers who were recruited through local organisations. Two were used by volunteers living with dementia living alone in their own homes, one by a married couple and the fourth was used in a bedroom and subsequently in a communal room of a nursing home. All were sent the prototype with set up and installation instructions. The prototypes were then used in daily life. An informal telephone review was carried out with carers one week after installation then a review of performance at three and six weeks.

The two older carers (in the married couple and the relative of the nursing home resident) were unfamiliar with digital picture frame technology and experienced difficulties with setting up and resetting the time on the clock whenever it was unplugged from the mains. This alerted us to the need for simple step by step instructions for the set up process and we revised the accompanying instructions accordingly. During the trial, poor reliability was highlighted as one volunteer was found to be referring to a clock that was showing the wrong day. Another user, a son, reported on sensitivity around the introduction of a reminder product for his mother. The approach the son took was deliberately low key and he set the Day Clock up in a prominent position in the kitchen. His mother later rang him to tell them about the clock in her kitchen; she said she did not know where it was from but it was, "*wonderful*". The clock was found to be beneficial as it helped her to be aware of the correct day and part of day so she could understand when to expect the carers and when to watch television, which she only liked to watch in the afternoons and evenings. This was a longstanding practice for her and one which she adhered to for as long as possible. This prototype is still being used, four years on in the same family with another relative. The couple also found the prototype Day Clock helpful as the husband could look at it daily and link it to their routine; if the day was disputed between them, they could refer to the Day Clock for confirmation. The Day Clock which was used in the nursing home was used in the day room for part of the evaluation was and valued by residents and staff. All participants used the Day Clock and all kept and used it after the end of the trial.

6 Development and Production of the Day Clock

Having seen the promising results of the home evaluations, we considered generating a free "How to" factsheet to enable people to create their own Day Clock using their own digital photo frame, just as we had done. This stemmed from Designability's charitable remit in which the aim is to help as many people as possible. However, it soon became clear that the purchasers were likely to be family carers, or in some cases professionals in care homes, most of whom would not have the time and/or the inclination to go through this process, however clearly described. A simple, minimum effort, standalone product was more desirable for the expected market, and the first market version of the Day Clock was produced in the in-house production unit using digital photo frames and memory cards. These first Day Clocks proved popular, and it was clear that a more sustainable supplier of the digital photo frames was needed. The accuracy of the 1-hour timer on some models of digital photo frame was also not consistent, and changed within and between models, so that the Day Clock display could lose or gain time. Although this was less critical for a Day Clock than for a clock that displayed the exact time, it was clearly undesirable for it to be an unreliable timepiece.

A commercial partner was identified as DFSales Ltd-who offered to engage with us to develop and supply a custom product to meet the growing customer need (www.digitalframesdirect.com). As a result of this input, we were able to upgrade the Day Clock to include tamperproof buttons (specific button sequences were required, so simple "fiddling" did not change or reset the Day Clock) and the use of a back-up battery so that once set, the internal clock did not need resetting even after being unplugged. Deliberately unplugging mains-powered items is a known issue in older people, including those with dementia, so this feature was a valuable change. However it is worth noting that early customers were prepared to tolerate the inconvenience of resetting the Day Clock because of the positive difference that the product made to their relatives with dementia. The images were stored within the clock firmware, obviating the need for external memory storage which could be vulnerable to damage. The production version of the Day Clock is shown in Figure 1.

Versions of the Day Clock were made available in seven languages, to accommodate the needs of a large number of users. This included not only a translation of the instructions and screen content, but locally appropriate time periods throughout the day to reflect how people in different countries think about the day, e.g. in Germany the period "Vormittag" is used to describe late morning so a direct translation of the English Day Clock display with just "morning" and "afternoon" would not be familiar or meaningful enough to a German user.

A dedicated product website was developed (www.day-clock.com), including the instructions, product information, suggestions on where to locate the Day Clock in the home, and a customer helpline.

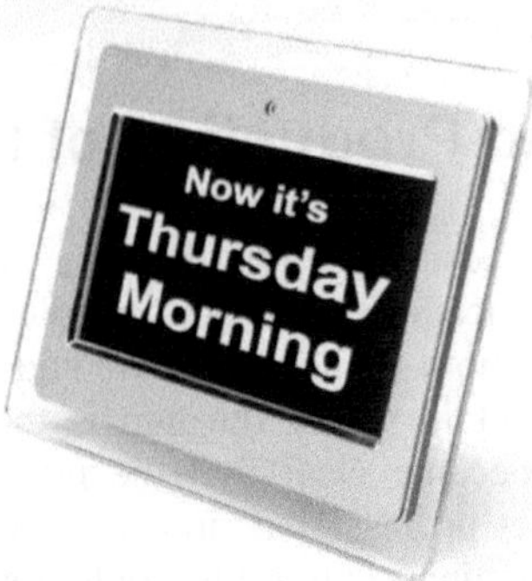

Fig. 1 Production version of the Day Clock

7 Memory Technology Library: Evaluation Phase

7.1 Background

A Memory Technology Library (Harris and Evans 2014) was established with the support of the South of England Dementia Challenge Fund and working in partnership with the Local Health and Social Care Provider and voluntary care providers in Bath and North East Somerset. The project, which ran for 12 months from March 2013, set out to raise awareness of low cost technology for people living with dementia and to look at the suitability and efficacy of available products. A range of low cost technologies was selected, including the Day Clock, and product training materials were developed and shared with community based 'librarians' at regular team meetings. A range of on-line and multimedia training resources to help promote the scheme were developed working with the media partner (www.designability.org.uk/researchproject/memory-technology-library/).

Referral criteria, and a pathway which allowed librarians and carers from within the partner organisations to request products, were established. The level of dementia of clients was assessed using a modified Clinical Dementia Rating Scale (CDRS) and all equipment loans were followed up after 4 weeks, using a goal attainment scaling (GAS) framework to assess outcomes and impact. GAS (Turner-Stokes 2009) uses personalised goal setting to establish outcome criteria before the intervention which can be measured as met, partially met or not met.

7.2 Clients Issued with Day Clocks

In total 181 Day Clocks were requested and issued to care homes, individuals, sheltered housing and community associations. Recipients were individuals living at home or in community settings and were identified as having difficulty with time orientation. All assessments were completed at issue and 123 reviews were received at follow up. The mean age of the recipients was 82 years old and almost two thirds were female. The level of dementia (modified CDRS) in the clients who were issued Day Clocks was: None diagnosed (27%), mild (19%), moderate (30%) and severe (24%).

7.3 Time Orientation Issues and Goal Setting

The key themes from the presenting problems of people living with memory loss and dementia who used the Day Clock were:

- Lack of awareness of day and time of day: *"He goes to the day centre but does not know what day it is"*
- Disorientation following sleep: *"Mr L often dozes during the day and when he wakes does not know the day it is"*
- Night time disorientation: *"K will get up at night and look for his wife in the next room and she has to tell him it is night time"*

The impact of these presenting problems on the person living with memory loss and dementia and their carers had themes including:

- Numerous questions and phone calls: *"She calls family at night thinking it is time to get up"*
- Anxiety, agitation, disagreement and anger: *"He will constantly ask his wife and gets very anxious about 'missing' something"*
- Impact on wellbeing of carer: *"Husband tries to manage confusion but needs respite and struggles"*
- Impact on wellbeing of person with memory loss and dementia: *"I rely on others to tell me the day and time and I feel dependent when others are busy"*

Goals of using the technology were identified for both the person with dementia and the carer. The key themes are summarised in Table 1.

The goals for the person with dementia were primarily about maintaining a daily routine; the carers' goals were about reducing repetition, dependency and conflict.

7.4 Were the Goals Met?

Figure 2 shows the overall results for all goals for the people with dementia (goals 1 and 2) and for carers (goal 3) at the review stage. The use of the Day Clock met the majority of goals set. This is evidence of efficacy of the product.

Table 1 Key themes from user and carer goals

Order of importance	Goals for person living with memory loss or dementia	Goals for carer
1.	Determine day/night	Reduce questions/phone calls
2.	Reduce missing events	Reassurance for user and carer
3.	Reduce prompting to do tasks / follow routine (food & medication) /enable independence	Reduce conflict
4.	Disorientation following sleep	Determine day/night (less time taken and more sleep for carer)
5.		Reduce missing events
6.		Reduce prompting to do tasks / follow routine (food and medication) /enable independence

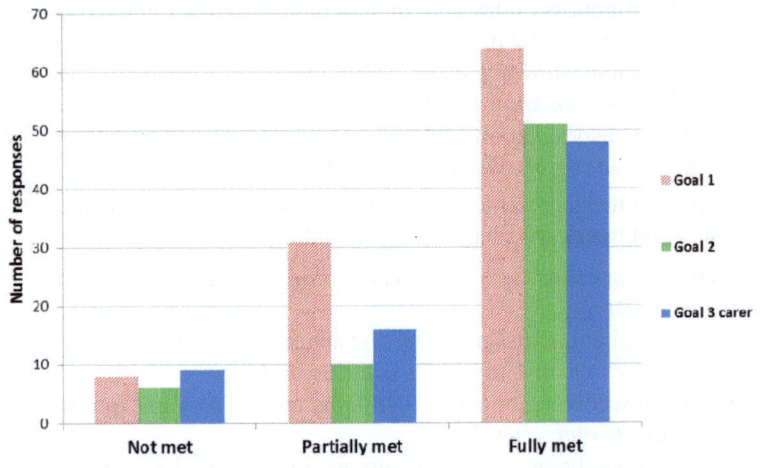

Fig. 2 Goal outcomes for the person with dementia and the carer

7.5 Was the Product Used?

It is known that products are sometimes purchased, or equipment issued, and subsequently not used. Some of the 123 reviews were incomplete, with data missing from some questions. Of those who responded to the question, most participants had used and were still using the Day Clock. Products were issued free of charge during the library project, but participants who chose to keep products at the end of the trial were asked if they would have considered purchasing them and 97% of those who responded to the question indicated that they would (Table 2).

Table 2 Use of the product and willingness to purchase

Was the equipment used?				Main reasons for non-use			
Yes	106	No	10	Poor vision (2) Lack of support (2) Not acceptable (2) Wrong room/not at home (2)			
Are you still using the product?				Yes	84	No	11
If the item wasn't free would you consider buying one?				Yes	94	No	3

7.6 Likes and Dislikes

Likes included positive comments about the Day Clock's operation and use. It was felt to have a clear display, was easy to use, and could retain its settings if unplugged. Dislikes included a requirement for additional or different information e.g. the time, month, or audio (including for those with visual impairment) and for a longer power cable.

8 Discussion and Conclusion

Time orientation products exist to support people with dementia, typically showing the time and date. A gap in the market was identified, where some people with dementia seemed to need a simpler display which showed only the day of the week and part of the day. A product was developed in consultation with people with dementia, carers and professionals, and was made available on the market. This Day Clock was then evaluated as part of a local technology lending library.

We used goal attainment scaling (GAS) to give personalised, individual goals that were specifically meaningful to each person with dementia and each carer, allowing analysis across the group. This method places strong emphasis on users' individual needs while allowing a quantitative outcome of how many goals were met. The effect of time disorientation on people with dementia was well understood before this evaluation, but the impact of time disorientation on the carers of people with dementia was greater than anticipated, and can be a significant source of anxiety and conflict.

A small number of Day Clocks issued were not used; most of the reasons given related to the context of issuing the Day Clock, where the product was not well-suited to the person rather than being inappropriately designed. One limitation of the evaluation was that although a good proportion of the issued Day Clocks were accompanied by a completed review (123 out of 181), it was not possible to gather the remaining data; some users' review data are therefore unknown. Some of the 123 reviews also had missing responses to some questions.

The simplicity and standalone nature of the Day Clock design, while queried by some critics, has been shown to be a valid approach which fits a specific market demographic (those with time disorientation who can still read but cannot make sense of the exact time or date). In people with dementia, the ability to read functionally can persist beyond the ability to tell the time, and should not be discounted when designing in this area. The negative impact of time disorientation on people with dementia and on their partners or relatives has been highlighted by the goals identified during the evaluations, and this impact can be reduced by using the right product.

The market evaluation has provided some of the strongest evidence available in this field about the efficacy of assistive technology products for people with dementia, and in particular the Day Clock, demonstrating that designing specifically for users' needs can lead to usable, effective products.

Acknowledgements

The authors would like to acknowledge Rob Austen and his colleagues at DFSales Ltd for their enthusiasm and support in developing and supplying the Day Clock; the technology library partners Sirona Health and Care, Therapeutic Media Company, Carer's Centre Bath and North East Somerset, Bridge Care and Bath Ethnic Minority Senior Citizens Centre (BEMSCA); and the people with dementia and their carers who tried the Day Clock.

References

Enable Project (2001) Can technology help people with dementia? Available at: www.enableproject.org/ (Accessed on 15 February 2015)

Harris N, Evans N (2014) A memory technology library – Using technology to support the cognitive and emotional needs of people living with dementia. In: Proceedings of the RAATE 2014, Birmingham, UK

Nygård L, Johansson M (2001) The experience and management of temporality in five cases of dementia. Scandinavian Journal Of Occupational Therapy 8: 85-95

Topo P, Saarikalle K, Begley E, Cahill S, Hagen T, Macijauskiene J (2007) I don't know about the past, or the future, but today it's Friday – Evaluation of a time aid for people with dementia. Technology and Disability 19: 121-131

Turner-Stokes L (2009) Goal attainment scaling (GAS) in rehabilitation: A practical guide. Clinical Rehabilitation 23(4): 362-70

Collecting Data for Inclusive Design: Emerging Tools and Methods

W. Ning and H. Dong

Abstract: Inclusive design aims to design for the widest range of users. In order to address people's diverse needs and accommodate their capabilities, it is important to establish users' database, including anthropometric, capability, psychological and social-cultural data, to support the practice of inclusive design. This paper discusses three emerging tools and methods that have the potential to be adopted for collecting user data: 3D scanners, photography and big data. Pros and cons of these tools are discussed based on literature review.

1 Introduction

There is an increasing awareness of the need to design for the widest possible range of users. The concept of inclusive design was raised to meet such a need. Inclusive design focuses on making products and services usable by as many people as is reasonably possible without requiring them to use specialized adaptations (Keates and Clarkson 2004). Traditional methods based on limited testing samples, such as user testing, are unable to reflect the variety of needs of the target user group (Sims 2003). For example, Johnson et al. (2010) concluded that in order to support designers in designing for the whole population, the full breadth of capability across domains couldn't be easily captured in any particular samples of users. General user-centered design methods and tools have been developed for inclusive design (Goodman-Deane et al. 2014). Projects such as HADRIAN (Porter et al. 2004), Exclusion Calculator (Clarkson et at. 2007), VERITAS (Kaklanis et al. 2015), MyUi (Edlin-White et al. 2012), GUIDE (Biswas and Langdon 2011) and VICON (Modzelewski et al. 2012) are also carried out to address the issues around designing for inclusivity, ranging from the development of simulation tools to the establishment of design guidelines. However, the above-mentioned design tools or methods all need the support of effective and adequate user data as they are currently developed on small size of user samples. Furthermore, there are still gaps that need to be filled in the existing databases

W. Ning · H. Dong (✉)
Inclusive Design Research Centre, College of Design and Innovation, Tongji University, Shanghai, China
email: donghua@tongji.edu.cn

P. Langdon et al. (eds.), *Designing Around People*,
DOI 10.1007/978-3-319-29498-8_15

(Johnson et al. 2010, Langdon et al. 2015) and future research should be conducted to find out more effective data collection approaches for capturing inclusive design user data.

Langdon and Thimbleby (2010) suggested that providing population's disability data based on a product and user perspective with its corollary functional capability and context information in formats suitable for designers' would 'have a direct effect on the design of products, services and work environments, leading to improved quality of life for the wider population'. Langdon et al. (2015) further described such data as 'accurate and up-to-date on impairment in the population', 'combined with a robust and complete model of human-product interaction with reference to environmental and social context'. These suggest that integrated anthropometric, capability, psychological and social-cultural data could be useful for designers.

There is a need for selecting, developing and combining different data collection methods and tools derived from different fields (e.g., human factors/ergonomics, psychology, sociology etc.) to collect such data. In this paper, we discuss three emerging tools and methods: 3D body scanner, photography and big data.

2 Methods

The three tools/methods were identified from the interview with four industrial designers, two design researchers and three human factors experts, and was further discussed based on literature review. In the interview, participants were asked about their experience of data use and data collection in design, their research processes, their views on current 'hot topics' for data collection and their future expectations. Based on a focused review of papers from 2005 to 2015, the potential application of these three tools for data collection was summarised in Table 1.

Table 1 Emerging tools and its expected application

Emerging tools	The corresponding data type
3D scanner	Anthropometric data
Photography	Social-cultural data
Big data	Capability, psychological and social-cultural data

3 Pros and Cons of the Emerging Tools

3.1 3D Scanner

Anthropometric data is an important type of dataset that designers often refer to during the design process. The role of anthropometric data is even more significant in the practice of inclusive design, as it represents physical capabilities of various groups of users (able/disabled, young/old), which is a fundamental dimension when designing for inclusivity (Nickpour and Dong 2011). Traditionally, these data are captured by a range of devices such as the Martin type anthropometer, sitting-height tables and the tape measure, but this process is time-consuming and usually only captures one-dimensional data. Additionally, data that is collected manually through traditional means is often presented with complex tables, which cannot match designers' preferences (Nickpour and Dong 2011).

3D body scanners offer the opportunity to harness new technology and remove some of the inaccuracies of traditional anthropometric measurements (Sims et al. 2012). Studies have been conducted to verify the application of 3D scan in collecting anthropometric data, ranging from whole body measurements (Han et al. 2010, Zwane et al. 2010) to specific parts, e.g. hand and foot shapes (Chang et al. 2007, Ran et al. 2009, Lee et al. 2012). Compared with traditional one-dimensional parameter measurements, the general advantages of using 3D scanners can be listed as follows (Chang et al. 2007, Ran et al. 2009, Han et al. 2010, Zwane et al. 2010, Lee et al. 2012):

- Much more surface information can be provided,
- The scanner measurements are generally more numerical in value,
- Fewer errors,
- Less measuring time is required, so participants like elder people who may suffer fatigue in traditional measurements could be involved in,
- Physical contacts between subjects and experimenters could be avoided,
- Scan data can be re-processed and other measures can be extracted after the event, without needing to rescan the subjects,
- Images of the whole body can be seen and assessed, removing the problem of traditional, anthropometry being seen to 'segment' people into univariate dimensions,
- Respondents' experience of the scanning process is better.

When 3D body scanners are used in collecting anthropometric data for inclusive design, it may offer a better data presentation and a more pragmatic data category.

More flexible and user-friendly presentation format: According to Nickpour and Dong (2011), Designers' main desired means of presenting anthropometric data was a 3D software capable of simulating the human body in various positions based on variables such as age, gender and physical capabilities, as well a flexible human body that is capable of producing new measurements from unmeasured body parts. They also wanted to be able to put this 3D model into CAD modeling software such as AutoCAD or 3DMax in order to see how the human and environment relate to the CAD modeling of the product. The methods of how 3D scan data is captured, stored and presented are expected to meet these requirements and even allow data users to create real, multivariate individuals.

More pragmatic data category: In real design contexts, 'functional' postures, rather than static standard postures, are more desired by designers. It is difficult to extract specific measures from existing anthropometric datasets and then apply them to real human-product interaction scenarios. Data based on functional postures may make it possible. For example, grip reach, a typical 'functional' posture, provides the length of the arm to the center of a grasping fist. This is a much more 'applicable' measure than the arm length to the fingertip of an outstretched hand, as for any given application how far someone can reach to grasp an object is much more useful than the maximum length of their arms (Sims et al. 2012). 3D scanners offer a faster and easier method to collect such data.

Despite the advantages, there are disadvantages of applying 3D scan to collecting anthropometric data for designers. Generally, there are significant differences between 3D scan data and traditional measurements (Han et al. 2010); it needs a larger space to set up the scanner and a longer time to calibrate, and experimenters should be well trained in advance. In additon, some groups of people could be excluded for technical reasons. Current scanning process has a comparatively strict requirement on participants' postures. They need to keep a 'standard' posture statically for a while (British Standards Institute 2005, 3D body scanning methodologies has regulated the procedure and postures in 3D body scanning), but postures like 'keeping legs close to each other and stretching arms at 90° to the body' means that the subjects should not suffer any stretching and reaching capability impairments. Furthermore, wheelchair users and those who are suffering from specific diseases (e.g. Parkinson) are excluded by current 3D scan trials.

3.2 Photography

Visual research methods are important in the design process (Boradkar 2011). Designers tend to be motivated by visual communication and like information to be presented with maximum use of graphics (pictures and color) and minimal texts; they ask for nuggets of information (short pieces of text) that can be easily digested (Lofthouse 2006). Photography, as an important visual method, has been widely used in the data gathering stage of different research projects by sociological, historical and anthropological researchers (Buckingham 2009), and it is often adopted in design, but often unsystematically.

Capturing 'hidden' information: A picture is worth a thousand words (Young and Barrett 2001). For people who are unable to participate in a survey verbally, photography can be seen as a supplementary method to collect information. For data collected through respondents' self-reporting, photography is also expected to fill the gaps between self-report and their real condition. Information 'submerged in verbal interviews' could be brought out by photographs (Collier 1957).

A more intuitive format to present information: Contextual data play an important role in helping designers get a deeper understanding of users. Visual methods such as photographs can provide insights and knowledge about the human condition and lead to a richer understanding of social, cultural, and other contextual factors (Wang and Dong 2013). Presenting these data visually is more preferred by designers. These images are more effective than words for delivering true feelings and concepts to a designer (Lee et al. 2002). Therefore, displaying user images could be an effective means of instilling greater empathy and encouraging more extensive use of human information (McGinley and Dong 2011).

The prime issue of applying photograph in inclusive design data is what types of images should be collected. Sanoff (1991) has explored visual methods for explaining the physical environment so that design researchers and designers can understand more about the form, action, and interpretations given to environmental settings. Ning and Dong (2014) collected three different hierarchies of photograph data of older people (i.e. images of the city/town where they live, images of the respondent and their living environment, and images relating to their capability and product interaction). But what types of photos can reflect users' social and cultural condition, preferences or even capabilities is yet to be explored. In a design context, in order to obtain better descriptions of the demands made by products and services on the user, photographs based on product-interaction scenarios are needed.

If photograph collection was applied to a large-scale survey, it would be important to ensure that the photos taken by different investigators to follow a unified standard. Given the reason that personal affection may have effects on photography, pictures are not always taken objectively, Wang (2015) has investigated how designers read and understand photographs. A toolkit which contains principles, skills and examples, was developed to help designers and researchers for collecting photographs. However, its effectiveness remains to be verified.

Ethics is another important issue when collecting photography data. Major ethical concerns were outlined by Wang and Redwood-Jones (2001). Ning and Dong (2014) found that because of privacy, the range of photos that could be captured was very limited. If the respondent was not familiar with the investigator, it was more difficult to get their permission to take photos. At the same time, it is challenging to present, and to sort out large amount of pictures in a user-friendly format.

3.3 Big Data

Big Data has become a ubiquitous term in business, industry and academic domain. According to Drury (2015), big data encompasses the collection, combining and analysis of datasets. De Mauro et al. (2015) give the following definition:

> *'Big Data represents the information assets characterized by such a high volume, velocity and variety to require specific technology and analytical methods for its transformation into value.'*

In the design domain, big data could be of great value when conducting design research. It can be applied to predetermine users' wish and group consciousness as well as contribute to the depiction of a clear user profile. It could also become an effective tool in defining scenarios, and refining design content (Qing 2015).

An 'ideal' sample size: The issue of 'size', i.e. 'volume' in the much-used '3 Vs' classification (volume, velocity and variety) proposed by Laney (2001), could be the first character of big data. Such whole-population-based datasets are usually much larger than traditional ones; there are tools available for compiling the database, analyzing it and turning the findings into useful information. Big data could be seen as an expansion of ergonomics/human factors research and could lead us to a point where we analyze data before formulating hypotheses (Drury 2015). It would change some research paradigms based on the flow of 'hypothesis, data collection and then verification'. When compared with traditional datasets in human factors/ergonomics domain, its advantage seems to be even more obvious. When it comes to big data, the term of 'sample' will not matter anymore, since big data are often based on the whole population, or at least a big 'sample' that traditional research can hardly reach. The capacity will be moved from a sample size (n) to close to the entire population size (N) (Mayer-Schönberger and Cukier 2013).

More user-friendly to designers: A feature of big data is that it presents not only in traditional structured data (traditional text/numeric information), which is not appealing or even confusing to designers (Nickpour and Dong 2011), but also in unstructured data (audio, video, images, text and human language) and semi-structured data, such as XML and RSS feeds (Russom 2011). These big datasets are in parallel development with the theories and techniques of data visualization. When converting information from massive datasets into insights, visualization can enable more intuitive and efficient results (Zhang 2014). And in fact, innovations in information visualization have demonstrated its great value in presenting a good user interface (Shneiderman 2014). So with more various types of data and more user-friendly means of data presentation, big data is expected to contribute to establishing a more designer-friendly database, which can take designers' preferences and habits into consideration.

More techniques with reference value: Although in traditional data collection and analysis, we cannot reach the scale of typical big data, data mining techniques could help out. Applications of big data in traditional ergonomics research range from using big data as the source to referring to the data mining techniques (Lin et al. 2007, Ghazizadeh et al. 2014, Lin et al. 2014).

However, it should be noted that, in the applications of big data, 'correlation' becomes more important and overtakes 'causality' as a way to make sense of trends and finally make decisions (Mayer-Schönberger and Cukier 2013). But in a complete design process, just knowing 'correlation' is inadequate to get deep understanding of the user. Although big data is equipped with a very large size, such abundant information does not always tell the truth. Auerbach (2015) and Harford (2014) have summarized that large datasets do not guarantee better data than small ones. Data may still be poorly collected, for example not having sufficient reliability or validity. Correlation-based analyses, even based on nearly the whole population, may still give spurious results.

Big data may be unable to offer necessary information and produce sampling biases because of the limits on its data sources. With the rapid development in smart devices, sensor technology and the pervasive usage of the internet, big data can be collected efficiently. Designers can rely on big data to get insights into users' wishes, preferences or specific habits, but it is difficult to get detailed data about users' exact features (e.g. psychological attributes). These data still need to be collected through other valid methods. As the sources of big data are mainly based on Internet technologies, it may produce biases even though in a large sample size. For example, research has proved that there are significant differences in technologies products usage between different age groups of users (Morris et al. 2006). Technologies by the younger generation may be seldom or even never used by elder people (Ning and Dong 2015).

Another problem is that big data often combines disparate datasets from different sources (Drury 2015). Based on big data, we can obtain specific information (e.g. hearing, vision, etc.) from a very large sample, and also people's preferences and habits. But it is difficult to match these different items together and then to form a clear user profile. For example, as illustrated by the broken lines in Figure 1, Benktzon (1993) proposed the Population Pyramid according to capability difference; by mining big data, we can obtain users' different levels of specific features, but we cannot correctly group these independent characters together, which may imply that it is impossible to attach these independent attributes to different groups of users. Furthermore, the 'variety' of the '3 Vs' means that big data-sets often combine disparate data from different sources, so even classifications that look similar are not in fact valid matches (Drury 2015).

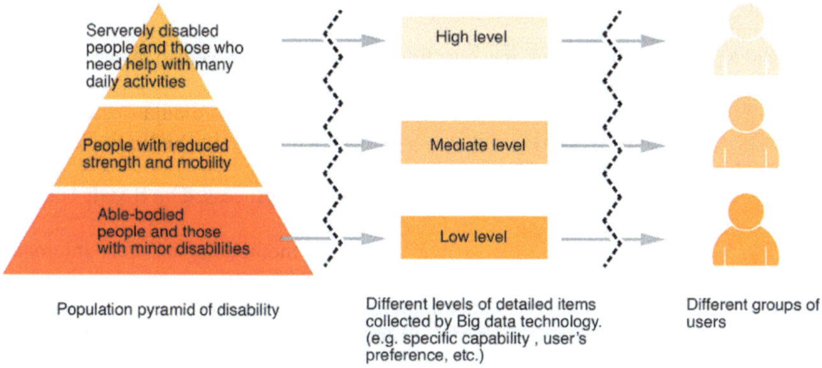

Fig. 1 The 'mismatch' of information based on big data

In addition, there are more privacy and ethical concerns about big data. Auerbach (2015) indicate that because of the lack of transparency of the 'black box' algorithms used in big data, these algorithms may have completely unforeseen consequences of ethics. The popularity of big data has brought serious threat to the security of individual's sensitive information (Xu et al. 2014).

4 Conclusion

In an inclusive design context, the pros and cons of three methods and tools are discussed in this paper. 3D body scanners can present anthropometric data in a more user-friendly format and it may provide more pragmatic data for designing. But the accuracy of data needs to be refined and there still exists specific groups of people who might be excluded by this technology. Photography is of great value in capturing contextual data. It can provide more intuitive information in line with designers' cognition and preference of data, and it can help designers detect useful information that might be difficult to obtain in traditional ways. Big data is expected to offer a large 'sample' and usually equipped with a good quality of data visualization. With its increasing popularity, inclusive design data could greatly benefit from the related techniques in big data mining. The limitations in these methods and tools need to be resolved in future research, especially issues that may lead to exclusion of groups of people. We have discussed the implications of the three emerging tools and methods theoretically, but the validity and feasibility are still to be verified through further research.

References

Auerbach D (2015) The code we can't control. Slate Magazine, Washington, DC, Washington Post, USA

Benktzon M (1993) Designing for our future selves: The Swedish experience. Applied Ergonomics 24(1): 19-27

Biswas P, Langdon P (2011) Towards an inclusive world-a simulation tool to design interactive electronic systems for elderly and disabled users. In: SRII Global Conference (SRII), 2011 Annual, pp. 73-82. IEEE

Boradkar P (2011) Visual research methods in the design process. The SAGE Handbook of Visual Research Methods, pp. 150

British Standards Institute (2006) 3-D scanning methodologies for internationally compatible anthropomteric databases, BS EN ISO 20685:2005

Buckingham D (2009) "Creative" visual methods in media research: Possibilities, problems and proposals. In: Hughes J (Ed.) SAGE visual methods 31: 227-247. SAGE Publications Ltd, London, UK

Chang C-C, Li Z, Cai X, Dempsey P (2007) Error control and calibration in three-dimensional anthropometric measurement of the hand by laser scanning with glass support. Measurement 40(1): 21-27

Clarkson P, Coleman R, Hosking I, Waller S (2007) Inclusive design toolkit. Cambridge Engineering Design Centre, University of Cambridge, Cambridge, UK

Collier JJ (1957) Photography in anthropology: A report on two experiments. American Anthropologist 59: 843-859

De Mauro A, Greco M, Grimaldi M (2015) What is big data? A consensual definition and a review of key research topics. In: Proceedings of the 4th International Conference on Integrated Information, Madrid, Spain

Drury CG (2015) Human factors/ergonomics implications of big data analytics: Chartered Institute of Ergonomics and Human Factors annual lecture. Ergonomics 58(5): 659-673

Edlin-White R, Cobb S, Floyde A, Lewthwaite S, Wang J, Riedel J (2012) From guinea pigs to design partners: Working with older people in ICT design. In: Langdon P, Clarkson J, Robinson P, Lazar J, Heylighen A (Eds.) Designing inclusive systems, pp. 155-164. Springer, London, UK

Ghazizadeh M, McDonald AD, Lee JD (2014) Text mining to decipher free-response consumer complaints insights from the NHTSA vehicle owner's complaint database. Journal of the Human Factors and Ergonomics Society 56(6): 1189 -203

Goodman-Deane J, Ward J, Hosking I, Clarkson PJ (2014) A comparison of methods currently used in inclusive design. Appl Ergon 45(4): 886-894

Han H, Nam Y, Choi K (2010) Comparative analysis of 3D body scan measurements and manual measurements of size Korea adult females. International Journal of Industrial Ergonomics 40(5): 530-540

Harford T (2014) Big data: A big mistake? Significance 11(5): 14-19

Johnson D, Clarkson J, Huppert F (2010) Capability measurement for inclusive design. Journal of Engineering Design 21(2): 275-288

Kaklanis N, Stavropoulos G, Tzovaras D (2015) Modeling people with motor disabilities to empower the automatic accessibility and ergonomic assessment of new products. Applied Ergonomics 51: 120-136

Keates S, Clarkson J (2004) Countering design exclusion. Springer, UK

Laney D (2001) 3D data management: Controlling data volume, velocity and variety. META Group Research Note 6: 70

Langdon P, Johnson D, Huppert F, Clarkson PJ (2015) A framework for collecting inclusive design data for the UK population. Appl Ergon 46(Pt B): 318-324

Langdon P, Thimbleby H (2010) Inclusion and interaction: Designing interaction for inclusive populations. Interacting with Computers 22(6): 439-448

Lee S, Harada A, Stappers PJ (2002) Pleasure with products: Design based on Kansei. In: Green W, Jordan P (Eds.) Pleasure with products: Beyond usability, pp. 219-229. Taylor and Francis, London, UK

Lee Y-C, Chao W-Y, Wang M-J (2012) Foot shape classification using 3D scanning data. Paper presented at the Network of Ergonomics Societies Conference (SEANES) 2012 Southeast Asian

Lin CJ, Wu C, Chaovalitwongsec WA (2014) Integrating behavior modeling with data mining to improve human error prediction in numerical data entry. In: Proceedings of the Human Factors and Ergonomics Society Annual Meeting 58(1): 854-858. SAGE Publications

Lin HF, Hsu CH, Wang MJJ (2007) An application of data mining technique in engineering to facilitate production management of garments. In: Proceedings of the 11th WSEAS International Conference on Computers, Crete, Greece

Lofthouse V (2006) Ecodesign tools for designers: Defining the requirements. Journal of Cleaner Production 14(15): 1386-1395

Mayer-Schönberger V, Cukier K (2013) Big data: A revolution that will transform how we live, work, and think. Houghton Mifflin Harcourt, Boston, MA, USA

McGinley C, Dong H (2011) Designing with information and empathy: Delivering human information to designers. The Design Journal 14(2): 187-206

Modzelewski M, Lawo M, Kirisci P, Connor JO, Fennell A, Mohamad Y et al. (2012) Creative design for inclusion using virtual user models. In: Proceedings of the 13th International Conference on Computers Helping People with Special Needs, Linz, Austria

Morris A, Goodman J, Brading H (2006) Internet use and non-use: Views of older users. Universal Access in the Information Society 6(1): 43-57

Nickpour F, Dong H (2011) Designing anthropometrics! Requirements capture for physical ergonomic data for designers. The Design Journal 14(1): 92-111

Ning W, Dong H (2014) Adapting a capability survey to collect Chinese old people's data for designers: A pilot study. In: Proceedings of the 5th International Conference for Universal Design, Fukushima and Tokyo, Japan

Ning W, Dong H (2015) Collecting old people's data for more accessible design: A pilot study. In: Zhou J, Salvendy G (Eds.) Human aspects of IT for the aged population. Design for aging, pp. 84-93. Springer International Publishing

Porter JM, Case K, Marshall R, Gyi D, neé Oliver RS (2004) Beyond Jack and Jill: Designing for individuals using HADRIAN. International Journal of Industrial Ergonomics 33(3): 249-264

Qing J (2015) Grand interaction design in big data information era. Packaging Engineering, 8: 002 (in Chinese)

Ran L, Zhang X, Chao C, Liu T, Dong T (2009) Anthropometric measurement of the hands of Chinese children digital human modeling, pp. 46-54. In: Proceedings of the 2nd International Conference on Digital Human Modeling. Held as Part of HCI International 2009, San Diego, CA, USA

Russom P (2011) Big data analytics. TDWI best practices report, Fourth Quarter, TDWI

Sanoff H (1991) Visual research methods in design. John Wiley & Sons Incorporated

Shneiderman B (2014) The big picture for big data: Visualization. Science (343): 730

Sims R (2003) Design for all: Methods and data to support designers. Ruth Elise Sims

Sims RE, Marshall R, Gyi DE, Summerskill SJ, Case K (2012) Collection of anthropometry from older and physically impaired persons: Traditional methods versus TC2 3-D body scanner. International Journal of Industrial Ergonomics 42(1): 65-72

Wang CC, Redwood-Jones YA (2001) Photovoice ethics: Perspectives from Flint photovoice. Health Education and Behavior 28(5): 560-572

Wang Y (2015) A method study on photo collection, analysis and interpretation in user research. Master's thesis, Tongji University, Shanghai, China (in Chinese)

Wang Y, Dong H (2013) Exploring photography as a method for research. Paper presented at the Design Management Symposium (TIDMS), 2013 IEEE Tsinghua International

Xu L, Jiang C, Wang J, Yuan J, Ren Y (2014) Information security in big data: Privacy and data mining. Access, IEEE, 2: 1149-1176

Young L, Barrett H (2001) Adapting visual methods: Action research with Kampala street children. Area 33(2): 141-152

Zhang C (2014) Research of big-data mining visualization application. In: Long S, Dhillon BS (Eds.) Proceedings of the 13th International Conference on Man-Machine-Environment System Engineering 259: 201-209, Springer Berlin Heidelberg, Germany

Zwane PE, Sithole M, Hunter L (2010) A preliminary comparative analysis of 3D body scanner, manually taken girth body measurements and size chart measurements. International Journal of Consumer Studies 34(3): 265-271

Part IV

Designing Cognitive Interaction with Emerging Technologies

Beyond Anthropometrics: Prehensile Control Analysis for Capability Assessment

R. J. Holt, R. O. Coats, G. P. Bingham and M. Mon-Williams

Abstract: How can we design objects that are better suited to people with disabilities? Finite Element Analysis is a useful technique for engineering physical objects, but optimal design must be informed by how the human interacts with objects. Our group is attempting to model the control of hand movements in order to create CAD packages that allow object design to be informed by an individual's sensorimotor control strategies (Prehensile Control Analysis). Prehension, the ability to reach-grasp-and-manipulate objects, is one of the most important human capabilities. Numerous activities of daily living (dressing, feeding, cleaning etc.) rely on dexterity, so it is perhaps unsurprising that impairment of prehension (through illness, injury or ageing decline) is often associated with disability. The kinematics of reach-to-grasp movements show high levels of stereotypicality in neurologically intact adults whilst impairment produces predictable kinematic changes in behaviour. Moreover, kinematics change lawfully as a function of the task and the properties of the object. These facts open up the exciting possibility of modelling prehensile kinematics so that a designer can determine the optimal object properties for an individual with a given impairment. This chapter presents a simple model for characterising an individual's quality of movement in a given reach-to-grasp movement. Our model is able to capture typical and atypical prehension and is the first step in the development of CAD for handheld objects: a tool that allows design around people.

1 Introduction

The study of ergonomics has traditionally focused upon anthropometrics; measurements of size, strength and dexterity (e.g. Dreyfuss 1967, Smith et al. 2000, Yoxall et al. 2007, Gonzalez et al. 2015). There is no doubt that this is extremely useful, but such models do not account for the dynamic nature of the tasks required in daily life: the ability to co-ordinate movements and generated forces. These affordances are not a simple binary can/can't do: there is a border region where success is probabilistic,

R.J.Holt (✉)
School of Mechanical Engineering, University of Leeds, Leeds, UK
email: R.J.Holt@leeds.ac.uk

R.O. Coats · M. Mon-Williams
School of Psychology, University of Leeds, Leeds, UK

G.P. Bingham
Department of Psychological and Brain Sciences, Indiana University, IN, USA

P. Langdon et al. (eds.), *Designing Around People*,
DOI 10.1007/978-3-319-29498-8_16

or where a task may be feasible but inconveniently slow. Computer packages such as HADRIAN (Porter et al. 2004) attempt to account for this by taking recordings of individuals to be replayed. However, these rely on pre-recorded data from exemplar individuals: similar to the use of personas. Again, a useful tool – but it is impossible to quantify from these approaches how different groups' capabilities differ.

Our aim is to develop a model for the control of prehension movements that can be used to characterise an individual's capabilties and the demands of a task - not only static measures of body-scale and strength, but also the dynamic ability to execute and control movements. Through examining the metrics commonly used in motor control studies (duration, velocity, etc.) and modelling the shape of the kinematic profile, we can characterise atypical reach-to-grasp movements by their goodness of fit to our model. The paper will start by discussing the structure of reach-to-grasp movements, and some of the challenges in attempting to model this behaviour. We then propose our approach to modelling reach-to-grasp movements and illustrate it with examples drawn from experimental data, before discussing future implications and the work needed to develop the approach further.

2 Reach-to-grasp Movements

Prehension – the act of grasping and manipulating an object – is one of the most important skills possessed by humans, and fundamental to the way we have designed the world around us. Accordingly, being able to assess the demands of manual tasks and an individual's abilities is extremely important, not only for ensuring ergonomic design but for identifying impairments and monitoring rehabilitation. A variety of tests exist for assessing various elements of prehension-related skills (such as the Purdue Peg Board test (Tiffin and Asher 1948), Box and Block test (Mathiowetz et al. 1985), Southampton Hand Assessment Procedure (Light et al. 2002)). These are useful for assessing general levels of capability and improvement or decline but they aren't very helpful in assessing how capabilities are affected by object form, and therefore have limited utility for design. Furthermore, they do not identify where a particular problem lies (e.g. is it a lack of strength, or poor co-ordination or limited mobility) which would be useful for identifying the particular source of the problems and therefore the sort of interventions that may be appropriate.While work has been done on assessing the control of grip strength, the pre-contact stage of reach-to-grasp actions has yet to receive the same level of attention. Yet this is an essential part in the execution of skilled actions – involving not only the efficient transport of the hand to the object, but also the positioning of the fingers to avoid collision and ensure an appropriate grasp (Mon-Williams and Bingham 2011).

The pre-contact stage of prehension can be divided into three components: a transport element, in which the hand accelerates towards the target, an orientation element, and a grasping component, in which the fingers close around the object. The hand's velocity and the intra-digit aperture must be co-ordinated by the motor system, and there is rich evidence to suggest that this involves feedforward and feedback control (Jeannerod 1988). This is studied in terms of the velocity profile, and is assessed in terms of the overall movement time (MT), peak speed (PS), time to peak speed (tPS) and normalised time to peak speed (the ratio of tPS to MT), as illustrated in Figure 1. It is also studied in terms of the grip aperture (the distance between thumb and index finger) which is characterised by Maxiumum Grip Aperture (MGA) and time to Maximum Grip Aperture (tMGA).

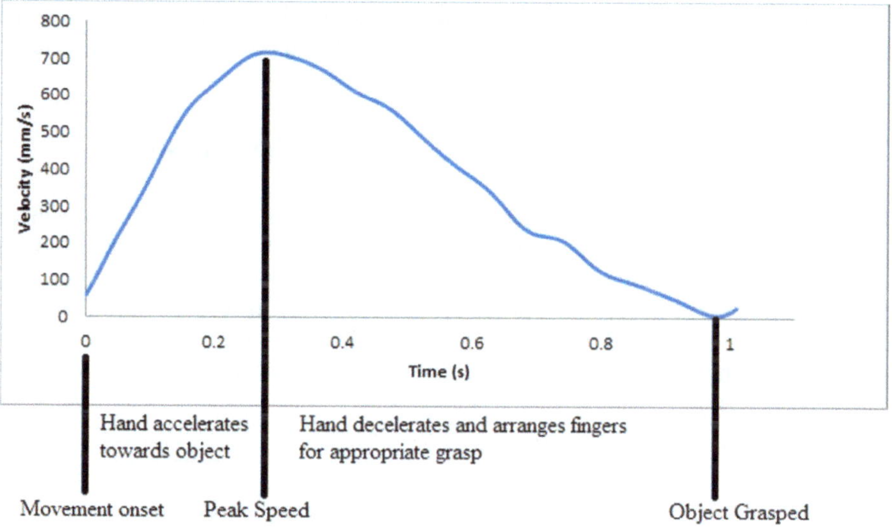

Fig. 1 The stages of a reach-to-grasp movement

These reach-to-grasp movements are stereotypical and change in predictable ways as a function of task. Larger objects produce shorter movement times, and larger grip apertures whilst small grip surfaces are associated with longer movement times (Mon-Williams and Bingham 2011). Wide objects and low coefficients of friction also cause a shift in behaviour as participants show a greater tendency to pause upon reaching the object, before closing the fingers onto the grip surfaces (Mon-Williams and Bingham 2011, Flatters et al. 2012). However, these effects also interact with individual factors – for example, Holt et al. (2013) demonstrated that age had a greater effect on the challenge of picking up wide, low-friction objects than on picking up either higher-friction objects with equal width, or narrower objects with equally low friction.

Modelling this presents significant challenges. The model presented in Figure 1 is a simplification – while velocity profiles *can* be as regular as this, they are often more irregular (as will be illustrated by the graphs in Section 3, below), as corrections are made during the movement in response to visual and proprioceptive feedback. Taking the lambda version of the Equilibrium Point Hypothesis (EPH – Feldman 1986), the motor system does not control muscle length directly, but rather adjusts the position and stiffness of the various joints by changing the recruitment threshold of alpha motor neurons. In this case, the hand is propelled towards the target by changing the equilibrium point of the shoulder, elbow and wrist joints. Analysing such a model is complex: it is possible to approximate its behaviour as that of a virtual mass-spring-damper system (Arimoto and Sekimoto 2006), but determining the biomechanical parameters related to the impedance of this is extremely complex, and will vary greatly between individuals (Mizhari 2015). Fortunately, while this is important for those studying the underlying neurophysiology of prehension, it is not necessary for those interested in characterising grip capabilities. Instead, we propose a "black box" approach that fits a model to gathered kinematic data, without the need to know the specifics of impedance or control signal. We outline the approach in the next section.

3 A Model of the Reach-to-grasp Movement

Rather than try to model the system from first principles, we have used a simple curve-fitting approach to approximate the amount of correction in a given movement. This supplements the existing metrics described in Section 2 for reach-to-grasp studies. We adopt a two-phase approach in order to account for the skewed nature of most speed profiles, partitioning the velocity profile at the point of peak speed, and fitting a Gaussian Curve to each section, as illustrated in Figure 2.

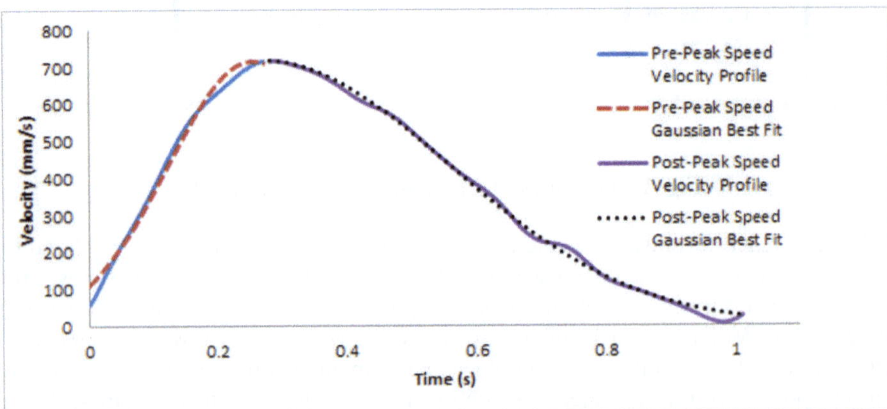

Fig. 2 Partitioned velocity profile, and Gaussian fits to pre- and post- peak data

A Gaussian Curve is the classic bell-curve used as the basis of the normal distribution, defined by three parameters: its amplitude, a, its peak location, b, and its standard deviation, c. The velocity curve, $v(t)$, as a function of time t is then given by the equation:

$$v(t) = a \exp\left(-\frac{(t-b)^2}{2c^2}\right)$$

Tools for finding the parameters of the best-fitting Gaussian curve for a data set are readily available in packages such as LabVIEW and MatLab. This provides for the fact that a well-executed action with little correction may still have a significant level of skew (such as where overshooting carries a significant risk – a wine glass balanced on the edge of a table, for example). We can then measure the amount of correction by using the R^2 value for each curve to measure its goodness of fit to the relevant part of the data. Significant deviations from the original movement can be identified by a poor fit to this model (represented by a low R^2 value) and represent either substantial corrections during the movement, or variability in the velocity itself. Each curve can therefore be described by a dyad $\{R^2_{pre}, R^2_{post}\}$ which summarises the goodness of fit of each gaussian curve to its corresponding partition of the data. Thus, a curve {1,1} would represent a movement that involved minimal correction - a perfectly planned and executed movement.

To provide an initial assessment of the model, we have applied it to sample velocity curves from Mon-Williams and Bingham (2011). In this case, National Instruments' LabVIEW was used to write a virtual instrument to partition the velocity profile at the point of peak speed, fit Gaussian curves to each part and calculate the R^2 value for each partition. Figure 3 illustrates different combinations of low and high values of R^2_{pre} and R^2_{post}, based on a single participant grasping a single object. This gives us some measure of the degree of correction taking place, and where in the grasp it takes place: for Curve A {1.0, 0.99}, there is relatively little correction; whereas B {0.99, 0.88} starts off smoothly, but has significant adjustments after peak speed, including two further lower peaks; C {0.88, 0.99} starts making corrections long before peak speed, showing a gradual build up – but the movement finishes smoothly. Finally, curve D {0.96, 0.98} makes corrections throughout.

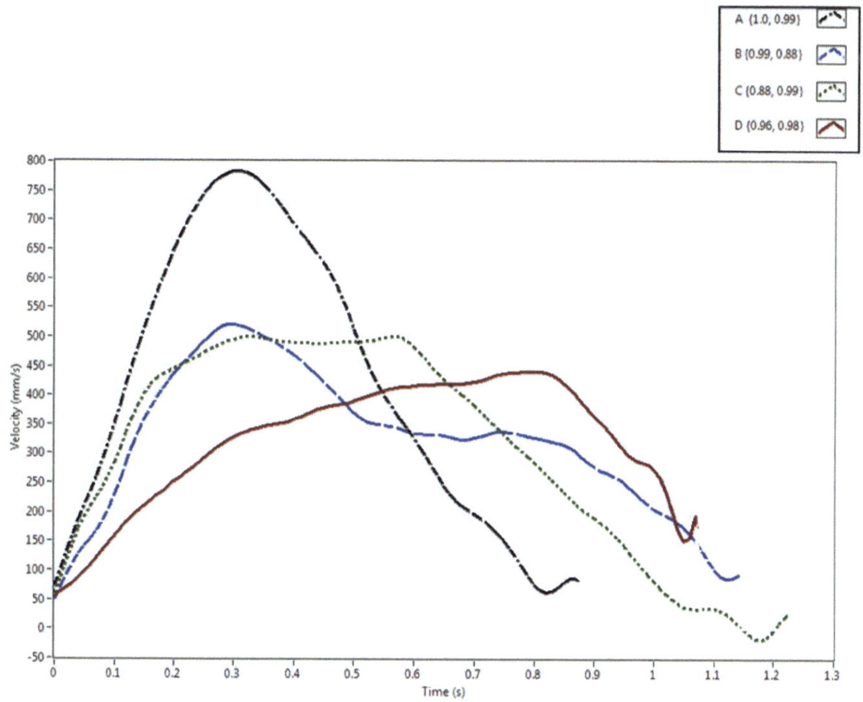

Fig. 3 Examples of curves with different dyads

These curves illustrate two important points not captured by the conventional metrics. Firstly, corrections can take place before peak speed, suggesting that the point at which feedback control begins is not *necessarily* the point of peak speed. Secondly, that even movements that have significant corrections in the early part may finish with few adjustments. Note that this does not necessarily imply that feedback control has ceased – simply that by the point of peak speed, corrections to the original movement have been sufficient to bring it back to the optimal trajectory. Under the lambda version of the EPH, this would imply that the system has now found the optimal combination of position and impedance signal to allow the momententum of the hand to complete the movement.

4 Discussion

A detailed examination of reach-to-grasp movements in neurologically intact adults shows that the movements are tailored beautifully to the task in hand. Thus, bigger objects cause a larger grip aperture (the distance between the thumb and the digits), with the maximum aperture occurring at around 70% of the movement duration. The maximum aperture is typically larger than the size of the object, providing a safety margin that ensures the digits do not collide with the object. The temporal features of the movements are likewise affected by the object charactersitics, so that decreasing the size of the grasp surface causes movements to increase in duration. It follows that larger grasp surfaces are associated with faster movements, with faster movements increasing the risk of the hand colliding with the object. It is therefore of note that the maximum grip aperture is larger when the grasp surface is smaller – providing a wonderful illustration of the precision with which the action is tailored to the object.

The pre-contact phase of reach-to-grasp movements is not only affected by the object but by the constraints of the task. It is a matter of common observation that adults reach more slowly to fragile and unstable objects than to robust and stable ones. Thus, the reach-to-grasp action is altered as a function of the costs of collision (colliding with a fragile object has a higher cost as it is more likely to fall over and break). The 'costs' associated with a variety of tasks can reasonably be assumed to be a function of the individual – with individuals assigning disperate costs (a fact often learned early in childhood with a parent's favourite ornament) and possessing different skills levels (meaning that the possibility of collision can be higher for one person than another). In support of these observations, Holt et al. (2013) showed that decreasing the difficulty of a task (where difficulty is defined as the information required to specify the task, Fitts 1954) caused qualititively different behaviour. In high difficulty tasks, Holt et al found that there was a greater probability of participants stopping the forward motion of their arm when reaching to lift an object from a tabletop. Notably, increasing the friction coefficient of the grasp surface raised the probabilty of 'fly-through' movements being recorded (movements where the object was grasped 'on-the-fly'). Holt et al. (2013) explored individual differences in the behaviour by studying the reach-to-grasp movements of healthly older adults. It was found that older adults showed quantitively and qualitively different movement patterns, reaching more slowly, showing a lower probability of 'fly-through' movements and being more affected by changes in the coefficient of friction.

The fact that reach-to-grasp movements are a function of the object and the individual means that the design of everyday objects needs to consider how a given individual will be affected by the characteristics of the object and task constraints. But how can the designer possibly predict the consequences of an object's properties on the behaviour of a wide range of individuals? It follows that there is an urgent need to produce models that are capable of predicting the impact of design decisions on human behaviour. To this end, we have created a model that is capable of providing a computer simulation of the reach-to-grasp action.

The process of creating the model has led us to new insights regarding the control mechanisms that must underpin these actions. It has long been recognised that prehensile movements are under feedforward and feedback control, with received wisdom suggesting that the first part of the movement (until the point of peak speed) is under feedforward control, with feedback mechanisms coming into operation in the deceleration phase of the movement. This conjecture has been questioned previously (Tresilian 2012) and our modelling endeavours suggest that the speed profiles observed empirically are best captured by an interplay between feedforward and feedback control throughout the whole movement. Implementation of such control mechansisms has allowed us to simulate the speed profiles observed in a range of measured prehensile actions. Moreover, our simulations allow us to identify deviations from the optimal behaviour (where optimal is defined theoretically as a maximally smooth movement with changes in speed following a Gaussian profile).

The fact that we can identify deviations from the optimal planned movements means we can quantify the effect of impairment (e.g. following stroke) on reach-to-grasp behaviour. In turn, this allows us to understand how the optimal design of a given object (e.g. a kitchen utensil) might be different for a given individual. This opens up the exciting possibility of designing objects that can decrease the levels of disability for an individual who has experienced neurological disease or the effects of older age (e.g. reduced mobility of the hand). Our modelling efforts have only just begun but we are optimistic that this process will provide a powerful tool for all those who seek to design handheld objects in an inclusive manner.

5 Conclusions and Further Work

Our model is still in its early stages. Its initial use in analysing existing data sets has illustrated some benefits over current approaches to characterising reach-to-grasp movements. The model has the advantage of generating metrics that can be readily extracted from a given velocity profile, in much the same way as peak speed, time to peak speed and movement time, and without the need for details of complex biomechanical parameters for the individual. It also goes some way towards characterising the variability within the curve, something not captured by existing models, and which is already allowing us to question the existing assumptions about reach-to-grasp control. The next step is to investigate the utility of this approach in assessing quality of control. Can it reliably capture changes with age or the trajectories observed following stroke? Can our model differentiate children with some level of motor impairment (developmental co-ordination disorder, for example) from typically developing children? Can we detect improvements in control, even where individuals still evidence deviations from normality? We now plan to apply our model to movements gathered from individuals with disabilities and to begin investigating the utility of the model beyond laboratory studies of human motor control.

References

Arimoto S, Sekimoto M (2006) Human-like movements of robotic arms with redundant DOFs: Virtual spring-damper hypothesis to tackle the Bernstein problem. In: Proceedings of the 2006 IEEE International Conference on Robotics and Automation, pp. 1860-66, Orlando, FL, USA

Dreyfus H (1967) The measure of man: Human factors in design, 2nd Ed. Whitney

Feldman AG (1986) Once more on the equilibrium-point hypothesis (λ model) for motor control. Journal of Motor Behavior 18(1): 17-54

Flatters IJ, Otten L, Witvliet A, Henson B, Holt RJ, Culmer P et al. (2012) Predicting the effect of surface texture on the qualitative form of prehension. PLoS ONE 7(3): e32770

Gonzalez V, Rowson J, Yoxall A (2015) Development of the variable dexterity test: Construction, reliability and validity. International Journal of Therapy and Rehabilitation 22 (4): 174-180

Holt RJ, Lefevre AS, Flatters IJ, Culmer P, Wilkie RM, Henson BW et al. (2013) Grasping the changes seen in older adults when reaching for objects of varied texture. PLoS ONE 8(7): e69040

Jeannerod M (1988) The neural and behavioural organization of goal-directed movements. Clarendon Press/Oxford University Press

Light CM, Chappell PH, Kyberd PJ (2002) Establishing a standardized clinical assessment tool of pathologic and prosthetic hand function: Normative data, reliability, and validity. Archives of Physical Medicine and Rehabilitation 83(6): 776-783

Mathiowetz V, Volland G, Kashman N, Weber K (1985) Adult norms for the Box and Block Test of manual dexterity. American Journal of Occupational Therapy 39(6): 386-391

Mizhari J (2015) Mechanical impedance and its relations to motor control, limb dynamics and motion biomechanics. Journal of Medical and Biological Engineering 3(1): 1-20

Mon-Williams M, Bingham GP (2011) Discovering affordances that determine the spatial structureof reach-to-grasp movements. Experimental Brain Research 211(1): 145-160

Porter JM, Case K, Marshall R, Gyi DE, Sims R (2004) Beyond Jack and Jill: Designing for individuals using HADRIAN. International Journal of Industrial Ergonomics 33(3): 249-264

Smith SA, Norris BJ, Peebles L (2000) OLDER ADULTDATA: The handbook of measurements and capabilities of the older adult – Data for design safety. Department of Trade and Industry, London, UK

Tiffin J, Asher EJ (1948) The Purdue Pegboard: Norms and studies of reliability and validity. Journal of Applied Psychology 32(3): 234

Yoxall A, Luxmoore J, Austin M, Canty L, Margrave KJ, Richardson CJ et al. (2007) Getting to grips with packaging: Using ethnography and computer simulation to understand hand–pack interaction. Packaging Technology and Science 20: 217-229

It's All in the Eyes: Designing Facial Expressions for an Interactive Robot Therapy Coach for Children

P. Cloutier, H. W. Park, J. MacCalla and A. Howard

Abstract: An important aspect for child and robot interactions in various therapy scenarios is the robot's ability to convey emotions to the child. Due to the fact that 93% of human communication is non-verbal, these socially interactive robots need to have the ability to mimic non-verbal cues to the child, particularly through the use of facial expressions. In this paper, we discuss the ability for a socially interactive robot to emote emotions through a minimal set of features, i.e. soley through the eyes. In a study with five participants, we evaluate participants ability to recognize emotions based on the Plutchik emotion scale and the universal emotions of happiness, sadness, anger, and fear. Results indicate that participants recognition of an emotion is maximum when the intensity of the emotion is not at the extreme ends of the Plutchik emotion scale.

1 Introduction

It is widely known that over 90% of human communication is non-verbal. Such forms of communication involve various cues from various facial expressions, some of which are understood around the world while others are learned and bear cultural significance. In particular, the universal emotional expressions include happiness, sadness, anger, fear, surprise, disgust, and interest (Ekman and Friese 1971). Although the intensity of certain expressions can carry different meanings across cultures and, in some cases, emotions such as fear and surprise are indistinguishable from one another (Ekman 1992), there lies a basic, cross-cultural understanding of the meaning of each of these universal expressions. One is able to display these emotions through the tension and relaxation of certain parts of the face, resulting in different facial movements (Bassili 1979). To express sadness, for example, people change their expression by moving their eyebrows inward and upward, while simultaneously moving their chin slightly upward. Anger is expressed through the tension of the mouth and lips to make a frown (Bassili 1979), as well as a furrowing

P. Cloutier · H. W. Park · A. M. Howard (✉)
Georgia Institute of Technology, Atlanta, GA, USA
email: ayanna.howard@ece.gatech.edu

J. MacCalla
Zyrobotics LLC, Atlanta, GA, USA

P. Langdon et al. (eds.), *Designing Around People*,
DOI 10.1007/978-3-319-29498-8_17

of the brows (Black and Yacoob 1997), while happiness involves raising the lips and the cheeks into a smile (Bassili 1979).

The role of emotions in social scenarios is to provide an inherent mode of communication between two parties. Emotions yield a natural form of communication, in that they can be shown visually through facial expressions, vocal expression, and actions/body movements. When emotions are properly employed and understood, people are able to respond appropriately, which further enhances the social interaction. In particular, when adults interact with children in therapy settings, effective emotion execution has the capability to build rapport, improve engagement, and optimize the interaction.

As the field of robotics continues to expand, an increasing number of robots are being introduced into settings involving therapy with children (Howard 2013). One of the key uses of emotions in these types of scenarios is to build a bond between robot and child. Typically, this bonding mechanism can be enhanced by having the robot exhibit forms of empathy. Empathy is a key factor used to enforce socially supportive behaviors (Tiberius and Billson 1991). In this vein, there have already been a number of research robots that use this type of empathy, or emotions, to communicate. Examples of such robots include the EU's iCub (Metta et al. 2008), the Nexi MDS (Delaunay et al. 2009), and the CMU GRACE (Simmons et al. 2003) robot. Each variant on facial expressions used on these robotic platforms has its own set of benefits, including ease of emotion conveyance and cost. Saerbeck et al. (2010) were able to implement empathy best by simply having a robotic agent smile (happy face) when a task was completed correctly and frown (sad face) when the task was completed incorrectly. During a case study involving a humanoid robot and children, Beck et al. (2013) were able to analyze the effects of upward and downward head movement relative to positive and negative emotion. The humanoid robot was programmed to have six different base poses: anger, sadness, fear, pride, happiness, and excitement. The results showed that moving the head up improved the identification of pride, happiness, and excitement, while moving the head down improved the identification of anger and sadness. Fear was identified well regardless of the head's position. In a similar study, Li and Chingnell (2011) analyzed how simple head and arm movements were able to communicate emotion in social robots. Here, they used a teddy bear to implement various arm and/or head movements. They concluded that when head movements were compared to arm movements, arm movements overall were perceived to be more lifelike. Finally, in Bennett and Šabanović (2014), a study was conducted that examined the use of minimal features for a robotic face achieved through actuating components. Their results suggest that actuated movement of the eyes, eyebrows, and mouth alone is sufficient to create reocgnizable facial expresions of affect.

In all of these scenarios, robots promoted effective human-robot communication through emotion conveyance. Following along the lines of prior research threads, we are interested in further exploring this concept of a minimal set of features that can be used to express emotions for social interaction. A reduced set of features is desirable since it can logically lead to a reduction in complexity of the hardware, and thus a more robust and affordable robot platform for in-home therapy. As such, in this paper, we focus on evaluating the ability of a robot to emote emotions soley through the eyes.

2 Approach

Although there have been various methods employed for expressing emotions on a robotic platform, by far, a digital interface, such as an LCD screen, is the least complex and most cost effective as it eliminates the use of servos and motors, as well as reduces the financial costs and building constraints of powering and wiring these actuators. To program an LCD screen to display emotions, it is beneficial to parameterize them. In this way, several emotions could be related to one another mathematically so that the change in one parameter of an emotion would have a predictable change and in turn display an equally predictable, new emotion. The research presented here sought to determine if various facial expressions could be understood using limited parameters and facial features. The facial expressions developed in this research focused solely on using the eyes. We focus on the eyes based on its validated use in children as a measure for recognizing the emotional state of people (Baron-Cohen et al. 1999). In this widely-used measure called the Reading the Mind in the Eyes Test for children (Baron-Cohen et al. 1999), a child's ability to recognize the emotional states of targets can be assessed by showing them photos of faces with only the eyes showing and asking them to choose from among four emotion state terms (e.g., friendly, sad, surprised, worried) which one best describes what the eyes show. This test was originally developed for children with Autism and has applicability to Traumatic Brain Injury. A modification of this test was also applied to adults, resulting in similar outcome measures.

Our facial expressions were implemented using a 128 x 128 Adafruit LCD screen and programmed using an Arduino Uno board. The facial expressions, represented by two eyes, were generated by parameterizing two ellipses for each eye – a primary ellipse which represented a *Neutral* facial expression (Figure 1) and a secondary ellipse that was used to evoke different expressions. The shape of each eye (primary ellipse) and each secondary ellipse was influenced by several parameters, including its x, y coordinates, width, and height. To generate various expressions, parts of the primary ellipse were obstructed by changing the parameters of the secondary ellipses. By covering various portions of the eye, the entire image is able to mimic the changes around the eye muscles associated with different expressions, including squinting and brow furrowing. By varying the amount of coverage, and the location of coverage (bottom, top), the eye can be designed to appear happy, afraid, angry, sad, or tired. For example, covering the top, inside corners of the eyes can exhibit the impression of one furrowing their eyebrows, thereby mimicking an angered expression (Figure 1b) whereas with the top, outer corners covered, the eyes can appear more downcast, thus mimicking a saddened expression (Figure 1c). Using this construct, there is a large variety of possible expressions. As such, it was essential that the options be narrowed down to a reasonable and testable size. Therefore, in this research we focused on selecting expressions based on the Plutchik (2011) emotion scale and the universal emotions of happiness, sadness, anger, and fear (Figure 2a). For each chosen emotion, five facial expressions associated with emotion intensity were designed covering from the inner to the outer boundary conditions of the emotion, giving a total of 20 different expressions to test.

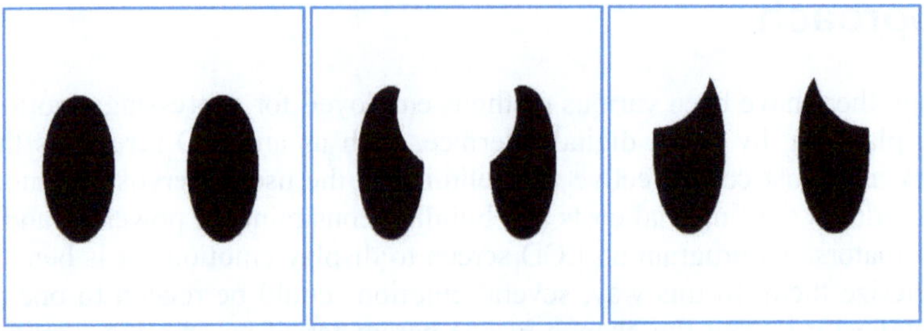

Fig. 1 (a) Left - neutral expression, (b) center - angry expression, (c) right - sad expression

To correlate emotion intensity to the depicted eye expression, we varied the percentage of the primary ellipse that the secondary ellipse would cover. The first expression of an emotion group had the least coverage and the fifth had the most. In this way, the emotions were intended to increase in severity as more of the eye was covered. Figure 2b depicts an example of an extreme for the happy emotion whereas 2c depicts the other extreme.

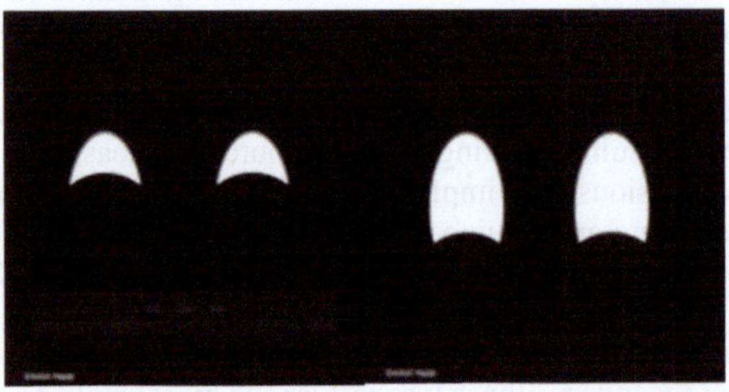

Fig. 2 (a) left - happy emotion at lower boundary, (b) right - happy emotion at higher boundary

3 Experimental Setup

Once the 20 expressions were created, they were displayed on the LCD screen for testing. The screen itself was mounted onto our interactive robot therapy coach so that the expressions could be tested in a realistic scenario. Emotions were grouped together and shown in increasing intensity, with one emotion displayed per case. To test the effectiveness of how well these emotions were conveyed, five participants were provided a survey and asked to observe each emotion and label their interpretation of the emotion on an image of the Plutchik emotion scale. In the current study, three male volunteers and two female volunteers participated, with a mean age of 29.6 and standard deviation of 7.2 years. For each survey question, a checkbox labeled "I don't know" was also placed next to each Plutchik emotion scale image so that if participants were unsure of an emotion, they could mark this box. Participants were able to move between emotions using two pushbuttons attached to the robot, a forward button and a backward button. When one of these was pressed, the program would switch forward or back to the next emotion in the sequence. This allowed for participants to be able to analyze each image and interpret it at their own pace.

In addition to evaluation of the 20 emotions, four additional faces were added to the end of the survey as a separate question (Figure 3). Each face progressed in feature complexity, starting from a pair of eyes to a fully-expressive face. This question was intended to assess what types of faces participants responded best to and what they found to be the most natural looking by having participants rank their preferred version of the face from 1 to 4.

4 Results

Given the pool of participants, the data was quantified for analysis. A polar graph was overlaid onto the Plutchik emotion scale and the radius and angle associated with each participant's mark on the survey was calculated. The angle, θ, which ranged from 0 to 2π, corresponded to the emotion and the radius, r, which ranged from 0 to 4.5, corresponded to the intensity of the emotion (Figure 4). A value of (r, θ) = (0,0) was stored for any "I don't know" labels selected by a participant. Each emotion group on the Plutchik scale was quantified to differ from other emotion groups by an angle of π/4 radians, or approximately 0.785 radians. Therefore, any difference between expected and response averages that was greater than this number signified a perceived emotion type that was entirely different from the hypothesis. The resulting averages and standard deviations are as shown in Table 1 and the resulting emotions are in Table 2.

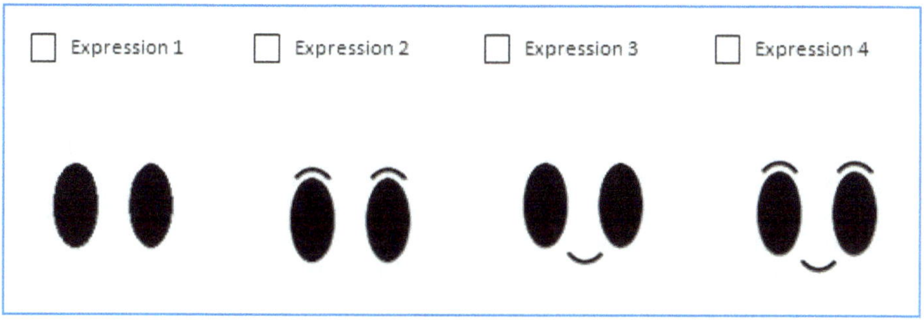

Fig. 3 Additional survey faces

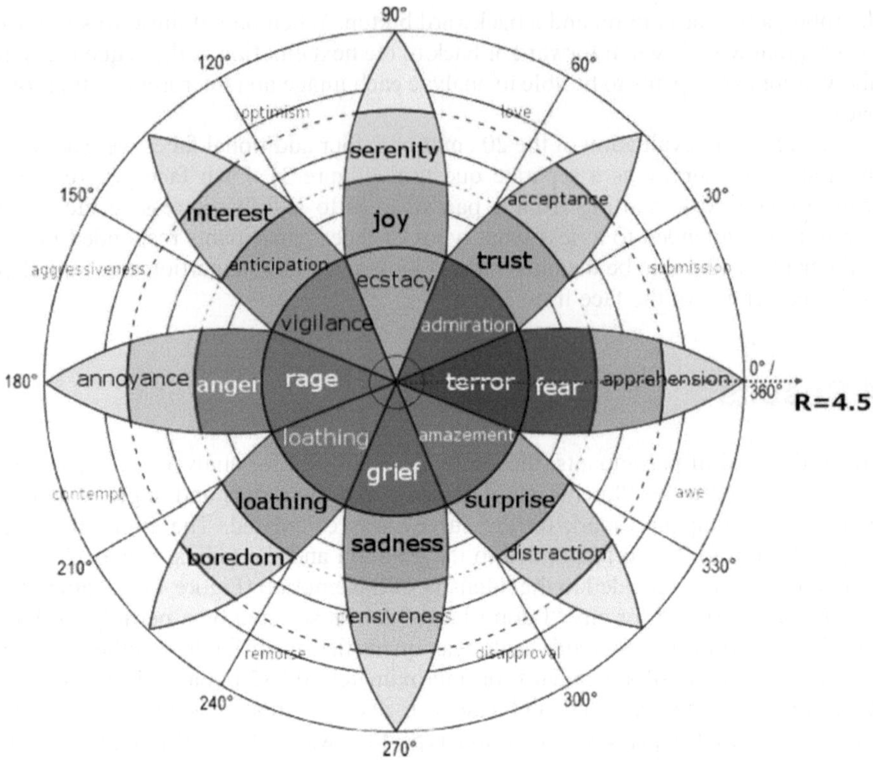

Fig. 4 Mapping of emotions to quantitative values (angle, radius)

From Table 2, it can be seen that the perceived emotion differed from the expected for nearly half of the emotions. Those that did not differ dramatically (i.e. the number of correct matches between the expected and the participants' perceived emotion was greater than 75%) mostly correspond to the middle-most emotions of each group, which suggests that the parameters corresponding to the intensity of these emotions were the easiest to determine when the emotion was in a middle state as opposed to on an extreme end of the emotion. In addition, the expected emotion of afraid was most matched by participants with surprise. This suggests that our depiction of the afraid emotion was not parameterized correctly

The second half of the survey (Figure 3) demonstrated the benefit of having a more involved facial display on the robot. Table 3 shows the ranking of participants' preferences, where a smaller number relates to a higher preference and a larger number relates to a lower preference (note: one participant did not complete the second part of the survey).

Table 1 Average and standard deviation of participants perceived emotion as compared to expected emotion

	Perceived		Expected/Programmed	
	Intensity (Radius) Avg (Stdv)	Angle (Position) Avg (Stdv)	Intensity (Radius)	Angle (Position)
Happy	1.7 (0.97)	2.36 (1.76)	2.5	1.57
	2.2 (0.27)	1.73 (0.86)	2	1.57
	1.6 (0.55)	1.88 (0.7)	2	1.57
	1 (0.71)	1.57 (1.11)	1	1.57
	2 (1.54)	2.2 (1.51)	1	1.57
Sad	2.4 (0.55)	5.02 (0.7)	4.5	4.71
	2 (0)	4.71 (0)	4	4.71
	1.5 (0.5)	4.71 (0)	2	4.71
	1.3 (0.45)	4.71 (0)	2	4.71
	1.6 (1.08)	4.4 (0.7)	1	4.71
Angry	2.5 (0.71)	3.3 (0.35)	4	3.14
	1.9 (0.22)	3.14 (0)	3.5	3.14
	1 (0)	3.14 (0)	2.5	3.14
	0.8 (0.45)	2.51 (1.4)	2	3.14
	0.6 (0.55)	1.88 (1.72)	1	3.14
Afraid	2 (0.71)	5.5 (0)	0	0
	1.8 (0.45)	5.5 (0)	0	0
	1.5 (1.66)	3.3 (3.01)	4	6.28
	1.4 (1.67)	3.3 (3.01)	4	6.28
	0.4 (0.55)	2.2 (3.01)	3	6.28

From the table, it can be concluded that the second and forth expressions (Figure 5) were equally the most favorable of the four expressions. Participants wrote that their preference for these faces was because of the natural impression and approachability of the eyebrows, as well as the clarity of expression in the mouth.

Table 2 Participants perceived emotion and recognition rate

Expected Emotion	Participant					Recog'on Rate (%)
	1	2	3	4	5	
Happy	Sad	Happy	Angry	Interested	Don't Know	20
Happy	Happy	Happy	Angry	Happy	Admiring	60
Happy	Happy	Happy	Angry	Happy	Happy	80
Happy	Happy	Don't Know	Angry	Happy	Happy	60
Happy	Happy	Interested	Angry	Don't Know	Bored	20
Sad	Afraid	Sad	Sad	Sad	Sad	80
Sad	Sad	Sad	Sad	Sad	Sad	100
Sad	Sad	Sad	Sad	Sad	Sad	100
Sad	Sad	Sad	Sad	Sad	Sad	100
Sad	Sad	Sad	Sad	Sad	Angry	80
Angry	Angry	Angry	Angry	Bored	Angry	80
Angry	Angry	Angry	Angry	Angry	Angry	100
Angry	Angry	Angry	Angry	Angry	Angry	100
Angry	Angry	Don't Know	Angry	Angry	Angry	80
Angry	Angry	Don't Know	Angry	Don't Know	Angry	60
Afraid	Surprised	Surprised	Surprised	Afraid	Surprised	20
Afraid	Surprised	Surprised	Surprised	Afraid	Surprised	20
Afraid	Surprised	Afraid	Afraid	Afraid	Surprised	60
Afraid	Surprised	Afraid	Afraid	Afraid	Surprised	60
Afraid	Surprised	Afraid	Afraid	Afraid	Surprised	60

Table 3 Participant ranking of emotions

	Expression 1	Expression 2	Expression 3	Expression 4
Participant 1	3	1	4	2
Participant 2	4	3	1	2
Participant 3	4	2	3	1
Participant 4	1	3	2	4
AVERAGES	3	2.25	2.5	2.25

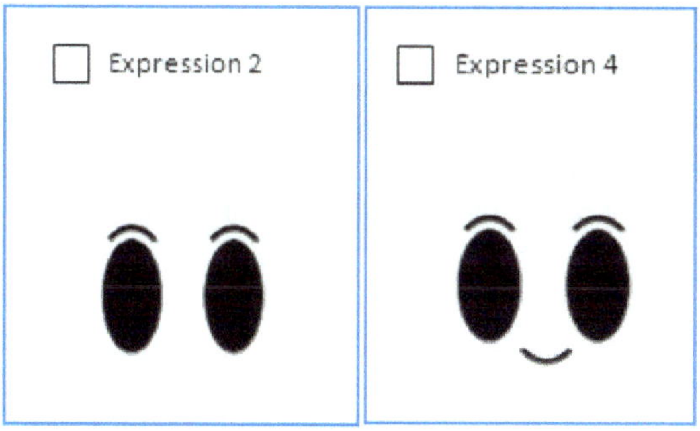

Fig. 5 Participant preference of faces

5 Conclusion and Discussion

Through the development, programming, and implementation of the emotions presented in this research, as well as through the testing and analysis of these emotions, it was found that eyes, as a minimum feature set, could be effective in communicating emotions on a physical robot. While the most extreme emotions had a higher variability in their interpretations than other emotions, overall it was found that the participants in this study were able to identify the general emotion that was displayed on the LCD screen. It should be noted that the results of the survey could have been affected by a variety of factors. For example, the survey may have negatively affected the results due to its wording. Many of the adjectives on the provided Plutchik chart used complex words, which could have made participant interpretations more difficult, especially for those whose first language was not English. The test itself could have had an influence on the findings, particularly with respect to the ordering of the expressions presented to the participants. The grouping of similar expressions in an order of increasing intensity may have influenced participants to choose a different expression than what they would have had the expressions been more randomized.

There are other ways in which this research could be improved upon. The ultimate goal of this research is to find a way to parameterize simple facial expressions on a robot. Therefore, in future work one of the next steps would be to develop a mathematical model that could be used to generate a variety of facial expressions. With respect to the study itself, in further iterations of this project it would be beneficial to attempt to randomize the facial expressions, as well as simplify the emotion graph. Ideally, the participant pool would be much larger as well, since the limited number of participants only suggest trends on the results. An additional study could also be developed to correlate any recognition differences found between a photo of eyes expressing emotion and a schematic rendition of eyes showing the same emotion.

Acknowledgements

This material is based upon work supported by the National Science Foundation under Grant No. IIP-1413850 and 0851643. The robot technology discussed in this research has been licensed to Zyrobotics, LLC. The terms of this arrangement have been reviewed and approved by Georgia Tech in accordance with its conflict of interest policies.

References

Baron-Cohen S, O'Riordan M, Stone V, Jones R, Plaisted K (1999) Recognition of faux pas by normally developing children and children with Asperger syndrome or high-functioning autism. Journal of Autism and Developmental Disorders 29: 407-418

Bassili J (1979) Emotion recognition: The role of facial movement and the relative importance of upper and lower areas of the face. Journal of Personality and Social Psychology 37(11): 2049-58

Beck A, Canamero L, Hiolle A, Damiano L, Cosi P, Tesser F et al. (2013) Interpretation of emotional body language displayed by a humanoid robot: A case study with children. International Journal of Social Robotics 5(3): 325-334

Bennett CC, Šabanović S (2014) Deriving minimal features for human-like facial expressions in robotic faces. International Journal of Social Robotics 6(3): 367-381

Black M, Yacoob Y (1997) Recognizing facial expressions in image sequences using local parameterized models of image motion. International Journal of Computer Vision 25(1): 23-48

Delaunay F, De Greeff J, Belpaeme T (2009) Towards retro-projected robot faces: An alternative to mechatronic and android faces. In: Proceedings of the 18th IEEE International Symposium on Robot and Human Interactive Communication, pp. 306-311, Toyama International Conference Center, Japan

Ekman P (1992) Facial expressions of emotion: New findings, new questions. Psychological Science (3)1: 34-38

Ekman P, Friese WV (1971) Constants across cultures in the face and emotion. Journal of Personality and Social Psychology 17(2): 124-129

Howard A (2013) Robots learn to play: Robots emerging role in pediatric therapy. In: Proceedings of the 26th international Florida Artificial Intelligence Research Society Conference, St. Pete Beach, FL, USA

Li J, Chignell M (2011) Communication of emotion in social robots through simple head and arm movements. International Journal of Social Robotics 3(2): 125-142

Metta G, Sandini G, Vernon D, Natale L, Nori F (2008) The iCub humanoid robot: An open platform for research in embodied cognition. In: Proceedings of the 8th Workshop on Performance Metrics for Intelligent Systems, pp. 50-56, Washington DC, USA

Plutchik R (2011) The nature of emotions. American Scientist 89: 344-350

Saerbeck M, Schut T, Bartneck C, Janse M (2010) Expressive robots in education: Varying the degree of social supportive behavior of a robotic tutor. In: Proceedings of ACM CHI 2010 Conference on Human Factors in Computing Systems, pp. 1613-1622, Atlanta, GA, USA

Simmons R, Goldberg D, Goode A, Montemerlo M, Roy N, Sellner B et al. (2003) GRACE: An autonomous robot for the AAAI robot challenge. CMU, Pittsburgh, PA, USA

Tiberius R, Billson J (1991) The social context of teaching and learning. New Directions for Teaching and Learning 1991(45): 67-86

It's a Curse … and a Gift: Developing the Own Input Alternative for Computer Interaction

T. Felzer and S. Rinderknecht

Abstract: The development process of any assistive computer interface for people with disabilities involves two, usually disjointed, groups of people. First, there is the so-called target population, i.e., potential end users of the interface. And second, there are the designers and developers who somehow became aware of particular interaction problems and are trying to solve them. This chapter is about the first author's work on an assistive computer interface that allows efficient text entry based on the supported usage of both thumbs. The interface relies on a small compact keypad which is able to do everything usually requiring a standard keyboard. The speciality is that the first author belongs to *both* groups mentioned above. He initially started to develop the keyboard replacement for himself, as using the normal keyboard for operating a PC became too slow and cumbersome. The outcome changed his life. It helps him a lot, and for about two years, he has used almost nothing else to work with a computer. The word 'initially' is very important here: he soon realized that if the tool works for him, it should work for others as well. Having Friedreich's Ataxia himself, his ultimate wish was to make life a little easier for people with certain neuromuscular diseases. This chapter talks about the interaction problems experienced every day by the first author and why it was necessary to develop a new alternative specifically adapted to his needs. It outlines the current results and discusses the advantages of being their own test subject.

1 Motivation (the "Curse")

Before his tenth birthday, the first author did not show any noticeable sign of a disability. He never was an outstanding athlete when it came to school sport, and he did not have the most beautiful handwriting among his classmates, but nobody thought that this had anything to do with a serious disorder.

Then, the real problems started, first with walking: he began stumbling, and he fell down more and more often. In addition, his writing skills decreased. He

T. Felzer (✉) · S. Rinderknecht
Institute for Mechatronic Systems in Mechanical Engineering, Technische Universität Darmstadt, Germany
email: felzer@ims.tu-darmstadt.de

P. Langdon et al. (eds.), *Designing Around People*,
DOI 10.1007/978-3-319-29498-8_18

became slower and it was increasingly difficult for him to get by with the amount of time normally granted for written exams in school.

At the age of fifteen, he was diagnosed with the hereditary neuromuscular disease Friedreich's Ataxia, which affects nerves and muscles, leading to problems in gait, motor coordination, and speech production. It also often causes various sorts of sensory deficiencies, such as loss of hearing and pathological nystagmus, as well as secondary symptoms like increased heart rate or cardiomyopathy (Lecky 1999). For the first author, the immediate consequence of this disease was that he became wheelchair-bound at age eighteen.

This challenge almost naturally led to some sort of vicious circle, as it was more or less the reason for his professional career: never wanting to be employed *because of* his disability, but *despite* his disability, he always aimed to be among the best, first in school, then later in university. His PhD degree in computer science was kind of a logical result. Today, he works as a researcher in the field of human-computer interaction.

The downside is that his occupation requires him to use a computer, but he has difficulty using the standard input devices for computer operation – keyboard and mouse. The main problem is that he constantly has to reposition the hands when using the large standard keyboard, in order to hit each key on the right angle. Due to impaired fine motor control, this takes a very long time and is very cumbersome. It is extremely frustrating for him that even after careful repositioning, he still makes lots of mistakes (which have to be corrected, *etc*., *etc*.). Since his disease is progressive, this trouble grows.

The dynamics become obvious when looking at the first author's entry rate with the regular keyboard. When he finished school, he achieved 12 wpm (*words per minute*) or more. 18 years later, this had halved to 6 wpm, and another eight years later – three years ago – it had halved again to less than 3 wpm. Therefore, the first author had to find a viable input alternative.

The next section justifies the necessity of developing a new alternative specifically adapted to the first author's needs. The section after that describes the basic structure of the resulting alternative *OnScreenDualScribe* (Felzer et al. 2014). What follows is a discussion of empirical results, before the chapter is concluded with a summary and some evaluating remarks.

2 Why an Own Alternative Was Needed

When his problems with text entry became more severe, the first author started to search for an alternative input method, at first solely as a member of the target population, i.e., among existing solutions. But alternatives that many others were able to use very efficiently exceeded his abilities by far.

A first example was *Automatic Speech Recognition* (ASR), which can be used (in principle) to enter text or issue control commands just by talking to the computer. Theoretically, it is even possible to enter text faster than manually, and almost effort-free. However, the first author's speech is dysarthric, meaning that there is a high variability in his speech. Therefore, it is impossible to recognize it automatically (even though the first author tried for weeks to train the utilized recognizer).

As the clear production of certain specific words is easier for the first author than that of most other words, the *CanSpeak* approach, providing a spelling interface based on the recognition of certain keywords (Hamidi et al. 2010), seemed to be a promising answer. But given the fact that their system used a normal recognition engine before filtering out the keywords, and since, even for this small set of words, the variability is rather large, this attempt did not yield the desired success either.

The first author still was not willing to give up the idea of controlling the computer using his voice completely. The paradigm of *Non-Verbal Vocal Interaction* (NVVI) deals with the production of humming or whistling sounds as input signals for the computer (Watts and Robinson 1999). Since the automatic recognition of corresponding sound patterns is much easier than that of speech signals, the first author was hoping to find the ultimate solution here. He co-implemented and evaluated the application *Chanti* which is based on the NVVI input idea (Sporka et al. 2011). The production of the required sound patterns turned out to be too laborious and error-prone to be a viable alternative.

Another approach for hands-free computer operation tested by the first author is the *Camera Mouse* (Betke et al. 2002). This system replaces the mouse by tracking an arbitrary point on the user's head (with the help of an inexpensive webcam) and moving the mouse pointer accordingly. In combination with an on-screen point-and-click keyboard, it is used by an ever-growing community of people with disabilities to effortlessly enter text. Since the first author's fine motor control is disturbed by an increasing amount of involuntary movements, this led to a very high error rate, and entry was slow and cumbersome.

Experiments involving an on-screen keyboard and a manual pointing device (e.g., Felzer and Nordmann 2006) showed that this combination was not what the first author was looking for either. Although text entry was almost error-free, the corresponding solution was hardly suitable for replacing the standard keyboard. On the one hand, there was no physical advantage, meaning that the demanded effort was about as high as before. On the other hand, entry was simply slowed down by a factor of about 3.

Semantic considerations are used in *Dasher* to accelerate mouse-based text entry (Ward et al. 2000). Words are entered by successively moving the mouse pointer into rectangular regions on the screen, associated with the individual characters of the word. Size and position of the region belonging to a particular character are dynamically adapted according to the probability that this character comes next, based on those entered previously. Usually, experienced users are able to achieve quite considerable entry rates, but since the first author's hand-eye coordination is extremely deficient, he was not able to usefully employ this tool.

Finally, the first author even tried several solutions based on *scanning,* where the computer cyclically suggests (sets of) options, and the user selects a suggested option by generating an input signal, e.g., the actuation of a switch, at the right time. For instance, the idea of a row-column scanning keyboard is to sequentially enter characters by consecutively selecting row and column of each character within a two-dimensional matrix (Simpson and Koester 1999).

He particularly evaluated own developments (though intended for a different user group), based on *intentional muscle contractions* as input signals (Felzer et al. 2009). Since he can do a lot more than just contract a single muscle, a large percentage of his true abilities were not being used. Thus, it was not surprising that the corresponding systems were no competitive alternative in comparison to his usual input method (e.g., Felzer and Nordmann 2006b).

On the whole, every solution tried by the first author either demanded too much or too little, meaning that he either was physically unable to use it, or he was limited to only a fraction of what he was able to perform. There was really nothing that was "just right". To fill this gap, the first author decided to develop his own alternative, something completely new, specifically tailored to his abilities. The outcome is based on the compact keypad (called *DualPad*) depicted in Figure 1.

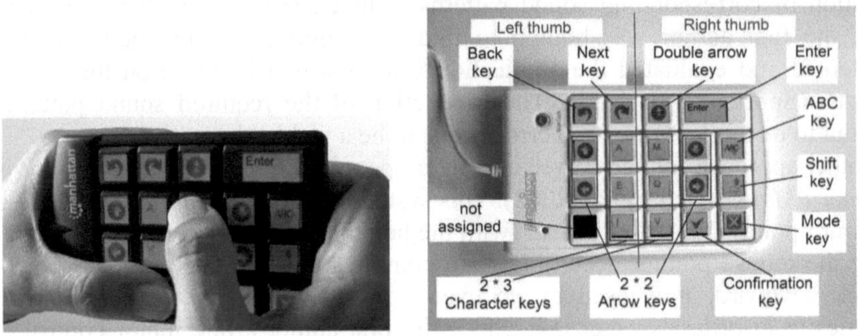

a b

Fig. 1 Input device *DualPad*: a. to be held securely with both hands and operated with the thumbs only; b. names of its 18 keys

The use of this keypad (in fact, just an off-the-shelf numeric keypad, rotated and equipped with keytop stickers) was directly inspired by the first author's experiences with the standard keyboard. He always liked typing the leftmost characters in each row of the full-size keyboard ("1", "Q", or "A"), since they allowed to type with the thumbs while stabilizing the hand by holding onto the left edge of the keyboard.

This line of action is normally only possible for very few keys, yet the *DualPad* allows it for every key. In particular, the right hand can be used in the same manner, almost doubling the entry speed. Besides, the keypad is small enough for every key to be reached from the same hand position. The software wrapper for this input device is briefly outlined in the next section.

3 Basic Ideas Implemented in *OnScreenDualScribe*

The purpose of *OnScreenDualScribe* is to turn the compact keypad depicted in Figure 1 into a universal input device, fully capable of emulating both keyboard and mouse, thereby assisting the user in efficiently operating a computer. Technically, the (Windows®) software intercepts physical keystrokes on the *DualPad* before they reach the active window, and computes virtual input events which are initiated instead.

To compensate for the smaller number of keys, this computation is not only based on the currently pressed key, but also on the current context, i.e., the history of keys pressed previously. Most keys do not result in directly emulating an input event, but in changing the context only. Moreover, the meaning of each key can vary with every keystroke, and the program window always displays an *avatar* of the *DualPad* reminding the user of the currently active key associations.

Integral component of the context is the program *mode*, which combines a set of similar input actions. Program execution is divided into twelve modes. Some are for text entry, some for mouse operation, and some for miscellaneous functionality. The default mode, which is reachable from every other mode with a single keystroke, is called *dual mode*. It implements a basic idea for text entry (see Figure 2).

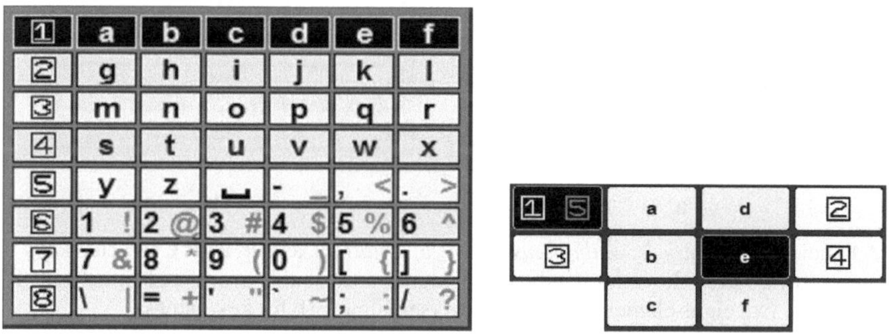

a b

Fig. 2 Basic text entry in *dual mode*: a. character matrix with eight rows and six columns; b. Arrow keys (labelled 1-4, to be pressed once or twice) for row selection and Character keys (labelled a-f) for column selection (see Figure 1b for key names)

Selectable characters are assigned to the cells of a two-dimensional matrix, and to enter any one of those characters, the user just selects the corresponding row and column. For the first 24 letters of the alphabet (i.e., the first four rows of the character matrix), this requires exactly two keystrokes, which would mean that the *KSPC* (keystrokes per character) for this input method would be around 2.0 (MacKenzie 2002).

Compared to the *KSPC* of the standard keyboard (1.0), this would mean a substantial overhead. However, while the user enters letter strings (which are interpreted as being the beginning of a word), the software inspects an internal dictionary for possible completions, and presents these candidates in a list, which is updated after every single letter. Once the intended word is in the list, the user may switch to *word prediction mode*, and select the corresponding candidate to save the remaining keystrokes (Koester and Levine 1994). Based on the used dictionary, this reduces the *KSPC* to a value slightly above 1.1.

Ambiguous mode provides a second, completely different method of text entry. The code is based on the first author's implementation of a *Scanning Ambiguous Keyboard* (MacKenzie and Felzer 2010) – albeit without the scanning part. The entire alphabet is distributed over just six keys, and to enter a word, the user composes a corresponding sequence of these ambiguous keys (see Figure 3).

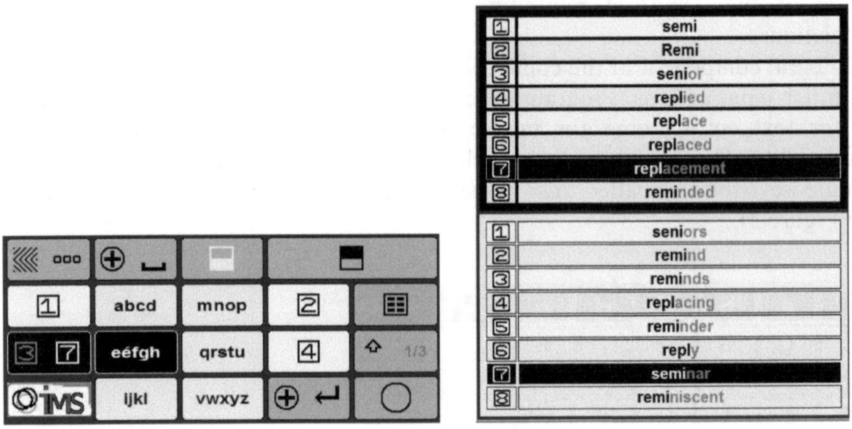

a b

Fig. 3 Efficient text entry in *ambiguous mode*: a. *DualPad* avatar with Character keys as ambiguous keys, Arrow keys for candidate selection, and Double arrow and Enter keys for finalization; b. two eight-element candidate lists (see Figure 1b for key names)

During composition of the sequence, the software looks through the same dictionary as before for possible matches or extensions of the prefix entered so far. Candidates are again presented in a frequency-ordered list, and can be selected to finalize the word. This technique – which may be regarded as "T9 on 6 keys" – is extremely efficient (with a *KSPC* of less than 0.9), yet it only works for in-dictionary words.

In order to be practically usable, *OnScreenDualScribe* offers a huge number of additional features facilitating input. In particular, and in contrast to many proof-of-concept implementations of other academically-motivated alternatives, it often allows multiple redundant ways to do the same thing, and the user has the option to choose the most efficient one for the current situation. For example, there are six ways to emulate a "TAB" keystroke, one in every other mode, just because it would be inefficient (though possible) to constantly change modes when tabbing through a document while performing arbitrary manipulations.

Other important topics involve checking the spelling (of single words or entire files), as well as updating the program dictionary (manually or automatically). In total, the tool is ready for practical, efficient use. It allows everything the standard input devices do (with very few exceptions). Plus, it offers a whole lot more.

4 Empirical Evaluation (the "Gift")

The abstract mentions two groups of people involved in the development process of an assistive interface: the target population and the developers. Both groups depend on each other. The developers are the ones with the expertise. They are able to manufacture the necessary hardware, and it is their job to implement corresponding software components. But all that would not be possible without the intended users iteratively expressing their needs and demands and evaluating the resulting system.

However, this loop can only be suboptimal. Users are hardly able to express their needs in source code form. And the developers therefore have to base their work on their own interpretation of the users' expressions – they are trying to find a "best match", particularly when multiple users with varying requirements are involved.

This is different for the first author. Being the intended user himself, he knows exactly what the target population needs and wants. Furthermore, after changing the software or adding a new component, he can immediately evaluate the change and decide whether to keep or modify it.

A second advantage of being their own test subject is that the first author is always familiar with the software. A novice user would always have to practice with the tool for quite some time. Instead, the first author is aware of what kind of input the program expects (or should expect) in every situation. He can spot bugs or circumvent them if necessary, and he has the internal knowledge needed to recover from any errors.

The third advantage is related to the first author's experience with *OnScreen-DualScribe*. To make full use of the program's power, the user has to be able to anticipate when it makes sense to look at the candidate lists, and he has to know how to handle out-of-dictionary words. How well a particular user performs is subject to a certain learning curve. After more than three years of experience, learning can almost be ruled out entirely for the first author, and especially numerical results evaluating peak performance solely depend on the quality of the interface (and the first author's current medical condition, of course).

Nevertheless, the example of the first author, proving that the idea really works, is just a start. It is of tremendous importance to conduct user studies involving participants other than the developer. The biggest drawback of *OnScreenDual-Scribe* is that recruiting participants for such a study is particularly challenging. The tool is rather comprehensive, and therefore complex and not easy to learn, and practicing takes long and is probably frustrating at first. However, the user gets a lot in return (if he is aware of how to use the power of the program).

If the user realizes that the software really helps them, he or she is more willing to "overlook" certain shortcomings (e.g., the graphics in *OnScreen-DualScribe* are rather "functional", as the developer, who implemented the entire source code alone, had other priorities). But to get to that point requires a considerable amount of time, and a prospective user of the system must be ready to invest that time. It is hoped that the more successful users and/or test participants there are, the easier it will be to convince other new users to give it a try.

Being able to develop one's own assistive technology is a curse and a gift at the same time. Needing to use the technology is definitely a curse, but having the opportunity to initiate and foster the development of something new that can help others as well, is a valuable gift.

5 All's Well that Ends Well (Well, Almost …)

This chapter talked about the development of *OnScreenDualScribe*, a very powerful tool to replace the standard input devices for computer operation – full-size keyboard and mouse – with a single number pad-like device, the *DualPad*, which is held in both hands, and operated with the thumbs only. The left and right edges of the input device (an off-the-shelf numeric keypad, rotated by 90 degrees, counterclockwise) serve as a guide, empowering the user to control the device with maximum confidence and reliability.

The software has been developed by and for the first author who has Friedreich's Ataxia (FA). He is able to employ both hands, but, due to unsteady movements has considerable problems moving from key to key on a regular full-size keyboard. Since his speech is subject to dysarthria, he is unable to compensate his problems with the help of speech recognition. A pathological nystagmus, a secondary symptom of FA, keeps him from using eye tracking. Other known alternatives, such as scanning-based ones which only require a single switch activation at certain times, do not make full use of his abilities. So, he always had to decide between either using a slow alternative or investing the effort demanded by the standard keyboard.

Until about three years ago, the first author mainly used the standard method for computer operation, but then, he decided to devise a new, efficient, helpful and viable computer interaction solution, considering the specific symptoms induced by his disease. Initially serving as his own test subject, he switched to the new input method, meaning that he uses almost nothing else to operate his computer (which consequently also applies to the authoring of this chapter).

It really changed his life. For example, he never liked writing emails as that was just "effortful work" for him – now he does, since the new method almost completely takes away the effort without decreasing the entry rate for composing an email. Quite the contrary: with about 6 wpm, he now is even faster than he was ten years ago (despite the progression of his disease).

For the future, the goal is to make the tool available to as many people as possible, especially users with similar symptomatologies as the first author. The next addition will be a point-and-click interface, allowing users to operate the system – instead of employing the *DualPad* – with a pointing device or a mouse replacement (e.g., Biswas and Langdon 2013) by clicking on the buttons of the onscreen avatar. The purpose of devising this pointing-based interface – which naturally represents a compact onscreen keyboard, incorporating all other advantages of *OnScreenDualScribe* – is to further expand the circle of prospective end users.

Acknowledgements

This work is supported by DFG grant FE 936/6-2 "EFFENDI – EFficient and Fast text ENtry for persons with motor Disabilities of neuromuscular origin".

References

Betke M, Gips J, Fleming P (2002) The camera mouse: Visual tracking of body features to provide computer access for people with severe disabilities. IEEE Transactions on Neural Systems and Rehabilitation Engineering 10(1): 1-10

Biswas P, Langdon P (2013) A new interaction technique involving eye gaze tracker and scanning system. In: Proceedings of ETSA'13, pp 67-70, ACM, New York, NY, USA

Felzer T, MacKenzie IS, Rinderknecht S (2014) Efficient computer operation for users with a neuromuscular disease with OnScreenDualScribe. Journal of Interaction Science 2:2. Available at: www.journalofinteractionscience.com/content/2/1/2 (Accessed in November 2015)

Felzer T, Nordmann R (2006a) Alternative text entry using different input methods. In: Proceedings of ASSETS 2006, pp 10-17, ACM, New York, NY, USA

Felzer T, Nordmann R (2006b) Speeding up hands-free text entry. In: Proceedings of CWUAAT'06, Fitzwilliam College, Cambridge, UK, pp 27-36, Cambridge Engineering Design Centre, Cambridge, UK

Felzer T, Nordmann R, Rinderknecht S (2009) Scanning-based human-computer interaction using intentional muscle contractions. In: Proceedings of HCI International 2009, LNCS 5615, pp 509-518. Springer, Heidelberg, Germany

Hamidi F, Baljko M, Livingston N, Spalteholz L (2010) CanSpeak: A customizable speech interface for people with dysarthric speech. In: Proceedings of ICCHP 2010, Vienna, Austria, pp 605-612, Springer, Heidelberg, Germany

Koester HH, Levine SP (1994) Modeling the speed of text entry with a word prediction interface. IEEE Transactions on Rehabilitation Engineering 2(3): 177-187

Lecky BRF (1999) Neuromuscular disorders: Clinical and molecular genetics. Brain, 122(4): 1-790

MacKenzie IS (2002) KSPC (keystrokes per character) as a characteristic of text entry techniques. In: Proceedings of Mobile HCI 2002, Pisa, Italy, pp. 195-210, Springer, Heidelberg, Germany

MacKenzie IS, Felzer T (2010) SAK: Scanning ambiguous keyboard for efficient one-key text entry. ACM Transactions on Computer-Human Interaction (TOCHI) 17(3): 11:1-11:39

Simpson RC, Koester HH (1999) Adaptive one-switch row-column scanning. IEEE Transactions on Rehabilitation Engineering 7(4): 464-473

Sporka AJ, Felzer T, Kurniawan SH, Poláček O, Haiduk P, MacKenzie IS (2011) Chanti: Predictive text entry using non-verbal vocal input. In: Proceedings of CHI 2011, Vancouver, BC, Canada, pp. 2463-2472, ACM, New York, NY, USA

Ward DJ, Blackwell AF, MacKay DJC (2000) Dasher – A data entry interface using continuous gestures and language models. In: Proceedings of UIST 2000, San Diego, CA, USA, pp. 129-137, ACM, New York, NY, USA

Watts R, Robinson P (1999) Controlling computers by whistling. In: Proceedings of Eurographics UK, Cambridge, UK

Designing Human Somatosensory System Interactions: Not Just for Haptics Any More!

M. Karam and P. M. Langdon

Abstract: We present an elaboration and application of a proposed framework highlighting the somatosensory system in our understanding of the design and development of computer interactions for the human body. The Somatosensory system encompasses the entire range of sensations, organisms, and mechanisms relating to the human sense of touch, and this framework is intended to serve as a tool for broadening our understanding of the multidisciplinary aspects that influence all interactions designed for the body. The framework illustrates a preliminary approach to organizing all touch-based systems into four categories of critical parameters that can enable the effective comparison of different technologies and systems applications, and approaches to human somatosensory system interactions (HSI). In this paper, the framework is applied to evaluate and compare four speech-to-touch (ST) systems towards informing the design of a novel system that uses tactile-acoustic devices to improve speech comprehension.

1 Introduction

We present a proposed framework developed to support research in human somatosensory system interactions (HSI) (Karam and Langdon 2015). This work further expands on proposed IEEE standards for haptic and tactile interactions (van Erp et al. 2010). This paper illustrates the HSI perspective through an evaluation and comparison of speech to touch (ST) display interactions. Using the framework, we classify ST displays to reveal critical parameters and their factors as a means describing and comparing interface across different applications, technologies, user experiences, and body site. The framework further aims to model and link research areas associated with physical interactions, offering new perspectives that consider the somatosensory system as crucial for the design of effective interactions that leverage the complex sensory capabilities of the body. This approach promotes the development and use of technology for our highly underused sense of touch, towards increasing the information bandwidth that can be effectively utilized for people with and without sensory, cognitive, or physical impairments.

M. Karam (✉)
Kings College London, London, UK
email: mkaram@tadsinc.com

P. M. Langdon
Cambridge Engineering Design Centre, University of Cambridge, Cambridge, UK

P. Langdon et al. (eds.), *Designing Around People*,
DOI 10.1007/978-3-319-29498-8_19

2 Background

The somatosensory system is a complex network of neural mechanisms, cognitive processes, and responses that are interconnected and relevant to all of human physical perceptions (Gault 1927). The myriad qualities, quantities, and connectedness of sensations known to be associated with the somatosensory system are critical factors to consider when designing displays for the body. People with sensory capability limitations can leverage this complex information processing system as a substitution, or augmentation to visual or auditory displays, in the same way fully sighted and hearing people can use the body to solve some of the problems of cognitive overloading of information.

Buzzers, vibrators, and motors are commonly used in haptic sensory substitution systems, but may be vastly underutilizing the human capacity to 'feel' by compressing, digitizing, and indirectly mapping sensory information to the body as signals, rather than exploring the natural mappings that may exist between the senses. The often 'one size fits all' approach to representing sensory information as patterns of haptic vibrations is clearly effective at communicating signals to the body. But this places additional cognitive load on the user, who must learn to identify and map signals to their associated meanings before it can be effectively understood. An alternative approach could leverage the multi-sensory nature of the somatosensory system and develop full body interactions to improve information access for people with and without sensory, cognitive, or physical impairments.

This paper demonstrates one instance of using the framework to compare four ST systems, towards informing design decisions on the development of a novel tactile-acoustic device aimed at enhancing speech comprehension for mobile phone interactions in noisy environments. Competing technologies are compared along the framework categories, focusing on the following critical parameters: interactions (application goals and constraints), technology (software, hardware), physiology (body site, form factors, receptors), and cognition (learning, perception and memory). The evaluation and analysis suggests potential hypotheses that can be tested in future experiments, towards better understanding the somatosensory system and the goal of improving the design of ST interactions.

2.1 Feeling Speech

One of the earliest recorded and effective speech-to-touch (ST) approaches is the Tadoma method, which demonstrates the inherent ability of the somatosensory system to detect and interpret the physical nature of speech (Reed et al. 1982). This is a haptic approach to speech sensory substitution, using both the cutaneous and kinesthetic receptors (cutaneous -> feeling vocal chord vibrations, kinesthetic -> feeling lips move while speaking) to support deaf-blind people in feeling speech.

This phenomenon informed the development of several devices that could aid in translation of speech to the body. The Teletactor (Popular Mechanics Magazine 1929). Developed by Bell Labs and Dr. Gault (Fig. 1, left) was shown to be effective at translating speech into tactile signals by presenting sounds from a telephone earpiece directly to the thumb and forefinger of a user. Tests showed that people who held the earpiece were able to feel sounds and recognize some elements of speech and of the voice by targeting the highly sensitive cutaneous receptors of the hand. This HSI approach leverages the innate similarities between the hearing senses, and the sense of touch. This phenomenon was further validated by Von Bekesy, whose work on modeling the human cochlea contributed to our understanding of hearing, and its relation to the skin. This is currently the dominant model used in ST interfaces (Fig. 1, right).

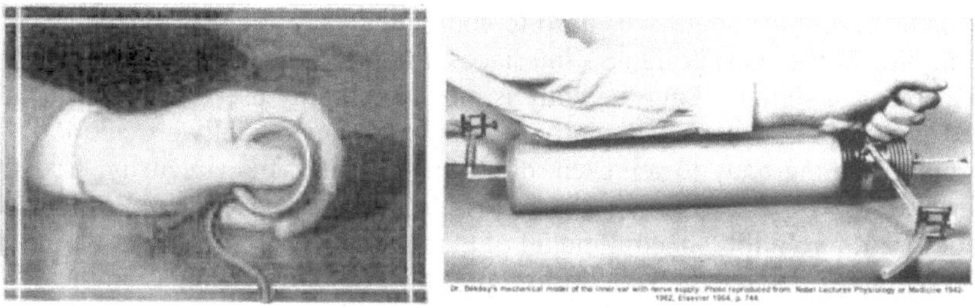

Fig. 1 Left: Teletactor - speaker device from an early telephone used for feeling speech. Right (Popular Mechanics Magazine 1929): Bekesy's inner ear model of sound waves travelling through liquid.

Further developments in this field led to different approaches to creating ST interfaces, using the more intense and targeted haptic receptors in the body. The tactile Vocoder uses both cutaneous sensors and bone conduction to convert sounds into 16 channels of low frequency or electrotactile signals. This uses an indirect mapping of frequency bands of sound as activation signals for the motors or vibrators to represent the bands of frequencies activated through speech sounds (Brooks and Frost 1983). This layout and distribution of signals leverages similar features as the human cochlea, and is referred to as the Spectral model of sound distribution (Reed et al. 1982). A linear arrangement of transducers represent the activation of sounds within the frequency range assigned to each channel, leveraging skin, bone, and muscle activation as a means of increasing the potential resolution available to emulate the distribution of sounds across the body, maintaining the relative activation of sounds that mimic the detection of sound waves through the cochlea.

3 Sound Systems for the Body

ST systems are one form of sensory substation that is essentially a sound system for the body. Physical devices used to support ST interactions come in many form factors, intensities, sizes, and sensations. This variation in technologies combined with the different sensitivities of body sites can influence our choice of device, given the physical effects we are specifically aiming to create. Understanding the effects of varying settings on devices is also essential in creating an effective HSI system that will maximize the full range of tactile receptors in the body.

Factors influencing how the user experiences the sensations of any device include signal intensity, signal distribution, device arrangement, layout, signal processing, signal source, and must additionally consider the physiological and cognitive effects they produce. For example, a voice coil can produce cutaneous, or haptic sensations depending on the intensity and nature of the signal it displays on the body: high-pitched tones (800Hz) at low intensity (10db) will barely stimulate the cutaneous receptors, while low frequency tones (100Hz) at high amplitude (80db) will lead to bone conduction, and deep tissue stimulation of the kinesthetic system, supporting haptic perceptions.

Spatial layout of the devices used to communicate to the skin is also critical in determining how to best design ST interfaces: the spectral model, based on the linear arrangement of signals along the body is most commonly used for ST applications (Reed et al. 1982), while the alternative grid layout can potentially provide additional information to the body to represent other features of sound (intensity, frequency, timing, etc.) (Wall and Brewster 2006, Novich and Eagleman 2015). While the grid layout departs from the Spectral model of mapping sound to the body, it affords the presentation of spatial data, which can support the display of images on the body as well as other information (Bach-Y-Rita et al. 1969). However, for sound translations, the grid approach may not be as natural as the spectral model in conveying the inherent relationships between sound and touch in ST applications, as mappings must be learned and memorized so that users can identify speech as vibrations patterned in grid formation.

Signal distribution, signal source, and signal processing models are equally critical in designing effective ST systems. Sounds may be separated and converted into motorized or electrotactile signals (Brooks and Frost 1983, Gemperle et al. 2001, Wall and Brewster 2006) or amplified to create sound vibrations on the body (Salminen et al. 2012), providing very different user experiences. While many approaches have shown some success in mapping word elements to vibrations (Gault 1927, Brooks and Frost 1983), there are other techniques that may offer improved information by better leveraging the body's ability to detect natural vibrations within the audible spectrum frequencies that make up sound.

3.1 Tactile-acoustic Devices

In 2007, the Model Human Cochlea (MHC) was developed to explore the potential of communicating music from movies to deaf and hard of hearing people (Karam and Fels 2008). Leveraging the similarities between the skin and the cochlea, the MHC represents a new model for translating sound into vibrations, using actual sounds in a manner analogous to the human cochlea. The MHC represents a model of sensory substitution that uses the full range of audible frequencies of sound to convey speech, music, noise, or other sensations to the body. The MHC is effectively a Spectral model that uses actual sound signals on the body (direct mapping), rather than using the frequency bands as activation codes for motors of vibrators (indirect mapping). We refer to tactile devices that support the display of the full range of audible frequencies on the body as tactile-acoustic devices (TADs). TADs enable sound signals to be directly mapped to the body, leveraging the naturally tactile nature of sound waves, and can be configured to map sounds onto different locations on the body. While both approaches show potential in ST applications, using the direct mapping of sound onto TADs have many advantages, not least of which is the inclusion of all sound signals, containing both specific (consonants, vowels, phonemes), and abstract qualities of speech including emotion, prosody, and voice characteristics (Nanayakkara et al. 2009, Ammirante et al. 2013).

3.2 Designing TADs for Mobile Phones

We are evaluating a new approach to designing a MHC for mobile phones and extending the concepts and methods from the original 4-channel MHC used in the Emoti-Chair (Karam and Fels 2008). An initial prototype was developed to explore the potential of adapting the original TAD system for a hand-held form factor (Figure 2). Mobile TAD system processes audio signals from the headphone jack, and separates the frequencies into 4-channels. These are directly mapped onto 4 TAD transducers, supporting thumb and forefinger access to the signals, drawing on the Teletactor interaction. Preliminary trials suggested that users could quickly detect voices, and emotional content presented in a five-minute sound bite from a radio talk show, featuring a male host and an angry female caller engaging in a heated debate. The four participants each correctly reported the sex of the speaker, and the intense emotion expressed through the vibrations. We decided to further explore other techniques to better validate our design.

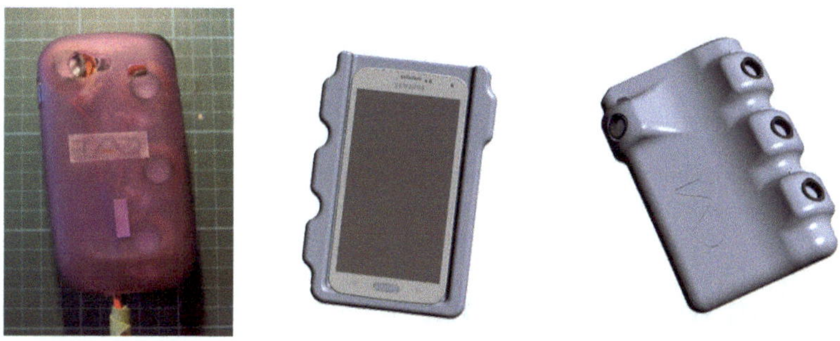

Fig. 2 The first TAD-mobile prototype (left, middle) and proposed new design (right)

4 Evaluating Speech-touch (ST) Interfaces

Using the framework, four systems are categorized and compared to inform and validate the design of the mobile-TAD device described in the previous section. Evaluation result and technical details of each system is organized across four critical parameters and factorized to reflect relevant characteristics of each system. Critical parameters and factors used in this work are presented in Fig. 3. The categories from Reed's review of tactile speech systems (Reed et al. 1982) are used to inform the selection of factors in the framework, based on system descriptions and experimental outcomes. The complexity of the somatosensory system and its mechanisms have motivated a qualitative approach to evaluating ST devices, which will consider each of the critical parameters and their relationship in different systems to support conceptual reconfigurations, physical relocations, and technology modifications in the design of new ST devices for mobile phones.

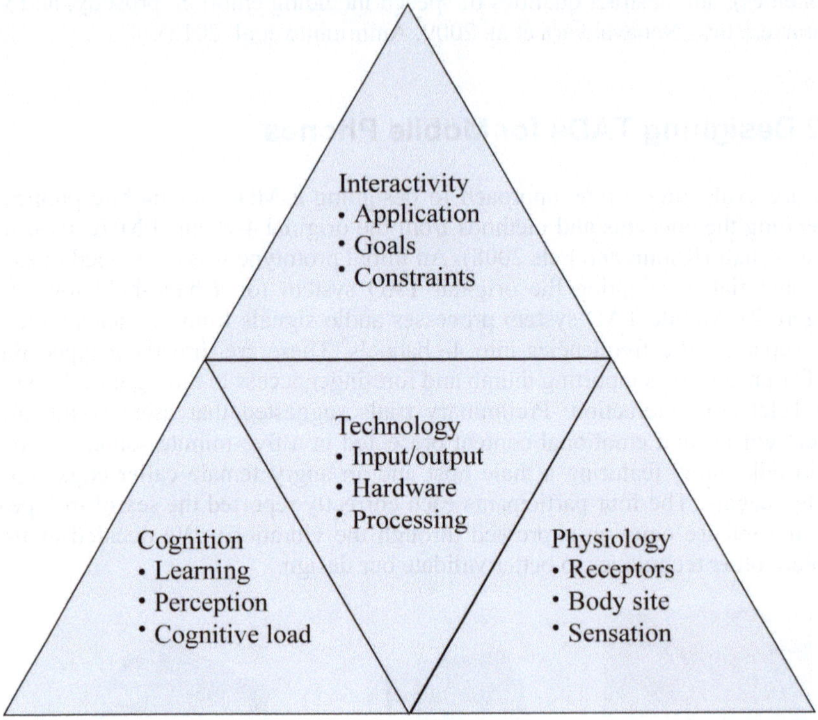

Fig. 3 Four critical parameters used as hierarchical categories with suggested factors relating to somatosensory interactions

5 Applying the Framework

To apply the framework, we organize device details and study results from four ST systems along the critical parameters, identifying several factors for each that are relevant to the translation of speech to touch. Results from past research are used to factorize the parameters to support cross-evaluation of the systems and exposing the HSI perspective. The four systems are: 16-channel Vocoder for the forearm, 1-channel Teletactor for the fingers (T1), a 2-channel Emoti-Chair for the back (T2), and a 4-channel TAD for the hand (T4). Each system is organized according to the framework, shown in Table 1 and Table 2. By comparing the factors across the different parameters, we reveal insights into the design of ST systems leading to hypotheses we can formulate by examining and codifying the data from the four systems.

Table 1 Research organized according to the framework, with some factors relating to speech sensory substitution filled in for the comparison and evaluation

Experiment	Goal	Approach	Constraints	Input	Processing	Output
MHC (Russo et al, 2013)	Speech Recognition - voice qualities	Substitition - users deafened - voice identification	Lab - prototype system	Recorded speech utterances from male/female speakers	Stereo - original signal amplified, direct.	Tactile-audio signals amplified - 2 channels
Vocoder (Frost, 1983)	Speech Recognition - words	Substitution - users deafened - word identification	Lab - commercial system	Live speech through microphone	Linear - sound split and processed as 100Hz signals	Solonoid activation and amplitude signal - 16 channels
Teletactor (Gault, 1923)	Speech Recognition - words	Augmentation - with lip reading/ hearing - word identification	Lab - Lip Reading + commercial system?	Live speech through microphone	Mono - Sound as vibration, amplified signal direct	Tactile-audio signals, amplified, 1 channel
TAD (2015) Pilot	Speech Recognition - voice qualities	Augmentation /residual sounds audible - voice, emotion detection	Public usability - prototype system	Recorded speech - talkshow, male/female speakers conversing	Quad - Sound as vibration, frequency split into 4 channels	Tactile-audio signals amplified, 4 channels

Table 2 Continued from Table 1

	Technology: Hardware		Physiology			Cognition	
Experiment	Contactors	Distribution	Body Site	Form factor	Targeted Receptors	Sensation	Recorded Effects
MHC (Russo et al, 2013)	Sound transducers 1 x 1 lower back lateral	Horizontal (stereo)	Lower back, equdistant between spine on left/right	Embedded into seat	Cutaneous - Pacinian. Tactile-audio	Subtle vibrations Feels like sound - bi-spinal signal	Word utterances & and voice matching
Vocoder (Frost, 1983)	Motor: Solonoids 100Hz range	Spectral (Linear) 16 channels	ventral median forearm	Plexiglass mount with arm resting atop	Haptic: Cutaneous & Bone conduction, muscle tissue	Buzzing motor at 100Hz Arm. Sounds like robotic speech.	Vowel & consonant recognition learning
Teletactor (Gault, 1923)	Sound transducer, single, finger, thumb	Mono	Hands - between thumb and forefinger	Held in hand, circular form, telephone speaker	Cutaneous - pacinian corpuscles - Tactile-audio	Actual sound through a single speaker/transducerAudible as sound	Vowels, consonant recognition learning
TAD (2015) Pilot	Sound Transducers, Quad, inner hand	Spectral (Linear) 4 channels	Hands - inner fingers, palm	Mobile phone case with transducer array embedded.	Cutaneous - pacinian corpuscles - Tactile-audio	Sound as vibrations 4 distinct signals Audible as sound	Emotion, context, voice detection

6 Analysis and Comparison

A general review of the systems within the framework organization can reveals important insights that can be used to better understand the strengths and weaknesses of each device in a given configuration or application. The critical parameters and their factors are discussed, towards the formulation of hypotheses that reflect insights into relationships as revealed through the framework.

6.1 Interaction Scenario

Each of the systems can deliver some element of speech to the body, as indicated by the results of the experiments. The Vocoder and the Teletactor were both effective at communicating speech elements, while the TAD and Emoti-Chair were effective at expressing voice qualities, and potential speech identification effects.

The Emoti-Chair and the Vocoder experiments used a sensory substitution approach and deafened participants for experiments, while the Teletactor and the TAD leveraged the low-sound output of the tactile-audio signals for sensory-augmentation. Observing that the single-channel Teletactor for the hand (T1) performed almost as well on the hand as the 16-channel Vocoder did on the arm, while the Emoti-Chair (T2) was effective at supporting the identification of speech elements to the back, we present our first hypothesis, which states that different application domains can reconfigure and rearrange ST systems to best support the user in achieving effective interactions given the specific interaction scenario (H1).

6.2 Technology

Two different signal mappings are used to display sound information to the body in the systems we compared (direct and indirect). Direct mappings process sound information into distinct frequency bands, which are amplified and used to directly drive a tactile-acoustic device (MHC). Indirect mappings similarly process sound into frequency bands, but the signal is used as triggers to activate corresponding motors or vibration devices used in the Spectral model approach. However, because sound includes all the components of speech that we can hear, the potential to access and extract relevant information chosen to represent speech to the body is built into the signal itself. To this end, our second hypothesis claims that the MHC approach is better for supporting ST tasks than haptic devices when using the same number of channels and frequency distributions (H2).

Signal intensity levels of TADs can also be increased, which can turn cutaneous stimulation into haptic sensations. For example, tactile-acoustic devices at low intensities will lightly stimulate the cutaneous receptors, while that same signal at a high intensity could be strong enough to produce kinesthetic sensations (bone conduction, deep tissue, etc.). This suggests another hypothesis, highlighting the advantages of using TADs over vibration motors or electrotactile devices for their ability to produce a wider range of sensations. (H3).

Physiology: The comparison of the four systems suggest that even without training, using a single tactile-acoustic channel, users can detect speech sounds almost as well as they can using the 16-channel Vocoder. This may be due to the higher sensitivity level of the hand (glabrous skin), and the complexity of signals that can be communicated through tactile-acoustic devices. Thus, while the hands represent the most sensitive location for cutaneous detection of sound (Pacinian corpuscles), it may be possible to achieve improved signal detection by moving the display to more sensitive areas of the body (H4).

Cognition: Haptic devices often require more earning and cognitive processing to identify, recognize, and memorize the vibration patterns that indirectly map speech onto the display channels. Recognition of speech elements requires significant training (Vocoder and Teletactor), while emotion and voice quality appear to be more intuitive (Mobile-TAD, Emoti-Chair). Emotion was not tested for the Vocoder, but we hypothesize that the abstract qualities of speech and sound (emotion, prosody, and voice qualities) will require more complex mappings of haptic signals than with the direct mappings used in TADs (H5). Finally, the single-transducer Teletactor suggests that even with only one TAD channel, it is possible to achieve similar word recognition rates as the 16-channel haptic Vocoder, suggesting that fewer tactile-audio channels can be used to deliver richer, intuitive information to the body than multi-channel haptic devices can offer (H6).

7 Conclusions

Observing four different ST systems through the lens of the HSI framework, we propose six hypotheses that can be evaluated and confirmed in upcoming studies to determine more effective approaches to designing ST interfaces, and specifically for designing a Mobile-TAD for ST. Improved comprehension may be achieved by increasing the number of channels (haptic devices or tactile-acoustic devices) or by using the glabrous areas of the skin to increase signal detection thorough TADs. This information may help to design a better ST device that won't constrain the user to using their hand to access the tactile sound. This would support users in accessing speech enhancements even while operating their mobile phones using Bluetooth headsets, or other hands-free interfaces required for phone use while driving. Further application of the HSI framework reveals additional relationships that exist between the factors we chose to compare ST systems, based on understanding the sensitivities of the different body sites (glabrous, non-glabrous), the number of transducers that can be used in the display (channels), and method of converting sounds to signals (direct or indirect). Additional information may be gleaned from the framework by including other systems in the tables, and expanding our understanding of the different ST interfaces, but the current results will improve design decisions made on the next version of Mobile-TAD. Future work will add additional systems to the framework, and continue testing our hypotheses towards increasing our ability to design effective HSI for communicating speech to the sense of touch.

References

Ammirante P, Russo FA, Good A, Fels DI (2013) Feeling voices. PLoS ONE 8(1): e53585

Bach-Y-Rita P, Collins CC, Saunders FA, White B, Scadden L (1969) Vision substitution by tactile image projection. Nature 221(5184): 963-964

Brooks PL, Frost BJ (1983) Evaluation of a tactile vocoder for word recognition. The Journal of the Acoustical Society of America 74(1): 34-39

Gault RH (1927) "Hearing" through the sense organs of touch and vibration. Journal of the Franklin Institute 204(3): 329-358

Gemperle F, Ota N, Siewiorek D (2001) Design of a wearable tactile display. In: Proceedings of the 5th IEEE International Symposium on Wearable Computers, IEEE Computer Society Washington, DC, USA

Karam M, Fels DI (2008) Designing a model human cochlea: Issues and challenges in crossmodal audio-haptic displays. In: Proceedings of the 2008 Ambi-Sys Workshop on Haptic User Interfaces in Ambient Media Systems, ICST, Brussels, Belgium

Karam M, Langdon P (2015) Seeing, hearing and feeling through the body: The emerging science of human-somatosensory interactions. In: Proceedings of the 9th International Conference on Universal Access in Human-Computer Interaction held as Part of HCI International 2015, Los Angeles, CA, USA

Novich SD, Eagleman DM (2015) Using space and time to encode vibrotactile information: Toward an estimate of the skin's achievable throughput. Experimental Brain Research 233(10): 2777-2788

Popular Mechanics Magazine (1929) Hearing through your fingers. Popular Mechanics Magazine 51(5). Available at: books.google.ca/books?id=wN4DAAAAMBAJ&pg= PA755 &source=gbs_toc_r&cad=2#v=onepage&q&f=false (Accessed in November 2015)

Reed CM, Durlach NI, Braida LD (1982) Research on tactile communication of speech: A review. ASHA Monographs 20(1982): 1-23

Salminen K, Surakka V, Lylykangas J, Rantala J, Ahmaniemi T, Raisamo R et al. (2012) Tactile modulation of emotional speech samples. Advances in Human-Computer Interaction 2012 (2012): Article ID 741304

van Erp JBF, Kyung K-U, Kassner S, Carter J, Brewster S, Weber G et al. (2010) Setting the standards for haptic and tactile interactions: ISO's work. In: Kappers AML, van Erp JBF, Bergmann Tiest WM, van der Helm FCT (Eds.) Haptics: Generating and perceiving tangible sensations, Part II, pp. 353-358. Springer-Verlag Berlin Heidelberg, Germany

Wall S, Brewster S (2006) Feeling what you hear: Tactile feedback for navigation of audio graphs. In: Proceedings of the SIGCHI Conference on Human Factors in Computing Systems, pp. 1123-1132, ACM, New York, NY, USA

Part V

Designing Inclusive Architecture: Buildings and Spaces

Ageing Engagement: Improving the Elderly Experience in Kitchen

Y. Afacan

Abstract: Being the most used rooms in any home, the kitchen has evolved for decades in response to older users' inclusive interaction. Therefore, understanding how older users engage with kitchens helps designers address inclusion of the elderly by eliminating physical, social and cultural barriers. This study further elaborates previously developed inclusive kitchen design factors (Afacan and Demirkan 2010) by adapting the 'Design Wheel' model proposed by Clarkson et al. (2011) with a focus on observations of 40 Turkish older users' kitchen needs. By creating personas and answering the four fundamental questions of the model (1. What are the needs? 2. How can the needs be met? 3. How well are the needs met? 4. What should we do next?), it aimed to gain more insight into an elderly way of thinking and acting in relation to the inclusive kitchen design. Depending on the findings of task analyses and observation of the participants, three personas are created and the three need categories with a total of 10 kitchen need attributes are listed. A mock-up kitchen environment is also created and tested with reference to these needs.

1 Introduction

The ageing population is increasing rapidly all over the world and it is inevitable that we should accept that being an older user does not mean individuals' characteristics remain the same throughout their lifetime. Responding to the diversity of ageing and engaging with their needs has become a prominent part of inclusive design (Afacan 2008, Goddard and Nicolle 2012, Afacan 2013, Cassim and Dong 2015). Inclusive design strives to create living spaces for the elderly that are more comfortable and sustainable with a focus on independent self-care. Most of the elderly want to continue to live independently, and feeding oneself is an integral part of self sufficiency (Holt and Holt 2011). Being the most used room in any home, the kitchen has evolved for decades in response to older users' inclusive interaction. Therefore, understanding how older users engage in kitchens helps designers and architects address inclusion of the elderly by eliminating not only

Y. Afacan (✉)
Bilkent University, Ankara, Turkey
email: yasemine@bilkent.edu.tr

P. Langdon et al. (eds.), *Designing Around People*,
DOI 10.1007/978-3-319-29498-8_20

physical, but also social and cultural barriers as well. But there has been a critical gap between the desire to provide inclusive kitchens and the actual situation in natural living environments. As most of the elderly prefer to avoid institutional living it is not easy to renovate, re-design or re-transform their existing kitchen spaces into inclusive spaces.

This study further elaborates previously developed inclusive kitchen design factors (Afacan and Demirkam 2010) by adapting the 'Design Wheel' model proposed by Clarkson et al. (2011) with a focus on the observed 40 Turkish older user kitchen needs. By answering the four fundamental questions of the model (1.What are the needs? 2. How can the needs be met? How well are the needs met? 4. What should we do next?), it is aimed to gain more insight into an elderly way of thinking and acting in relation to the inclusive kitchen design. It should be noted that this study does not aim to provide information about well-known kitchen design standards or ergonomic requirements for the elderly needs, rather it highlights the significance of user involvement and implication of the wheel model in the Turkish culture context.

2 Inclusive Kitchen Design

The demand of creating an inclusive kitchen, which is a multi-parameter task, has been increased tremendously as the demographic patterns of societies have been changed all over the world (Afacan and Demirkan 2010). Unlike 50 years ago, today kitchens are not only used by women, but also by all family members as a social interaction space (Mullick and Levine 2001). Kitchens have also become technologically smart, using information and communication technologies to support meal planning and preparation and also social connectivity and enjoyment (Kerr et al. 2014). Assistive technologies in kitchens for the elderly include using robots to assist the cooking process with visual recipes (Sugiura et al. 2010); sensory cameras to remind the user of the next step in the recipe (Olivier et al. 2009); smart appliances to allow healthier, safer and more energy-efficient cooking (Luo et al. 2008); social navigation systems that allows online shopping, sharing of digital recipes (Lagomarsino 2007) and interactive kitchen counters combined with eye tracking systems (Bradbury et al. 2003). However, it was claimed that not enough attention has been paid to diverse user capabilities when concerning usability of those smart-kitchen designs (Kerr et al. 2014). Many of the elderly have visual difficulty in reading and understanding the information written on control panels. Also mobility impaired elderly or those with hand deformities find it difficult to grasp knobs (Mullick and Levine 2001).

All these above-mentioned changes in kitchen design force designers, researchers, industry professionals and firms to develop a number of different types of kitchen features that are defined as accessible, adaptable and universal. Although these kitchens provide inclusive solutions with various cabinets, fixtures, appliances and materials, many of the elderly do not want to live in accessible living spaces because of their clinical apearance, and "the clearances for the able bodied were considered as lost spaces, for example, using clearance under the counter instead of base cabinet storage space in the kitchen" (Demirkan 2007, p. 34). Thus, understanding elderly needs, capabilities and expectations requires a flexible approach based on successive cycles of exploration, creativity and evaluation (Clarkson et al. 2011).

3 Research Methodology

3.1 Sample

A total of 40 Turkish elderly users (25 female and 15 male, between ages 65-90 with a mean age of 74.3) participated in the study. Participants were chosen by a stratified sampling among user clusters in urban areas with the same income level in Ankara, Turkey. With reference to the inclusive user involvement techniques described in the inclusive design toolkit (Clarkson et al. 2011), to obtain useful and accurate feedback from the participants, five user clusters were identified: 1. Broad user mix: eight healthy elderly with normal musculoskeletal system with regard to age; 2. Boundary users: seven physically impaired elderly using prostheses (n = 4) and cane (n= 3) as mobility aids; 3. Extreme users: five visually impaired elderly with total loss of sight and five elderly with mild loss of sight and have difficulty to walk without an aid; 4. Mixed experience users: eight healthy elderly with different levels of experience with similar brand of appliances and cabinets; 5. Community groups: seven elderly users with mild loss of sight who share experience of interacting with similar brand of appliances and cabinets. These five types of users are vital to uncover incorrect assumptions that could be made when selecting all the participants from highly skilled or minimally able users (Clarkson and Keates 2003).

3.2 Procedure

The major focus of the study is to implement the 'Design Wheel model' with the previously developed six inclusive kitchen design factors: 1. Operation of appliance controls with low effort; 2. Appropriate counter heights and spaces; 3. Operation of appliance controls with clear information; 4. Adequate illumination; 5. Ease of reach to oven; 6. Ease of reach to base cabinets (Afacan and Demirkan 2010). Figure 1 illustrates how each activity of the wheel is integrated into these factors.

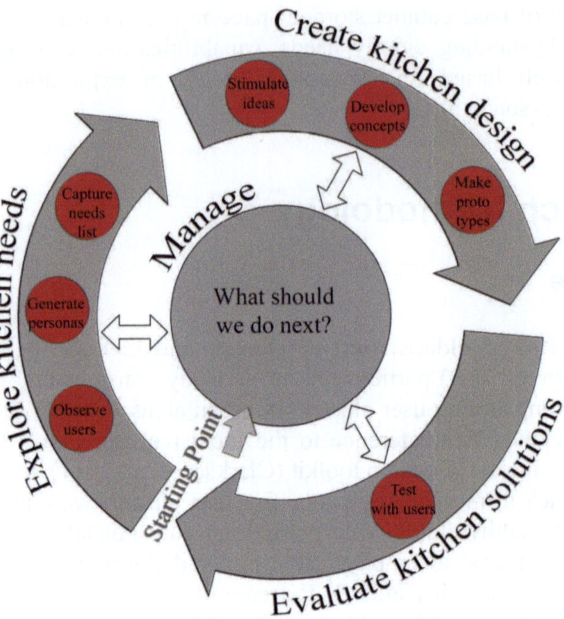

Fig. 1 'Design Wheel' model adapted from Clarkson et al. 2011

The first activity, 'explore', is conducted in the kitchen of each participant. Visits were arranged to suit participant's availability. Each participant was informed about the research, and task analyses have begun after giving informed consent. 40 participants were observed based on the five tasks corresponding to six factors over a three month period: T1. Operation of appliance controls (whether oven, fridge, cooktop and dishwasher controls require too much force or not); T2. Using the counter for cutting or preparing functions (whether it provides adequate clearance, inclusive access and reach; T3. Reading the information provided on each appliance control (whether they are easily readable and confusing or not); T4. Using the oven (whether it provides inclusive access and reach); T5. Using the below and above cabinets (whether they provide inclusive access and reach). The fourth factor 'adequate illumination' was observed based on the natural and artificial light comfort of each participant, i.e. her/his demand to open and close of a lighting fixture during these five tasks. Two researchers were present during the tasks. One researcher took notes and observed, while the other researcher conducted an unstructured interview about a task and then, watched the task be executed. Unstructured interviews were conducted individually after each task to gain data about what the users think about their own behaviour. Depending on the observation of the participants, three personas were created regarding each user type group that are mentioned in the previous section (Figure 2). Then, with reference to the three personas a total of 10 kitchen need attributes were listed. During the second activity called 'create', a mock-up kitchen counter was created with reference to the needs listed. In the third activity 'evaluation', the study focused on the user testing. A total of three representatives from each persona have been selected to use the mock-up kitchen counter with the same five tasks defined in the exploring activity. Because of the limitations of the study, only an oven is constructed and evaluated for the mock-up. The fourth activity called 'manage' is left as a further step of the study.

Guler, "healthy user"

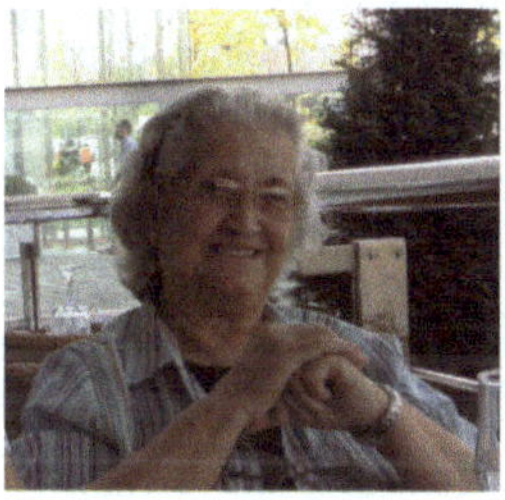

- 83 year old widow with two grown up children
- Relatively healthy
- Wears glasses
- Uses her kitchen actively
- Has a very active social life
- Enjoys cooking
- Cooks weekly for her children and grandchildren
- Has accessible kitchen cabinets
- Wants to have controls with less force and readable information
- Wants to use technology, such as meal planner

Gunseli, "user with a lack of acceptance"

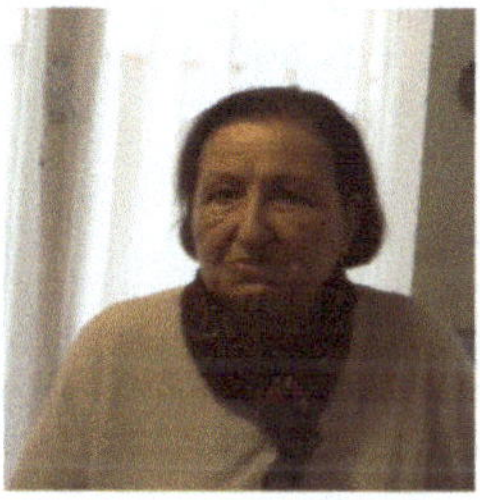

- 80 years, married with three grown up children
- Wears prostheses
- Uses her kitchen very happily despite her poor mobility and despite cooking tiring her
- Has inaccessible cabinets
- Her work top lacks adequate space and clearance
- Kitchen has little daylight and artificial lighting is required at all times
- She is satisfied with the existing kitchen and resist renovating it to become inclusive kitchen

Izzet, "extreme user "

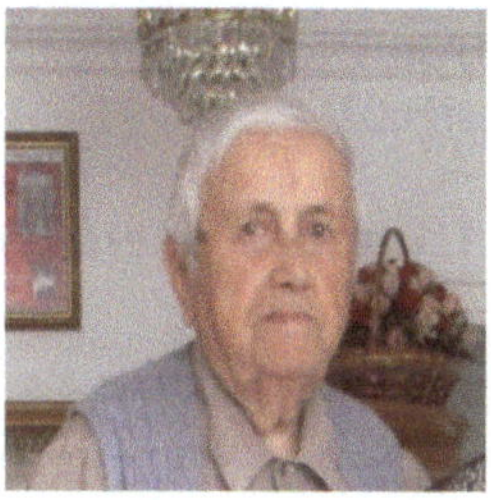

- 90 years, married with three grown up children
- Has an active social life
- Visually and physically impaired, which limits his kitchen usage
- Has difficulty in operating and reading all the appliance controls
- Has inaccessible cabinets and work top
- Wishes to have an usable kitchen with less force and readable information

Fig. 2 The three personas

4 The 'Design Wheel' Model

4.1 Explore: What Are the Needs?

The common finding while researchiung the elderly's needs is that they have a poor awareness of their own behaviour. Before doing each of the five tasks, all of the participants stated that they are capable of doing the task comfortably and were satisfied with their kitchen features. However, the majority of participants (37 of 40) struggled to articulate their needs and were unable to imagine what could be designed.

4.1.1 Active Users- Guler (83)

Active users are users that don't have any severe health problems. They have normal musculoskeletal and visual systems with regard to age. Since an active user uses her/his kitchen very actively, the counter heights and cabinets have been renovated according to easy and effective usage. Active users have accessible counters for cutting and preparing food so that the cabinets do not cause any physical strain and insure ease of access. Moreover, these users experience less difficulty because of specialized kitchen tools, such as rotating corner base cabinets and pull-out work surfaces. They are also capable of operating appliance controls. However, an active users find the simplicity issue more important. Operation should be simple and straightforward so that an untrained kitchen user can operate the controls and access the most important features of the controls easily. The ovens of active users are located at accessible heights to reduce reach distances and be comfortable. However, active users want to have temporary landing surfaces, such as rolling carts that act as a safe transfer for hot pot and pans. The following are some quotations obtained from their observation sessions: "I am happy to use my cabinets without deep bending" (User #5); "I have recently bought a cooktop, whose operation controls are coloured and simplified. I love using it" (User #11); and "I have diffuculty perfoming my everyday kitchen tasks because I need a temporary landing surface very often for cutting, removing hot pots and pans" (User #8).

4.1.2 Users with Lack of Acceptance- Gunseli (80)

Users with a lack of acceptance are the users, who have mobility impairments and share experience of interacting with similar brand of appliances and cabinets. Although they experience difficulty with food preparation, cooking and storing, they want to stay in their existing kitchens and do not want to renovate them into accessible kitchens for financial and social reasons. Generally, they have small kitchens with poor daylight and tasklighting. However, for an adequate indoor air quality both artificial light and daylight is essential to maximize legibility of essential information at working surfaces and reduce errors and hazards at cook-top. Because of their mobility impairments, sometimes they must sit while performing counter facilities. Therefore, appropriate counter spaces should be designed that remain within a safe distance without any accidents (Goldsmith 1997).

Although their ovens are located at accessible heights, because of insufficient kitchen space there is a lack of an appropriate counter space at least one side of the oven to manipulate hot pots and pans easily. This type of persona is very common in Turkey in every aspect of daily life and may be not be representative in other parts of the world. Rather than specialized/assistive/ inclusive housing environments, most of the older people today are aging in their own home environments with barriers where they lived in when they were younger (Afacan 2008). Below are some exemplary quotations from their observation session: "I know that I experience difficulties in reading text on oven and cooktop controls, but I do not want to buy any technologically new appliance. I found them strange" (User #1); "I am happy with my inaccessible kitchen counter. The counter height is too high for my comfortable usage, but I get used to using it from a seated position" (User #19), and "I am not able to access my above cabinets at all, but I am old and have not enough energy and money to renovate them" (User #12).

4.1.3 Passive Users- Izzet (92)

Passive users are the extreme users, who do not use their kitchens as active as the other two personas. Because of their mobility and visual impairments, they have difficulty to use the kitchen independently, but have an active social life with their relatives and friends. Unlike users with a lack of acceptance, they are willing to change their existing kitchens. Unlike the other two personas, they have difficulty reading and operateing the oven, cooktop, dishwasher and refrigerator controls. They want to use enhanced appliance controls with less force and legible information that is made appealing to all users and provides safe means of use regardless of user experience and knowledge. A passive user could not also use counters for food preparation, baking and cleaning up functions because of their uncomfortable and inaccessible counter heights and spaces that cause physical strain. They also want to reach to oven easily. For cabinets, a passive user wants to have alternative storage options to compensate for limited reach ranges and allow features to be used by both standing and seated users. Moreover, since their appliance controls did not provide any compatibility with a variety of techniques, such as color-contrasts, braille markings, large-print readouts, audible and tactile feedbacks, different than two personas, a passive user experiences more difficulty to read text on appliances to recognize warning features or know where and how the controls are set. Thus, they highlight the importance of adequate illumination levels and provision of helpful feedback from cook-top controls. They also prefer to have more task lighting options above and below cabinets: "I would like to be indepent and enjoy cooking as opposed to a limited kitchen usage" (User #27); and "I am open to new experiences. I would like to have an accesible kitchen, where I could cook comfortably and use all the appliances without any assistance" (User #3).

4.2 Create: How Can the Needs Be Met?

The personas and participants' responses to task analyses provide valuable inputs for the development of kitchen need attributes and a mock up kitchen counter.

Based on the requirements gathering and observation during these task analyses, it is possible to identify the three need categories with the following set of inclusive kitchen needs (Table1). Simplicity, comfort and safety are the key considerations to better inform the design decisions.

Table 1 The three need categories with the set of inclusive kitchen needs

I. Comfort	
1.	provide alternative storage options to compensate for limited reach ranges and allow features to be used by both standing and seated users;
2.	provide specialized kitchen tools, such as rotating corner base cabinets, pull-out work surfaces to improve quality of kitchen life;
3.	provide sitting choices while performing counter facilities;
4.	provide task lighting options above and below cabinets.
II. Simplicity	
5.	be simple and straightforward in appliance controls so that an untrained kitchen user can operate the controls;
6.	provide compatibility of appliance controls with a variety of techniques, such as color-contrasts, braille markings, large-print readouts, audible and tactile feedbacks;
7.	provide task lighting options above and below cabinets.
III. Safety	
8.	provide an adequate indoor air quality both artificial and daylighting for maximizing legibility of essential information at working surfaces and reducing errors and hazards at cook-top;
9.	provide temporary landing surfaces, such as rolling carts to act as a safe transfer for hot pot and pans;
10.	provide an appropriate counter space at least one side of the oven to manipulate hot pots and pans easily.

Depending on the above list, a mock-up kitchen counter with a knee space, a prototype oven and a rolling cart is constructed from a wooden material. The limitation of the mock-up is its material and lack of a sink. The main objective of this mock-up environment is to provide quick and simple testing environment compared to the expensive user trials. A total of 3 representatives from each persona used the mock-up kitchen counter with the same five tasks defined in the exploring activity, but in a different order to avoid any biases.

4.3 Evaluate: How Well Are the Needs Met?

The main objective of testing with the three personas is to evaluate how inclusively the participant can perform the tasks. The active user has performed all of the tasks effectively and stated that the inclusive features increased not only her usability, but also her satisfaction. The user with a lack of acceptance was more satisfied with the sitting option while performing counter facilities. The significant issue with this type of persona is that the mock-up environment provides insights into what design alternatives can be done and how they affect the user performance. Although this persona did not identify the need of legibility at controls, she found the legibility issue at controls very effective. In that sense, this mock-up environment is also significant in terms of observing the actual needs of users, if they have a poor awareness of their own behaviour. The passive user was very satisfied to be able to use the features of a kitchen environment independently. He effectively performed all the five tasks at a seated position. While performing the tasks in the mock-up environment, regardless the ability the three personas highlighted commonly the importance of rounded corners and using contrast colours in the floor and counter material. So, the mock-up environment is important to uncover hidden requirements as well.

5 Conclusions

Better solutions could be developed if real users and business needs could meet with stronger evidences of user involvement techniques. To overcome the challenges of inclusive kitchen, this study adapted the 'Design Wheel' model which is composed of successive improvement cycles of understanding the true diversity-exploration, applying the knowledge-creativity and evaluating the rough prototypes-evaluation. The personas assisted to identify need areas and holistic insights. Although the identified three need categories have been already known and stated in the literature previously by other studies, the personas help focus on who is the target user and how it could be further elaborated within the successive improvement cycles of the 'Design Wheel' model in the Turkish context. Getting the right needs with the right design decisions are vital to reach a wider market, increase user satisfaction and engage the ageing population (Heylighen and Bianchin 2013). In that sense, this study focused on a goal directed research through the model and personas to better concentrate on elderly needs and generate empathy for their experienced difficulties. As a future study, a full mock-up kitchen could be designed with real materials and all the prototypes of the appliances.

References

Afacan Y (2008) Designing for an aging population: Residential preferences of the Turkish elderly to age in place. In: Langdon P, Clarkson PJ, Robinson P (Eds.) Designing inclusive futures, pp. 241-252. Springer, London, UK

Afacan Y (2013) Elderly-friendly inclusive urban environments: Learning from Ankara. Open House International 38: 52-62

Afacan Y, Demirkan H (2010) A priority-based approach for satisfying the diverse users' needs, capabilities and expectations: A universal kitchen design case. Journal of Engineering Design 2: 315–343

Bradbury JS, Shell JS, Knowles CB (2003) Hands on cooking: Towards an attentive kitchen. In: Proceedings of the ACM CHI 2003 Human Factors in Computing Systems Conference, Ft. Lauderdale, FL, USA

Cassim J, Dong H (2015) Interdisciplinary engagement with inclusive design and the challenge workshops model. Applied Ergonomics 46: 292-296

Clarkson PJ, Coleman R, Hosking I, Waller SD (2011) Inclusive design toolkit, 2nd ed. Available at: www.inclusivedesigntoolkit.com (Accessed in May 2015)

Clarkson PJ, Keates S (2003) Investigating the inclusivity of digital television set top box receivers. In: Digital television for all. DTI, London. Appendix E. Available at: www.digitaltelevision.gov.uk (Accessed in May 2015)

Clarkson PJ, Waller SD, Cardoso C (2015) Approaches to estimating user exclusion. Applied Ergonomics 46: 304-310

Demirkan H (2007) Housing for the aging population. European Review of Aging and Physical Activity 4: 33-38

Goddard N, Nicolle C (2012) What is good design in the eyes of older users? In: Langdon P, Clarkson PJ, Robinson P, Lazar J and Heylighen A (Eds.) Designing inclusive systems, pp. 175-183. Springer- Verlag, London, UK

Goldsmith S (1997) Designing for the disabled the new paradigm. The New Paradigm, Oxford: ArchitecturalPress

Heylighen A, Bianchin M (2013) How does inclusive design relate to good design? Designing as a deliberative enterprise. Design Studies 34: 93-110

Holt RC, Holt RJ (2011) Gerontechnology: Kitchen aids. European Geriatric Medicine 2: 256-262

Kerr SJ, Tan O, Chua CJ (2014) Cooking personas: Goal-directed design requirements in the kitchen. International Journal of Human-Computer Studies 72: 255-274

Lagomarsino A (2007) Kitchen album: Concept based on progressive user research. In: Proceedings of the 2007 Conference on Designing Pleasurable Products and Interfaces, pp.423-428, Helsinki, Finland

Luo S, Xia H, Gao Y, Jin JS, Athauda R (2008) Smart fridges with multimedia capability for better nutrition and health. In: Proceedings of the International Symposium on Ubiquitous Multimedia Computing, pp. 39–44, Hobart, Australia

Mullick A, Levine D (2001) Universal kitchens and appliances. In: Preiser FEW, Ostroff E (Eds.) Universal design handbook, pp. 41.1-41.18. McGraw-Hill, New York, NY, USA

Olivier P, Xu G, Monk A, Hoey J (2009) Ambient kitchen: Designing situated services using a high fidelity prototyping environment. In: Proceedings of the 2nd International Conference on Pervasive Technologies Related to Assistive Environments, pp. 47, ACM Press, New York, NY, USA

Sugiura Y, Sakamoto D, Withana A, Inami M, Igarashi T (2010) Cooking with robots: Designing a house hold system working in open environments. In: Proceedings of the ACM CHI 2010 Human Factors in Computing Systems Conference, pp.2427–2430, Atlanta, GA, USA

How Do Older Residents Experience a Recently Built Innovative Housing and Care Facility?

K. Coomans, P.-W. Vermeersch and A. Heylighen

Abstract: Housing for older people in Flanders evolves toward small-scale, homelike environments. As population ageing puts pressure on the affordability of this tendency, architects are challenged to design innovative living schemes that offer the advantages of smale-scaleness in an affordable way. Little is known, however, about how people use and experience these schemes. Therefore we analyse how a recently built innovative housing and care facility is experienced by its residents. Analysis of interviews and guided tours suggests that the contemporary architecture is not criticised, but that its materialisation should offer a more homelike atmosphere. The generic layout is experienced as highly confusing and should offer more differentiation. The study confirms the importance of furnishing a place in making it "your own", and shows how architects can facilitate this. While the design incorporates qualities of small-scale, homelike living schemes for people with dementia, the facility lacks some of the underlying ideals. It is therefore unclear whether the intended benefits for people with dementia are still present in this specific set-up. Together the findings illustrate the importance of follow-up studies since architects might take such an innovative concept as an example without knowing its actual benefits and deficiencies. They also highlight the added value of qualitative case studies for such unique housing and care projects.

1 Introduction

In Flanders, housing and care for older people is evolving toward small-scale, homelike environments with more attention for residents' quality of life (Verbeek et al. 2009). At the same time, population ageing (and silvering) puts pressure on the affordability of this tendency (Coomans et al. 2011). Architects are therefore challenged to design innovative living schemes that allow offering the advantages of small-scaleness in an affordable way.

K. Coomans · P.-W. Vermeersch · A. Heylighen (✉)
KU Leuven, Department of Architecture, Research[x]Design, Belgium
email: ann.heylighen@kuleuven.be

K. Coomans
D E architecten, Belgium

P.-W. Vermeersch, (Full) Scale architecten, Belgium

P. Langdon et al. (eds.), *Designing Around People*,
DOI 10.1007/978-3-319-29498-8_21

In designing such schemes, architects typically interact directly with the client (management), while future users (residents, staff, visitors) remain absent or hypothetic. Architects thus conceive of buildings with the aim of offering users a specific experience, without having direct knowledge of their motivation, values, or prior experiences. How people eventually use and experience the buildings may correspond to, but also significantly differ from architects' design intentions (Barnes et al. 2002, Crilly et al. 2008).

As currently no obligation exists to compare architects' intentions with users' actual experience, unexpected effects are not systematically fed back into the value chain. This lack of consistent learning mechanisms in architecture is becoming increasingly problematic in the context described above. In an attempt to contribute to more systematic learning, this paper investigates how a recently built, innovative housing and care facility is experienced by its primary users, i.e. its residents.

2 Context

The evolution toward small-scale, homelike environments in housing and care for older people originates in dementia care (Verbeek et al. 2009). In this context, small-scale, homelike or so-called "normalized" living refers to a small group of people who live together like a household or family (Van Audenhove et al. 2003). The group's size is subject to discussion: pioneers of small-scale living mention six people (who can sit and eat at one table, like in a household), others expand it to even 17 or 18 (Wijnties 2003, Declercq et al. 2007). The Dutch Trimbos Institute formulated six imperatives of small-scale living (Boekhorst et al. 2007): (1) a resident remains a resident for good or ill; (2) an ordinary household is run; (3) the resident directs the set-up of his/her daily life; (4) the staff is part of the household; (5) residents form together a group; (6) a small-scale living scheme occurs in an archetypical house. As these imperatives are arranged in order of importance, one might conclude that keeping the group's size limited is important since running an ordinary household becomes difficult otherwise. Less importance seems to be attached to the housing environment, leaving the possibility for novel schemes.

Such a scheme was designed for the housing and care facility studied here, referred to as Fairfield Home. The concept evolved from designing a large scale facility, as described in the brief dating from 1998, over incorporating qualities of small-scale living, to balancing both because of budgetary concerns. The final building, which was completed in 2012, ended up as an innovative in-between solution. It consists of four compact six-story buildings at the edge of a town centre, conceived by the architects as four towers amid greenery, connected at the basis by a dug-in public service centre and cafeteria (Figure 1). Each group of about 10 residents shares a sitting area, dining area and balcony. Kitchen and nurse station are shared with a second group of about 10 residents on the same floor, so that both groups' staff can help each other if necessary. The private rooms of the first resident group are positioned below the floor with communal spaces, those of the second group on top of it. The different levels are stacked on top of each other into a tower. This tower is multiplied by four around a central courtyard and garden. The towers' floor plans are identical, but rotated and mirrored so that all dining areas face the central courtyard and each other. These four compact buildings accommodate 154 residents in total, 38 per building. Fairfield has been conceived as a dementia friendly facility, i.e., a facility with no specific wing for people with dementia. This means that, unlike in the former facility, residents do not have to move to a different group when their condition worsens.

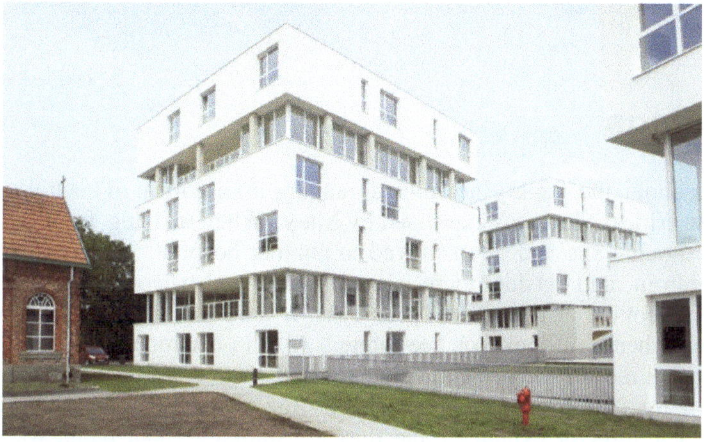

Fig. 1 Housing and care facility conveiced as four towers around a courtyard and garden © the architecture firm

3 Methods and Material

To gain insight into how the facility is experienced by its residents, a combination of methods was used. Central to the study were face-to-face interviews, combined with accompanied walks, with three residents of Fairfield (referred to by pseudonyms Albert, Edward and Mary). Participants were selected by the staff, mainly because of their good mental health, and their ability to express themselves well and guide the authors around the facility. Residents with severe dementia were therefore not interviewed in this research (Interviewing people with dementia is not impossible (Nygård 2006), but would have required much more time than available for the present study.). The interviews took between one and two hours. They started with an in-depth, semi-structured conversation in the resident's private room and continued with a tour around Fairfield's communal spaces and in some cases the surroundings and cafeteria, guided by the interviewee. To contextualise residents' perspective, extra data were collected. On the one hand, a two-hour focus group interview was conducted with the director, the coordinating and advising doctor, a nurse, a volunteer, a resident's wife, and a technician. Afterwards, the director guided the authors around part of Fairfield, further explaining the management's vision. On the other hand, face-to-face interviews (also one-to-two hours) were conducted with residents of the service flats located next to Fairfield on the same site (pseudonyms Herman & Betty, Frank & Louise, Alice, and Irene), and with neighbours still living in a private house who are on the waiting list to move there (pseudonyms Carlos and Anna). Some of these interviewees know Fairfield only from the outside, others make use of its public facilities or have been in there for a tour or visit.

Together this variety of perspectives offers a nuanced and comprehensive view of Fairfield. The notes made during the tours and the interviews' extensive content logs were analysed qualitatively based on the following questions: how is the facility experienced by the residents? And what role does architecture play in this experience?

4 Findings

Opinions about the facility are mixed, ranging from critical to neutral to positive. The most critical view was expressed by Mary. When arriving from the hospital, she first thought she had been moved to another hospital. She dislikes the white colour, both in- and outside: there is no life in it and when the sun is shining on the towers, looking at them hurts your eyes. It looks too much like a hospital for her: "everywhere you look you see white." Also in her room more colours would make her feel more at home. The volunteer and nurse confirmed that the corridors are very bare. The former always feels an urge to hang up posters, which is not allowed. The director explained that they are thinking about paint, wall paper or artwork. Anna finds the buildings too big and too high; Carlos calls them "towers" in a rather negative tone. On the other hand, several interviewees complimented the large windows and nice views outside thanks to the tower concept. Irene, who lives in a service flat and whose sister lives in Fairfield, thinks it is a very nice and modern concept. Albert and Edward have few comments on the building. Albert contends that he is not a difficult person and does not need luxury. For Edward it is good enough: "perhaps others have complaints about it, but I don't". Below we discuss in more detail how different aspects of the building are experienced.

4.1 Spatial Organisation

4.1.1 Orientation

The facility's organisation into different towers is evaluated both positively and negatively. The main functions in the building seem clearly located and easily reachable by the residents interviewed. The separation between public functions in the basement and residential areas in the towers is clear and seems to work well in terms of outer recognisability and internal navigation. Problems seem to occur in relation to locating the building block, floor or room within the whole.

Although the residents interviewed seemed to be in a good mental condition, in the beginning they all had problems finding their way in the facility. Albert and Edward forgot to look at the floor numbers and regularly left the elevator on the wrong floor. Mary had difficulty too, so she started memorizing certain points on her route: only her corridor has a fire extinguisher at the end, and her room is two doors away from that point. Edward and Mary notice that other people frequently have problems finding their way; both mentioned often helping other residents to find their room; mostly people with dementia, but during a tour through the building Mary too got confused. She took the researchers to the elevators of block A, where she had not been herself before, and had trouble locating the block in which she lived herself.

All focus group members agreed that repeating, rotating and mirroring almost identical buildings creates considerable confusion, for residents but also for themselves, family members and deliveries. Due to the mirroring the buildings have a similar but not identical layout, and all interviewees are regularly confused when walking around in them.

4.1.2 Social Contact and Reaching Out

Positioning the residents' private rooms on a different level than the communal space offers a high level of privacy, but appeared to compromise social contact, the staff's overview and sometimes even residents' security.

According to the doctor, the corridors in the former facility created long walking distances, but the rooms' open doors contributed to a certain community feeling. Now residents can stay all day in their room without seeing someone. This might be the residents wish, but he noticed that some people are waiting for others to pass by and get in contact.

Carlos assumes that the "tower-concept" negatively impacts on the nurses' response time. The focus group confirmed that staff have limited visual and acoustic control. E.g. between 5:30 and 6:30 pm, most residents start retreating to their room. At that time, less nurses are available than in the morning and they have to work on several floors at once. A resident's wife explained that around that time her husband becomes very restless, and fell a few times because there was no nurse on the communal floor to calm him down. The nurse said she sometimes feels powerless because she cannot always quickly see or help when important medical emergencies occur.

4.2 Personal Room

Carlos and Anna, who visited Fairfield on different occasions, and Alice, who lives in a service flat next doors, described the private rooms as very small or minimal. Mary on the other hand described her room as cosy and large. When you are alone you do not need much, she said. Albert again does not really have an opinion, he would not change anything. The director considers the "spacious rooms" as a quality of the new buildings, yet acknowledges that many people moving into the facility have difficulty with the room size.

The residents interviewed mentioned not being able or allowed to bring much furniture or other items from home. Albert used to be a real *collectionneur* and misses many of his belongings. He brought some small closets and his old sewing machine is displayed in the living room on the second floor. Edward did not bring any of his own furniture. His family wanted to bring an extra closet, but the staff said not enough room would be left to move around. Mary wanted to bring a closet with a display window, filled with many small items that have memories attached to them; because it was too high she was not allowed to bring it. Residents can bring only closets as high as a table. Mary brought her own recliner as the one offered in the facility was uncomfortable for her. She also wanted to bring her own TV and would want an extra chair for when she has visitors. The director clarified residents are only allowed to bring their own recliner if it is washable, because recliners made out of fabric are very unhygienic. Carlos and Anna also plan to bring some of their own furniture, but are still in doubt about which pieces, since the available space in Fairfield is limited.

All three residents interviewed have some pictures and small items that bring up memories for them. Albert likes talking about earlier times and has several pictures in his room to help him with that and remind him of those times. Mary had several pictures and paintings hanging up, some of them taped on the bathroom door. Edward's room contained less personal items.

4.3 Communal Space

Anna thinks that the rooms in Fairfield are made small deliberately, because residents are expected to live in the communal space, also for daily activities like reading, watching TV, having breakfast. She was reluctant to such a concept.

4.3.1 Dining Areas

Meals are organised in groups to promote social contact, also for more passive people. Only residents who are too ill eat in their room. The (potential) downside is that the meal times are fixed and residents have to adopt the day rhythm of the organization. Only in the morning is the time frame flexible. Breakfast is around 8am, lunch at 11:30am and dinner at 4:30pm. Albert and Edward seemed to have few problems with that, Mary found these times way too early.

During meal times, the two dining areas on one floor are mix-used for both resident groups. According to the staff meal times were originally organised in two groups divided by care needs (in practice often coinciding with having dementia or not). But, also according to the staff, residents ask to keep the same table mates and help take care of them. A resident's wife confirmed that residents help each other out: her husband cannot find the dining table by himself, but she is confident that, when she is not around, the staff and other residents will show him his place. Mary confirmed that the dining area is divided into a subgroup needing help when eating and a more independent one. She describes the former as "the people they need to help, who are a little disabled". Over time this division became indeed less strict as people's behaviour and capacities evolve, and they stay at their own table. In Edward's group, men and women eat on different sides.

The director highlighted that during meal times there is always a sense of calm in the groups, which she considers positive. During the tour, however, the atmosphere at mealtime seemed to be rather tense. This impression was confirmed by the residents. During meals nothing is said at Mary's table and nobody answers when she greets them. On her way from the elevators to the table she can hear a mouse running. The head nurse already asked whether she would like to change tables, but it is the same everywhere, she said. Albert mentioned knowing the people at his table, but has little contact with the others. Edward liked the dining area better in the rehabilitation centre where he stayed for a while. There the entire group gathered for meals, while here there are only seven men and 13 women who eat on opposite sides of the kitchen. In the rehabilitation centre getting to know others was easier because of the larger group.

4.3.2 Sitting Areas

Each communal floor features two sitting areas. According to the staff, the smaller area is used by couples who want more privacy, or to separate someone from the group. During the tour through the building, the director explained that, thanks to the large windows, you can separate a resident e.g. a shouting resident can be moved into such a corner from the rest of the group, without making him or her feel isolated.

During the tour, however, we witnessed that one sitting area was always used by people who seemed to be in a worse mental condition while the other one was empty. The residents interviewed never sit in the communal sitting areas. Instead they go to their own room to sit, read, watch TV. Albert blames his bad hearing: "and here with the people, I don't do that … I don't hear all that well", he tries to explain that it is difficult for him to communicate with them. When Edward showed us the first sitting area he explained: "now you can see how the people are here" and "that's why I never go sit here", "you can't talk with them". At the other, empty sitting area he said: "you see how many people there are here, so you sit here alone as well". Mary explained that "those people understand nothing from a movie" and "those who can't go upstairs anymore stay here". The volunteer knows a resident who definitely does not want to sit in the living room, but often goes to the cafeteria. The director thinks it is her personality, while the doctor believes that she does not like to sit amongst the other residents because people would think that she is also "like that".

In general everyone was in silence when sitting in the living room. The group of residents with dementia seemed to be stigmatized and isolated, especially because of the lack of interaction and their inability to participate actively in conversations. In more than one case their presence represents the reason why other residents avoid the living room during the day.

4.3.3 Balconies

Most activities for the residents are organized on the balconies. Albert and Edward join all activities they can. Mary used to, but stopped, possibly because of the tense atmosphere in her group. Edward likes that through these activities you get to know everyone. It is the main reason why he likes living in the facility so much.

Except during these activities, none of the residents interviewed use the balconies. Edward comes there twice a day to water the plants, but never sees anyone sitting on them. He sees no point in having two such balconies on the same floor. The interviewees cannot explain why they are not used: Albert mentioned there is not too much draft; Edward thinks the view on both balconies is ok; Mary told that it can be hot there before noon but nice in the evening. Yet, rather than go sitting there, she prefers to go outside. "Perhaps I will when I'm like those", she said, referring to the people with dementia who stay on this floor all day. A resident's wife confirmed that the terraces are hardly used; one balcony should do and the other one may just as well be part of the interior space to accommodate indoor activities.

5 Discussion and Conclusion

The facility studied in this paper was conceived as a large scale care facility with qualities of small-scale, homelike living schemes. This led to an innovative building and care organization fitting budgetary norms while applying small-scale ambitions. How is this facility experienced by its residents?

The generic layout of the plans (multiplying, rotating and mirroring a single unit to create one floor, duplicating this floor to create a building and multiplying, rotating and mirroring the building itself) results in a spatial configuration that is experienced as highly confusing on different levels, by older people with cognitive problems and also by staff. This should be interpreted not necessarily as a critique on the concept of a generic layout, but as a call for more differentiation within the same concept.

The outspoken contemporary architecture in itself is not criticized, e.g. the large windows are very much appreciated. What is criticized, however, is the materialization. Especially the walls' white colour, both inside and outside, is subject of discussion and plans are made to change it. There are complaints that the walls are too hospital-like, that the building is too bare, it lacks a little homelikeness. Combining the benefits of this contemporary architecture with materials and colours that offer a more homelike atmosphere and differentiation seems to be a major challenge when designing a new facility.

With regard to this homelikeness, furnishing a place can help to make it "your own" (Van Steenwinkel et al. 2012). Although not everyone attaches high importance to this, the interviews suggest that most interviewees do. For reasons related to hygiene and the habitation's temporary nature, the management limits this appropriation to some extent, often causing frustration for the residents. The building design can also influence this process by offering (often simple and small) opportunities to appropriate the space. We could observe that the suspension systems were used to hang up paintings, and that open shelves and tables were intensely used to display personal items. As the example of Albert's sewing machine suggests, the appropriation of the communal spaces is also important in residents' experience.

Concerning the size of personal rooms, this study does not allow neither positive nor negative general conclusions to be drawn. Larger spaces would allow residents to bring more of their own furniture and personal objects when moving in. On the other hand, having to reorganise and consider what (not) to bring is inherent to moving to a smaller space. Moreover, two out of three residents interviewed did not comment on it; the third thought their room was large.

In our opinion the size of the personal room cannot be discussed in isolation from the size and concept of the communal space. In a (real) small-scale living scheme, where people spend most of their time in the communal area, investing more space in the communal areas might be justified. In contexts where privacy is more important, people are likely to spend more time in their own personal space and thus the size should be adjusted accordingly.

In the context of the facility studied, we witnessed during tours and interviews, that some of the ideals of small-scale, homelike living are absent. Although director and staff did refer to the community feeling of a small-scale living group, interviews with residents suggest that this feeling is lacking, and that a strong reluctance exists to interact with the residents with dementia. Residents who have no mental problems avoid the communal living areas and have few other places to go besides the outside environment and the cafeteria.

Since we did not interview people with dementia or their family members, we have no insight into how they experience the current situation. From other studies and literature we know that small-scale living can indeed be a valuable alternative for people with dementia (Boekhorst et al. 2007, Declercq et al. 2007). Thus we see the previous not as a critique on small-scale living itself, but rather as related to the specific set-up in this facility.

In terms of organization, we noticed that both groups are actually combined into one group of 20, which is far from the "ideal" number of six and thus not really stimulating a situation of small "households". The two dining areas on one floor are used not for each individual "household", but to separate residents who do not need help from those who do. Residents with dementia (from both groups) stay in the largest sitting area during the day, while the others avoid it and the smaller sitting area seems hardly used. Activities are mostly organised for both groups together on one balcony, while the other remains underused. During our visits, small-scale principles like cooking per "household" or staff without uniform could not be observed. Furthermore, by locating the private rooms on different floors than the communal areas, residents' privacy may increase whereas the communal feeling and connection with "their" living room seems somewhat lost.

We would therefore indeed characterise Fairfield as something in between actual small-scale living and the more traditional group living in large-scale residential care facilities. Perhaps such a combination is possible, but in this specific set-up we could see how residents without dementia start redrawing from the group, and yet have few other places to go to. We also wonder whether the intended benefits of small-scale living for people with dementia are still present in this set-up. Future research should therefore include their perspective as well.

Our findings confirm that how people eventually use and experience a building, may significantly differ from designers' intentions (Barnes et al. 2002, Crilly et al. 2008), e.g., the floor plan could be interpreted as a small-scale living scheme of two groups of 10 residents, who only share a kitchen and nurse station, but turned out to function mainly as one group of 20. Without this kind of follow-up research, architects might consider this case as an ideal example of a small-scale layout, and reproduce (parts of) it without knowing the actual benefits and deficiencies.

Our findings also show the added value of in-depth case studies in this context. When conducting a large-scale study about housing and care facilities, particular benefits or deficiencies might not surface, as they are very specific for this case and thus not comparable with others, e.g. the tower concept is unique in Flanders for such a facility. The appreciation of the views from such a height, or staff's lack of overview due to private rooms and communal spaces located on different floors, are quite unique for this facility. This kind of in depth case-studies are thus important to identify the specific benefits and deficiencies of unique and innovative concepts.

Acknowledgements

The authors thank all who contributed to this study: Simone Pizzagalli, the architecture firm, the director and staff of Fairfield, all interviewees for sharing their time and experiences, and the reviewers for their valuable comments.

References

Barnes S and the Design in Caring Environments Study Group (2002) The design of caring environments and the quality of life of older people. Ageing & Society 22: 775-789

Boekhorst S, Depla MFIA, De Lange J, Eefsting JA (2007) Kleinschalig wonen voor ouderen met dementie. Tijdschrift voor Gerontologie en Geriatrie 38:17-26

Coomans K, De Smet H, Heylighen A (2011) In search of a future for large-scale care homes in Flanders. Journal of Housing for the Elderly 25(4): 329-351

Crilly N, Majer A, Clarkson PJ (2008) Representing artefacts as media. IJDesign 2(3): 15-27

Declercq A, Van Audenhove C, Mello J, Demaerschalk M (2007) Stapstenen naar kleinschalig genormaliseerd wonen: Eindrapport. Lucas, Leuven, Belgium

Nygård L (2006) How can we get access to the experiences of people with dementia? Scandinavian Journal of Occupational Therapy 13(2): 101-112

Van Audenhove C, Declercq A, De Coster I, Spruytte N, Molenberghs C, Van den Heuvel B (2003) Kleinschalig genormaliseerd wonen voor personen met dementie. Garant, Antwerpen, Belgium

Van Steenwinkel I, Van Audenhove C, Heylighen A (2012) Home in later life: A framework for the architecture of home environments. Home Cultures 9(2): 195-217

Verbeek H, van Rossum E, Zkwahalen SM, Kempen GI, Hamers JP (2009) Small, homelike care environments for older people with dementia. International Psychogeriatrics 21(2): 252-264

Wijnties M (2003) Wordt kleinschalige zorg groot? Aedes-Arcares kenniscentrum Wonen-Zorg, Utrecht, The Netherlands

Adjusting an Older Residential Care Facility to Contemporary Dementia Care Visions

I. Van Steenwinkel, E. Verstraeten and A. Heylighen

Abstract: Older residential care facilities are increasingly confronted with an incongruity between contemporary visions on dementia care and outdated infrastructure. In this context a case study analyses how the architecture of such a facility hampers or supports the implementation of its dementia care vision. Interviews, participant observation and document analysis offer nuanced insights into the interplay between care vision and architecture. The latter's limitations include its spatial organisation, lack of high-quality communal areas, authoritarian character and hospital-like atmosphere, while potential lies in using adaptable lighting, homelike materials and furniture, and small spatial interventions. These interventions can be framed within a major renovation in the long term, which would allow to realize far-reaching improvements in the ward. Since many older facilities display similar features, the case study's approach and outcome can help them in adjusting their outdated infrastructure to increase the autonomy of people with dementia and support their individuality and emancipation.

1 Introduction

In the 1970s, attention grew for integrating people with dementia in society, increasing their autonomy, and supporting their individuality and emancipation. However, these objectives were not yet translated into architectural design practice (Mens and Wagenaar 2009). The residential care facilities (RCFs) built at that time often have an institutional, hospital-like character (de Rooij 2012). Today it is even more emphasized that, since dementia is currently irreversible, focusing on its medical aspects contributes little for the patient. Contemporary visions on dementia care put patients' experience and quality of life centre stage (Finnema et al. 2000). In this experience, an important role is played by the physical environment (Calkins et al. 2001, Van Audenhove et al. 2003, Sternberg 2009, Van Steenwinkel et al. 2014). Yet, because the existing infrastructure cannot always be replaced, often an incongruity exists between a RCF's dementia care vision and its outdated architecture. This paper addresses this incongruity between care vision and

I. Van Steenwinkel · A. Heylighen (✉)
KU Leuven, Department of Architecture, Research[x]Design, Belgium
email: ann.heylighen@kuleuven.be

E. Verstraeten
Architectenbureau Lowette & Partners, Belgium

P. Langdon et al. (eds.), *Designing Around People*,
DOI 10.1007/978-3-319-29498-8_22

architecture in the case of a particular RCF, referred to as Hilltop (pseudonym). We analyse what Hilltop's care vision implies within its architectural context. Central in this study is the question to what extent the architecture hampers, or holds potential for, the implementation of dementia care concepts considered important at Hilltop.

2 Context

Dementia is a syndrome associated with progressive memory impairment and loss of other cognitive functions (American Psychiatric Association 2000), with far-reaching consequences for patients and their environment. There are several types of dementia and different, not clearly discriminated stages in the dementing process, which may succeed each other at different rates.

Hilltop can be situated in the recent evolutions of visions on dementia care. Whereas this care used to focus on the underlying pathology, in the 1970s attention shifted towards the psychological and emotional well-being of people with dementia (Finnema et al. 2000). For Hilltop's directors the most prominent features of dementia are disorientation in time, space and identity, inability to perform daily activities and, as a result, loss of dignity. To cope with these features, the directors consider it essential to offer **structure** in both environment (space) and schedule (time), guarantee **safety and security**, and stimulate **autonomy**.

This evolution in visions on dementia care has implications for the care architecture. A transition is taking place from hospital-like RCFs to housing schemes directed at normalisation and well-being, like small-scale normalised living (Verbeek et al. 2009). The latter denotes a housing and care type where six to 16 persons with dementia, with professional guidance, form a household in a for them familiar and homey environment (Van Audenhove et al. 2003).

Due to the ageing population, however, the demand for high-quality housing comes with a demand for *more* housing. Since the latter cannot be met with new built projects only, pressure on older RCFs increases. These are often confronted with an outdated infrastructure (Coomans et al. 2011), as is the case for Hilltop. Although it adopts a contemporary vision on dementia care, the implementation of this vision is not always straightforward due to the RCF's architecture. Hilltop accommodates two wards for people with dementia, situated in a building from 1994, designed with a focus on offering efficient care. This can be derived from the central kitchen for all seven wards, long monotone corridors leading to nursing stations, and small living rooms. Moreover, the building was designed not specifically for people with dementia and due to later extensions, most wards are difficult to reach. Like several other RCFs in Flanders, Hilltop is thus confronted with a demand for more and higher-quality housing for people with dementia.

3 Methods

The case study presented here combined multiple methods: participant observation, interviews and document analysis.

To gain insight into daily life at Hilltop, the second author (henceforth 'the researcher') volunteered in one ward, one morning per week for two months. This allowed her to become familiar with the ward through **participant observation**. The ward was selected in consultation with the directors. Of the two wards for people with dementia at Hilltop, it is the more problematic because there is less space for the same number of residents. Participant observation started at 8am, when part of the residents had already been woken, and ended at 12:30pm, during or after lunch. The researcher's tasks included assisting caregivers in preparing and serving breakfast, assisting residents in taking their meal or using the toilet, accompanying them and listening to their stories, etc. Because most residents spend most of the day in the living room or central hall, most observations were done there. Yet, the researcher also spent time with residents in their private rooms. Assisting bedridden residents with their meal made sure that they were not overlooked. During the fieldwork notes and sometimes pictures were made. These were processed in a report on the day they were made.

The researcher also conducted **interviews** with the management (general director and director resident care, quality coordinator, palliative referent, and psychologist/referent dementia) and the ward's residents. All interviews were semi-structured around open questions. The interviews with the management aimed at getting to know the RCF, their vision on dementia care and its impact on architecture. The interviews with residents tried to gain insight into what is important to them. Interviewing people with dementia comes with several challenges. For some of them, finding words and following complex conversations is difficult or impossible. Moreover, they often have difficulty to stay focused on the conversation and topic and process questions. For this reason, the researcher conducted multiple shorter informal conversations with several residents. She listened to their stories and asked short questions when possible.

All interviews (except for two) were audio-recorded and transcribed verbatim. Based on the transcripts a content report was made that summarizes the interview's major points, followed by a narrative report that addresses its storyline more elaborately. Subsequently, themes from each interview were abstracted, based on which the interviews were analysed and conceptualised.

The observations and interviews were complemented with a **document analysis** of Hilltop's website and vision statement, the building plans, as well as pictures, notes and sketches made during the fieldwork. The plan analysis started from spatial themes that address the impact of the built environment on people's experience (Nylander 2002, Ching 2007, Unwin 2014). Examples include spatial organisation, materiality, light, and circulation.

4 Findings

This section describes the limitations and potential of Hilltop's architecture for realising its vision on dementia care.

4.1 Limitations

To start with, the **spatial organisation** suggests that the building was designed from a vision that gave priority to efficient care, rather than to residents' perspective and daily activities. The layout seems to be conceived to **limit** staff's **walking distances**: a central nursing station from which corridors with private rooms depart (Figure 1). This spatial organisation hampers hominess and security and offers residents little normalisation and spatial structure.

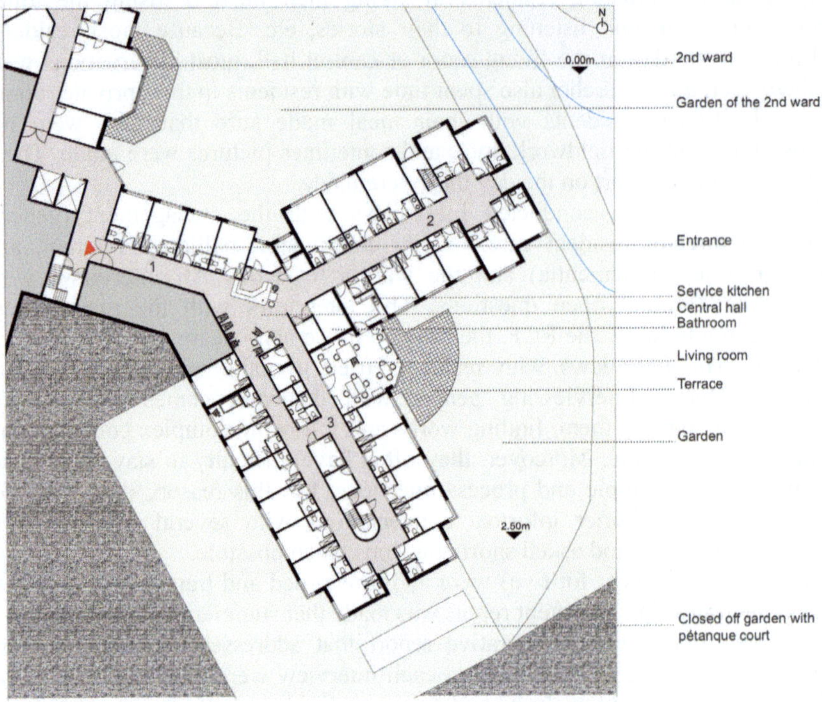

Fig. 1 Floor plan of the ward's current situation

Second, the focus on staff's **circulation** results in little attention for spaces where residents can reside. Judging from the ward's layout, the designers assumed that residents would stay most of the time in their private room. The living room accommodates only 15 of the 30 residents, the others sit in the central hall. The latter shows little flexibility since the staff's run lines need to be kept clear (Figure 2). As the **communal rooms lack** an **adequate arrangement**, the ward fails to offer residents all facets of life. For instance, there is neither a kitchen where residents can be involved in preparing meals nor a sitting area — two places that are closely linked with normalisation and hominess. Residents can sit only at a table or in a row against the wall, and have few opportunities for variation in the interior and use of spaces. As no other options are available, except for the private room, residents rarely change places in between meals, which reduces the structure in their day. In summer the terrace offers more opportunities for variation in the use of spaces. In winter this is not an option, however.

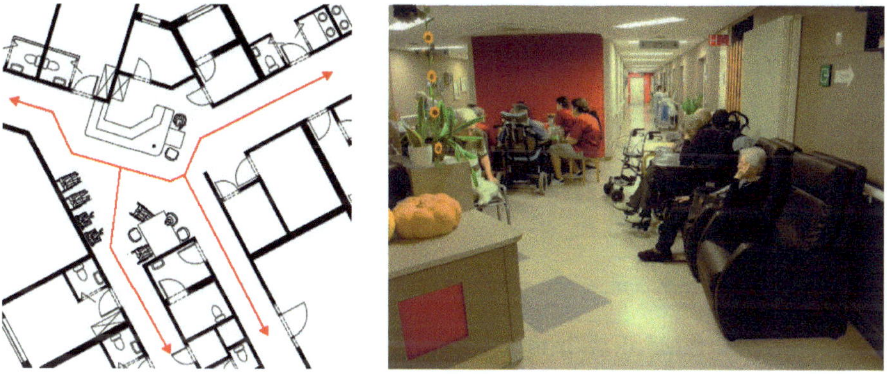

Fig. 2 Circulation dominates the central hall

Because the building was designed for efficient care, whereby residents seemed to be of secondary importance, the spatial organisation radiates an **authoritarian character** towards them. This third limitation is exemplified by the central nursing station which acts as a control point. The authoritarian character contributes little to a homelike and secure atmosphere. Moreover, it contradicts Hilltop's care vision, in which residents are equal to the staff and every resident should be treated and cared for as an individual and with respect.

Fourth, the **materials** used give the ward a **hospital-like character** while the **similarity** between the corridors contributes to **disorientation**. Everywhere the same materials are used while few landmarks are present. This is especially the case in the corridors, which are long, identical in terms of material use, and radiate a hospital-like atmosphere (Figure 3).

A final limitation is the fact that **daylight** is present only in the living room and private rooms. By consequence, residents seated in the central hall cannot benefit its advantages and the **structure in time** it offers. Since different activities overlap, they do not offer much structure in time either. Also due to the staff's busy schedules and limited spaces, meals usually lack a clear start and ending, which reduces their value as a structuring element.

4.2 Potential

Despite the architecture's limitations, several adaptations are possible to improve the residents' quality of life. To start with, much can be improved through small and medium interventions, which can be implemented relatively simply, quickly and cheaply. They can be framed within larger and more radical renovation works in the long term. The following should be considered as lines of thought, not as concrete design proposals.

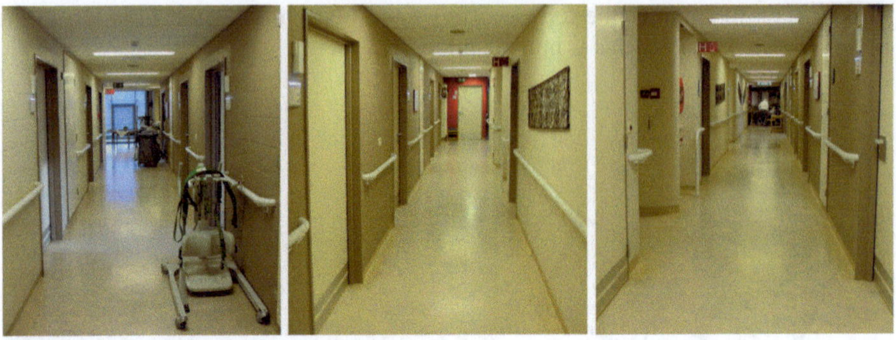

Fig.3 The three corridors are long, identical and hospital-like

4.2.1 Small and Medium Interventions

The institutional light fittings that are currently used in the corridor (Figure 3) could be replaced by more homelike fittings. Furthermore, using higher intensity ambient bright light and offering a view outside is very likely to improve the day-night rhythm and orientation in time for residents (Day et al. 2000, Thorpe et al. 2000, van Hoof et al. 2009), especially for those who reside in the central hall. In addition, the staff could look for ways to better delineate structuring activities, such as the organisation of meals.

Wall and floor furnishings in corridors and rooms could be adjusted to create a warmer atmosphere. Material use could also address residents' disorientation in space, e.g., by distinguishing corridors through colour or decoration. Individualising the doors of the private rooms with pictures, objects or colours would assist residents in locating their own room (Lawton et al. 1984).

The furniture could be improved too. By using tables of a more appropriate size in the living room, more space would become available for residents to sit in the living room or another function; e.g., a reminiscence corner. The chairs and sofas could be replaced by furniture with a more homelike character, without losing sight of criteria related to maintenance and ease of use. The built-in closets in the rooms can be substituted by personal closets.

Technology might offer a solution to lock the private rooms and other spaces for people not allowed to enter. Introducing personal bracelets would ensure that residents can enter their own room, but not that of others. This could increase residents' security, privacy and autonomy (Godwin 2012). Currently, most doors to the private rooms are locked during the day to avoid residents entering the wrong room. As a result, residents who want to go to their room have to ask the staff first.

The bathroom in the private rooms could be renovated to be more user-friendly. The door opening could be adapted such that it is directed at the room. If the door occupied a slanting side of the bathroom, the room would look larger and residents would no longer have the feeling of entering through a narrow corridor – between the closet and bathroom wall – before reaching the actual room. The direction of rotation would ensure that residents' privacy is guaranteed when staff enters.

Finally, opportunities exist to create more space through small interventions. For instance, the entrance hall where the elevator arrives is rather big for its role as passageway and could be partially used to create a sitting area (see Figure 4). Circulation would still pass through this hall, so the solution is not perfect. But more differentiated places would become available to residents, e.g., those who eat in the central hall could be brought there in the afternoon. Staying there would be more pleasant than staying in the central hall as it is less busy and daylight enters through the big window. Because the corridor joins onto the hall, residents would no longer be confronted with the closed door at its end (Although the problem might move to the door of the entrance hall.).

Furthermore, the central nursing station could be removed. It strongly contributes to the central hall's authoritarian character and is rarely used. Most tasks now executed there could also be done at a table among residents. For tasks that do require isolation, the staff could use the small table in the administrative room. By removing the desk, the central hall's authoritarian character would be reduced and the staff would mingle more with the residents. Also, more space would become available in the hall, allowing for a more flexible configuration.

4.2.2 Major Renovation

The smaller interventions mentioned above can be framed within a major renovation in the long term, which would allow far-reaching improvements in the ward to be realized. Figure 4 shows a possible intervention; Figure 1 shows the current situation by way of comparison. Note that the smaller interventions are integrated in this proposal. By working in this way, one can avoid a certain intervention being nullified by another intervention a few years later.

The rationale behind the proposal is the following: why would residents and visitors need to enter the building through the main entrance, if they could just as well go directly to the ward's front door? The far end of corridor 2 is situated close to the street. Currently there is an emergency exit, which could be renovated into an effective front door of the housing unit. Through this door, visitors would enter a big living room with an open kitchen, a sitting area, and eating area. This room could be created by removing four private rooms at the far end of the corridor and constructing a new extension. By transforming the old kitchen and living room into three new private rooms, only one room would be lost. The new living room would offer a comfortable place to reside during the day, providing enough space for all residents and allowing a flexible set-up. Because of the large number of residents, preparing complete warm meals in the open kitchen would remain impossible. Yet, soup and dessert could be made within the ward, allowing residents to assist. This intervention would add a living room with much daylight and differentiate day and night zones, which would benefit residents' orientation in time.

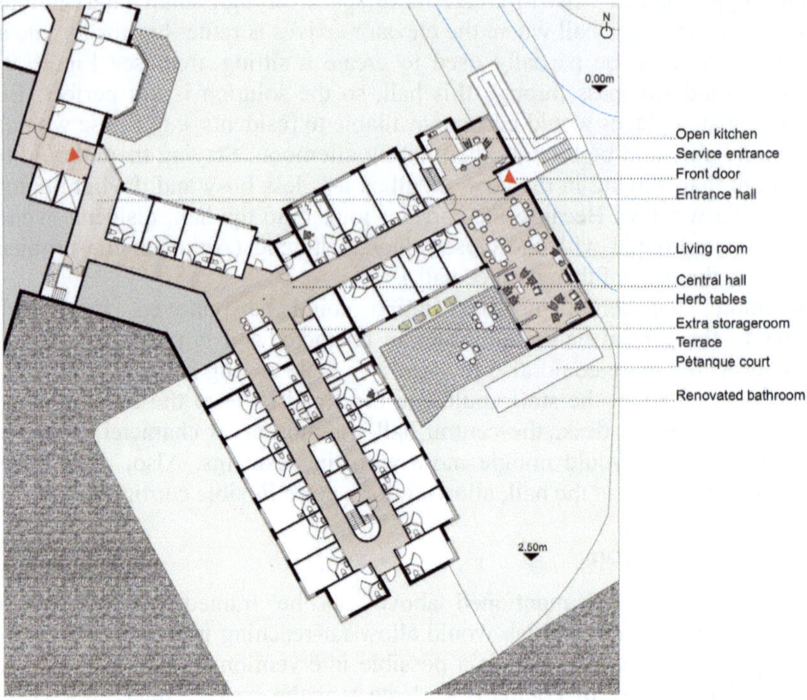

Fig. 4 Floor plan proposed renovation

The old entrance would become a service entrance through which the meal trolley is brought and staff can reach other wards. Also residents and visitors could keep using this entrance when they want to take the elevator to the cafeteria. Because the central hall would no longer serve as extension of the living room, much space would become available. This would allow extending the nave of corridor 3 with extra storage room. Next to it a table or sofa could be installed for residents who like to retreat or a reminiscence corner could be created.

Enabling residents to go outside in a safe and comfortable way, also in winter, would enhance autonomy and health (Chalfont 2005). In Figure 4 a door is foreseen from the living room to the garden. Through the use of technology, the door could be always accessible for residents who are allowed to go outside independently. Not having a doorstep would make it easier for residents to go outside and hanging coat hooks with coats against the wall could prompt residents to do so. Also the garden could be improved so that residents could better enjoy it. Activities could be offered by laying out paths or a small vegetable garden. A vegetable or herb garden is laid out best as a 'herb table' so that it can be reached easily by residents, including wheelchair users (Kamp 2005). Finally, in the part of the garden that is accessible for the residents, the pétanque court or other play equipment could be installed to encourage enjoyment and human relationships (Chalfont 2005).

5 Conclusion

This paper explored through a case study how an older RCF's outdated infrastructure influences the implementation of its contemporary care vision. The study was motivated by the challenges the ageing population poses and the evolution toward higher-quality and person-oriented care for people with dementia. We analysed to what extent the RCF's architecture holds limitations or potential for a better implementation of this care. A combination of fieldwork and document analysis offered insight into the daily routine in one ward and architecture's influence on it.

The analysis suggests that the architecture's major limitations include its spatial organisation, lack of adequate communal areas, and authoritarian character. The latter seems to suggest that residents are of secondary importance. Despite the staff's efforts this character cannot be hidden. Due to the lack of space there is little flexibility and few facets of daily life can be accommodated. Nevertheless there is considerable room for improvement through different interventions. These are expected to contribute to a better implementation of the RCF's contemporary care vision and to a higher quality of life. At the same time, we should not forget that the physical environment is but one factor that plays a role in residents' quality of life. Other efforts made by the directors and caregivers are at least as important.

A limitation of the study is that residents and staff were not involved in co-designing the improvements. This is because the study was originally intended as an exploration and preparation for the actual work. However, Hilltop's management considered the results so valuable, that some of the suggested changes have already been implemented. The floor material has been replaced by parquet-like laminate, creating a more homelike atmosphere. The desk of the central nursing station has been removed and part of the entrance hall has been annexed. Removing the desk resulted in more space in the central hall. Because extra space has been added at the end of the first corridor, less residents sit all day in the central hall or stand waiting at the front door until someone opens it. For Hilltop it is important to continue trying to improve the residents' quality of life through small and large interventions. The case study's results offer a basis to understand the different dynamics in the ward and make targeted interventions in the future. At the same time it is also important that Hilltop continues to work on aspects that are less dependent on the architecture (relationship between residents and staff, activities offered) as these can help counterbalance the building's authoritarian character.

Since many older RCF's share similar features with Hilltop – long, hospital-like corridors attached to a central area with nursing station; lack of daylight and high-quality communal areas; authoritarian character; hospital-like materials – this case study can help to identify limitations and potentials of their architecture. Both the approach and the outcome of the case study might offer inspiration to other RCFs who want to adjust their outdated infrastructure to contemporary care visions.

Acknowledgements

This study received support from the Research Fund KU Leuven (OT/12/051). Thanks are due to the management, staff and residents at Hilltop for sharing their time and experiences.

References

American Psychiatric Association (2000) Diagnostic and statistical manual of mental disorders: DSM-IV-TR. American Psychiatric Pub, Washington, DC, USA

Calkins M, Sanford JA, Proffitt MA (2001) Design for dementia. In: Preiser WFE, Ostroff E (Eds.) Universal design handbook, pp. 22.1-22.4. McGraw-Hill, New York, NY, USA

Chalfont GE (2005) Building edge. Alzheimer's Care Quarterly 6(4): 341-348

Ching FD (2007) Architecture-form, space & order. John Wiley & Sons, Hoboken, NJ, USA

Coomans K, De Smet H, Heylighen A (2011) In search of a future for large-scale care homes in Flanders. Journal of Housing for the Elderly 25(4): 329-351

Day K, Carreon D, Stump C (2000) The therapeutic design of environments for people with dementia. The Gerontologist 40(4): 397-416

de Rooij AHPM (2012) Living with dementia in small-scale and traditional longterm care settings. DekoVerdivas, Tilburg, The Netherlands

Finnema E, Dröes RM, Ribbe M, van Tilburg W (2000) A review of psychosocial models in psychogeriatrics. Alzheimer Disease and Associated Disorders 14(2): 68-80

Godwin B (2012) The ethical evaluation of assistive technology for practitioners. Journal of Assistive Technologies 6(2): 123-135

Kamp D (2005) Beyond the view: A collaborative approach in creating useful outdoor spaces for aging populations. Alzheimer's Care Quarterly 6(4): 335-340

Lawton MP, Fulcomer M, Kleban M (1984) Architecture for the mentally impaired elderly. Environment and Behavior 16: 730-757

Mens N, Wagenaar C (2009) De architectuur van de ouderenhuisvesting: Bouwen voor wonen en zorg. NAi Uitgevers, Rotterdam, The Netherlands

Nylander O (2002) Architecture of the home. Wiley-Academy, Chichester, UK

Sternberg E (2009) Healing spaces: The science of place and well-being. Belknap Press of Harvard University Press, Cambridge, MA, USA

Thorpe L, Middleton J, Russel G, Stewart N (2000) Bright light therapy for demented nursing home patients with behavioral disturbance. American Journal of Alzheimer's Disease and Other Dementias 15(1): 18-26

Unwin S (2014) Analysing architecture. Routledge, Abingdon, Oxon, UK

Van Audenhove C, Declercq A, De Coster I, Spruytte N, Molenberghs C, Van den Heuvel B (2003) Kleinschalig genormaliseerd wonen voor personen met dementie. Garant, Antwerp, The Netherlands

van Hoof J, Aarts MPJ, Rense CG, Schoutens AMC (2009) Ambient bright light in dementia: Effects on behaviour and circadian rhythmicity. Building and Environment 44(1): 146-155

Van Steenwinkel I, Van Audenhove C, Heylighen A (2014) Mary's little worlds. Qualitative Health Research 24(8): 1023-1032

Verbeek H, van Rossum E, Zkwahalen SM, Kempen GI, Hamers JP (2009) Small, homelike care environments for older people with dementia: A literature review. International Psychogeriatrics 21(2): 252-264

Designing Inclusive Architecture: Facilitators and Barriers of the Healthcare Environment for Rehabilitation at Stroke Units

A. Anåker, L. Von Koch and M. Elf

Abstract: The significance of inclusive and enriched environment for persons with stroke is strongly emphasized by various international studies. This study aimed to explore how architecture can support or hinder rehabilitation for persons with stroke. The result shows that specific training facilities are only used to a small extent. This point to conclusion that there is an essential need for architecture that promotes rehabilitation at stroke units.

1 Introduction

Is the architecture of stroke care units inclusive? Inclusive or universal architectural design is about designing more accessible spaces for the widest possible range of users, regardless of age and capabilities (Clarkson et al. 2007). It requires better understanding of all potential user needs. In stroke care, inclusive design can be described as a space that is available, functional and comfortable for promoting rehabilitation activities for all persons with stroke. Promoting independence in everyday life for stroke survivors is an important goal for the rehabilitation in stroke care. Thus, rehabilitation should start early, already at the acute phase (Brainin et al. 2004, Langhorne and Dennis 2004). Studies have shown that an enriched environment with access to meeting places and possibilities for individual activities can promote the well-being for persons with stroke (Indredavik et al. 1999, Askim et al. 2012).

Observations of patient location, interaction and physical activity has shown that patients at stroke units are inactive and alone (Bernhardt et al. 2004). In order to achieve an inclusive design there is a need of studies focusing on facilitators and barriers of the physical healthcare environment in stroke units. In this presentation we report from a case study where persons with stroke were observed and explored regarding where the persons were placed (location), what they were doing (activities) and with whom they interacted (interaction). The aim of this study was

A. Anåker · L. Von Koch · M. Elf
Department of NVS Division of Occupational Therapy, Karolinska Institutet, Sweden
email: anna.anaker@ki.se

P. Langdon et al. (eds.), *Designing Around People*,
DOI 10.1007/978-3-319-29498-8_23

to explore how architecture can support or hinder rehabilitation for persons with stroke.

2 Method

A case study, using quantitative and qualitative data was used. Observation of patient activities, locations and interactions at a new built stroke unit was executed in order to obtain information of how the design facilitated or hindered the rehabilitation.

3 Results

Preliminary results show, as in other studies, that in the therapeutic day the patients were alone in their room and lying in bed most of the time. They were only involved in a few training activities. This is contrary to the recommendations in stroke guidelines. The specific training facilities were used to a small extent. Instead corridors were used as a training space. The unit was designed with many single rooms and that might cause that the patients were not visible in the public areas. The conclusion drawn from this study is that the architecture did not promote rehabilitation.

References

Askim T, Bernhardt J, Loge AD, Indredavik B (2012) Stroke patients do not need to be inactive in the first two-weeks after stroke: Results from a stroke unit focused on early rehabilitation. Int J Stroke 7: 25-31

Bernhardt J, Dewey H, Thrift A, Donnan G (2004) Inactive and alone: Physical activity within the first 14 days of acute stroke unit care. Stroke 35: 1005-1009

Brainin M, Olsen TS, Chamorro A, Diener HC, Ferro J, Hennerici MG et al. (2004) Organization of stroke care: Education, referral, emergency management and imaging, stroke units and rehabilitation. Cerebrovascular Diseases 17: 1-14

Clarkson J, Coleman R, Hosking I, Waller S (2007) Inclusive design toolkit. Cambridge Engineering Design Center, Cambridge, UK

Indredavik B, Bakke F, Slordahl SA, Rokseth R, Haheim LL (1999) Treatment in a combined acute and rehabilitation stroke unit: Which aspects are most important? Stroke 30: 917-923

Langhorne P, Dennis M (2004) Stroke units: The next 10 years. The Lancet 363: 834-835

An Evaluation of Public Space Accessibility Using Universal Design Principles at Naresuan University Hospital

C. Phaholthep, A. Sawadsri and H. Skates

Abstract: The objective of this research is to study how well Naresuan University Hospital complies with the requirements of seven Universal Design (UD) principles in relation to the requirements and physical restrictions of deaf, blind, mobility impaired and elderly users. To achieve this the requirements and physical obstacles of the facilities within the public zone of the hospital were analysed. The research uses qualitative and quantitative methods to implement a heuristic evaluation method (HEM) along side a scenario access audit which required a participation of a group of people with different types of disabilities, experience the level of accessibility of the service functions in public areas of this hospital. The UD principles investigated were: equitable use; flexibility in use; simple and intuitive use; perceptible information; tolerance for error; low physical effort; size and space for approach use. The results of this research present a specific summary of the observations, which found that significant obstructions occurred in the main communication and circulation spaces. This problem has been classified into two parts consisting of: (1) Obstructions to general service accessibility caused by inappropriate use of space, and (2) insufficient and inappropriate facilities covering all types of disability.

1 Introduction

In the twenty-first century in developing countries, design should incorporate the important paradigm that gives due consideration to the widest range of users including people with disability. This is consistent with the democratic concept of equality and the concept of continuous improvement. These fundamental concepts not only apply to a service facility but also to all types of operations related to design including product, interior, architecture, urban, traffic even communication and information technologies (Preiser and Ostroff 2001).

C. Phaholthep (✉) · A. Sawadsri
Faculty of Architecture, King Mongkut's Institute of Technology Ladkrabang (KMITL), Bangkok, Thailand
email: yummer308@hotmail.com

H. Skates
School of Environment, Griffith University, Gold Coast Australia

P. Langdon et al. (eds.), *Designing Around People*,
DOI 10.1007/978-3-319-29498-8_24

UD is the name ascribed to design with an emphasis on social sustainability and a belief that differing physical abilities are a regular occurrence of the human condition and so encourages equal access for all to all service functions. This being the case, UD principles should be applied to healthcare facilities, being projects that contain the widest range of requirement of accessible conditions for different groups of people with different physical abilities. The World Health Organization's Definition of Disability International Classification of Functioning (IFC), IFC2001 refers to seven principles of universal design as a measurement method of the accessibility level of service facilities (Sahachaiseri 2011).

In today's society, the role of the hospital is not merely to be responsible for the quality of medical treatment, but also to serve society in matters of people's health rights and security. In order to supply 'right to health' such facilities should be easy-to-access, and give equal priority to all people inclusively. Right to health, as such, belongs to social rights, not expressed simply as the distribution of state benefits, but on social life as it happens in places such as the built environment and in buildings (Longo 2012, cited by Setola et al. 2013). Functional spaces require spatial management to support activities and effectively connect different activities, to provide satisfactory experiences for users. According to Sahachaiseri (2012), in healthcare building design, space usability should be based on the user's activity and behaviour. Unfortunately, the majority of measurements and evaluations of the service quality in healthcare organizations are conducted in terms of medical service quality, despite the importance of the physical functioning of buildings (Preiser et al. 2009). The built environment is an important factor to provide or prevent access (Imrie 1995).

In Thailand, hospital buildings should comply with policy and rules and regulations of law, e.g. 'The ministerial regulations regarding facilities for the disabled and elderly of Thailand 2005' (Department of Empowerment of Persons with Disabilities 2012). These regulations refer to physical features e.g. signage, ramps, lifts, parking, building entrances and the connection between buildings, doors, toilets, tactile characters etc. Despite this, problems are evident in some hospitals. From simple observation, way-finding/way-showing systems, sizing and clearance of passageways and overcrowding are just some of the problems encountered.

2 Aim and Methods

The purpose of this research was to investigate the physical features of Naresuan University (NU) hospital in relation to seven UD principles for a variety of impaired users.

This research uses qualitative and quantitative methods to implement an heuristic evaluation method (HEM) and scenario access audit, as follows.

A literature review was conducted on the concept and theories of UD and international best practice of hospital design (Adler 1999, DoH 2013, DoH 2014). A preliminary study was then undertaken observing the flow of outpatients and the physical features of each service point on the main hospital public communication and circulation spaces as per Table 1. An access audit was conducted consisting of simulated deaf, blind, vision impaired, wheelchair user, walking stick and armless person as per Table 2. Obstacles were identified that contributed to disadvantaging the simulated user group. The hospital public zone was evaluated within the heuristic evaluation method (Afacan and Erbug 2009) by experienced designers including a product designer, interior designer and two architects.

Table 1 The physical feature evaluation checklist for accessibility

No.	Feature and design considerations	Review of physical appropriation		
		good	fair	poor
1	Clearly visible		/	
2	Identifiable and cognitive		/	
3	Easily accessible, covered setting-down point from cars			/
4	The colour of around area not detracts from important signs.		/	
5	The color can be used on floors to help identify routes bring to the reception, waiting area ,lifts and departments			/

Table 2 Physical evaluation checklist of the hospital public zone specifically base on the seven principles of UD (person with disability)

No	Evaluation criteria	Review of physical appropriation within 7 UD principle and type of disability						
		UD1,D	UD2,D	UD3,D	UD4,D	UD5,D	UD6,D	UD7,D
1	Main entrance is clearly visible	/	/	/				
2	Easily accessible, covered setting-down point from cars	/	/	/				
3	A quick and ease of access	/	/	/				
4	The reception, information or help desk immediately apparent.	/	/	/				
5	The pathways can come and go affects utilization	/	/	/				

UD1=Equitable Use, UD2= Flexibility in use, UD3=Simple and intuitive use, UD4=Perceptible information, UD5= Tolerance for error, UD6= Low physical effort, UD7= Size and space for approach of use, D= 6 type of Disability

The results were analysed to show the source and extent of the problem areas and suggestions made to improve service accessibility.

3 Results and Discussion

The results of this research indicate that major obstructions occur in the communication and circulation spaces. The problem can be classified into two parts as follows: Firstly, the obstruction to general access consisting of congestion caused by people standing in communication spaces as shown in Figure 1. People standing in the queue at the reception point, where the line goes across the main hospital access corridor causes congestion and reduces easy access to other important departments in the hospital. This congestion creates a barrier to the passage of wheelchairs, patient trolleys, people with disability and ambulant people as well. In addition, the location and position of furniture shown in Figure 2, presents a barrier to communication spaces and access to other departments. Consequently, the visually impaired as well as wheelchair users face great difficulties in way finding, passing through spaces and accessing service points.

Poor way finding exacerbates the problem and slows down users who are unable to identify their present location or destination direction as seen in Figure 3.

Secondly, further obstructions are caused by inappropriate facilities for all types of disability; such as navigator devices for the blind, visual monitors for the deaf, inappropriate height of counters which causes difficulties wheelchair-users when communicating with staff etc. Interestingly, in some instances there are various devices present complying with compulsory regulations but because of the congestion problems these cannot be used effectively.

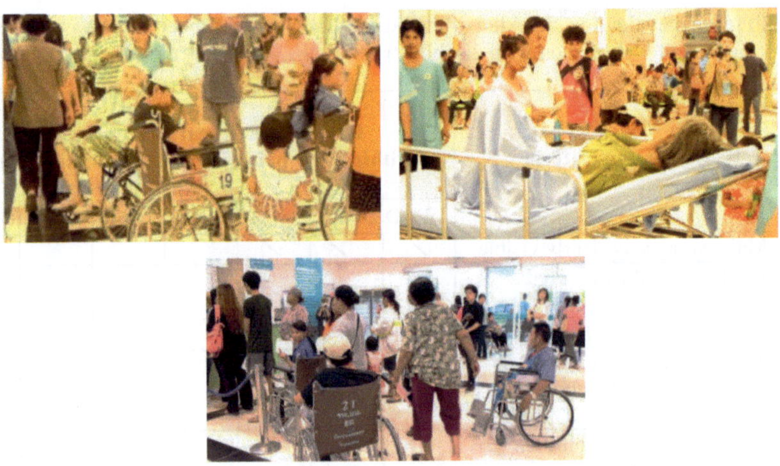

Fig. 1 Overcrowding at the main entrance area

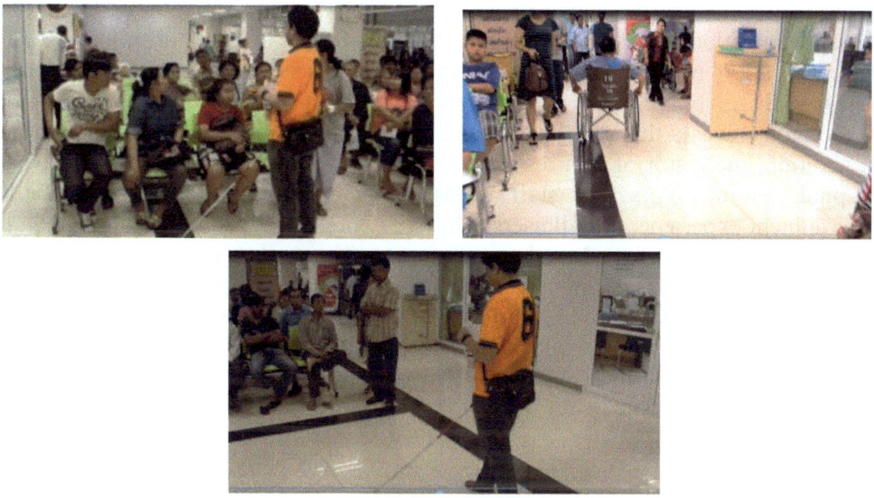

Fig. 2 Location of the waiting area (including seating)

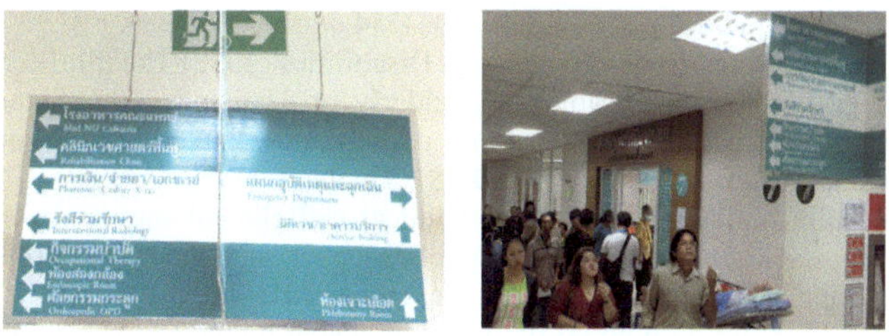

Fig. 3 Signs with small text in inappropriate locations

4 Conclusions

Imrie (2015) suggests that successful UD consists of the understanding of foundation concepts: institutionalization and practice; technical, product-base rationalities; and (disability) politics. This research has identified and classified potential problems and barriers to universal access in relation to persons with disabilities within the hospital public zones of the case study. On the face of it, the main problem appears to be overcrowding leading to congestion, but on further investigation, and given that the problems occur in spaces that conform to international best practice standards, it appears that operational issues (participation and technical, product-base practice)is, if not the main cause, at the very least contribute to access problems. These have been identified as: having queues crossing main communication routes; and having seated waiting areas immediately adjacent to communication routes, causing those unable to find a seat to stand and wait in the communication routes. This causes additional problems for disabled users with regard to physical passage and also inhibits easy wayfinding and restricts pedestrian flows. Better management of people using the space could easily rectify both of the above issues. Organizing queues so that they run parallel to communication spaces and providing waiting areas that do not obstruct the main communication routes could achieve this. The observations from this scenario access audit gives valuable information regarding the level of accessibility and furthermore reveals the additional requirements of users with physical limitation. In addition, the result of this research is able to highlight the issues identified to hospital administrators and staff to assist them in providing a better built-environment experience for all users. This study presents a process of evaluation to identify requirements for a broad range of users. The method operates by using the opinion of experienced designers and user participation. The results from this study provide important data for the in-depth investigation of the potential sources of access problems and solutions for future hospital design.

References

Adler D (1999) Metric handbook: Planning and design data. Architectural Press

Afacan Y, Erbug C (2009) An interdisciplinary heuristic evaluation method for universal building design. Applied Ergonomics 40: 731-744

Department of Empowerment of Persons with Disabilities (2012) The ministerial regulations regarding facilities for the disabled and elderly of Thailand 2005. Sample models of facility design for a person with disability and all ages, 2nd Edition. Ministry of Social Development and Human Security (MSDHS), Thailand

DoH (2013) Health building note 00-03: Clinical and clinical support spaces, pp. 66-68. Available at: www.gov.uk/government/publications/design-and-layout-of-generic-clinical-and-clinical-support-spaces (Accessed in November 2015)

DoH (2014) Health building note 00-01: General design guidance for healthcare buildings, pp. 27-46. Available at: www.gov.uk/government/publications/general-design-principles-for-health-and-community-care-buildings (Accessed in November 2015)

Imrie R (1999) The body, disability and Le Corbusier's conception of the radiant environment. In: Butler R, Parr H (Eds.) Mind and body spaces: Geographies of illness, impairment and disability, pp 25-45. Routledge, London, UK

Imrie R (2015) Socializing design and equitable living: Towards an assessment of the relevance of universal design. Lecture given on 20 October 2015 at Griffith University Queensland College of Art, Australia

Longo E (2012) Le relazionigiuridiche nel sistema dei diritti sociali. Profiliteorici e prassicostituzionali. CEDAM

Preiser WFE, Ostroff E (Eds.) (2001) Universal design handbook. McGraw-Hill, New York, NY, USA

Preiser WFE, Verderber S, Battisto D (2009) Assessment of health center performance: Toward the development of design guidelines. International Journal of Architectural Research (3)3: 21-44

Sahachaiseri N (2011) Universal design. Teaching documentary. King Mongkuk's Institute of Technology Ladkrabang, Thailand

Sahachaiseri N (2012) Sustainable design paradigm. Teaching documentary. King Mongkuk's Institute of Technology Ladkrabang, Thailand

Setola N, Borgianni S, Martinez M, Tobari E (2013) The role of spatial layout of hospital public spaces in informal patient-medical staff interface. In: Proceedings of the 9th International Space Syntax Symposium, Sejong University, Seoul, South Korea

Better Supporting Blind Pedestrians and Blind Navigation Technologies Through Accessible Architecture

M. Williams, B. Dubin, C. Amaefule, L. Nguyen, A. Abdolrahmani, C. Galbraith, A. Hurst and S. Kane

Abstract: Many assistive technology researchers motivate their blind navigation work based on navigation being difficult due to one's visual impairment. However, through our extensive navigation-related studies with 46 visually impaired adults we learned that architectural details and environmental designs are primarily what make navigation difficult, not one's disability. In this paper we expound on the ways that architecture both aids and hinders blind pedestrian navigation. We also propose architectural and environmental changes that would better support navigators and future technologies through accessible and standardized architecture. With this we also make a case for collaborations between technologists and architects (especially those focused on accessible architecture).

1 Introduction

There have been several proposed navigation technologies to aid people with severe visual impairments that are promisng and exciting for end users, for example, drones that guide a navigator and computer vision solutions that identify landmarks and obstacles (Cang et al. 2014, Folmer 2015). In proposing these solutions assistive technology researchers often present their motivation as if one's visual impairment is the sole reason navigation is difficult. While there are certainly physical impacts as a result of blindness, many of the reasons navigation is difficult are architectural design features and environments that lack inclusive and universal designs for people with vision impairments.

Exploring the design of navigation technology for people with vision impairments, we as technology and user interface researchers first conducted many qualitative exploratory studies to understand the current navigation strategies employed. Through phone interviews, real-world observations, focus groups, and diary studies with 46 adults with severe visual impairments we learned how people with vision impairments gather pertinent information about the environment

M. A. Williams (✉) · B. Dubin · C. Amaefule · L. Nguyen · A. Abdolrahmani · C. Galbraith · A. Hurst
University of Maryland, Baltimore County, MD, USA
email: mawilliams@umbc.edu

S. K. Kane
CU-Boulder, University of Colorado Boulder, CO, USA

P. Langdon et al. (eds.), *Designing Around People*,
DOI 10.1007/978-3-319-29498-8_25

through architectural details, often without the use of technology. However, we also noticed how architecture was as much a hindrance as an aid (such as Figure 1).

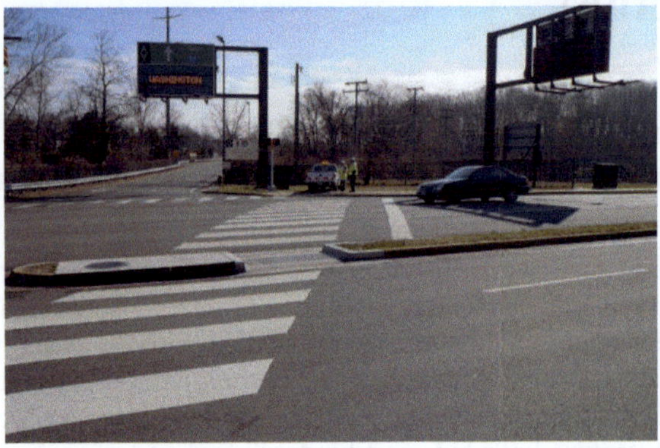

Fig. 1 Wheelchair accommodation in median seen during participant observation that makes street crossing difficult for blind navigators. An architectural change to remove/change this would more easily alleviate this tripping hazard than a technology built to detect and announce it.

Reflecting upon our findings, we also recognized that not only would accessible architecture aid pedestrians but also the technologies designed to assist them. Many technologies such as computer vision experience difficulties in development because of the overwhelming variations in what they detect. Accessible architecture would alleviate the need for certain technologies all-together by making the environment more discernible physically, and would help with detecting perpetually visual aspects, such as signage, by creating uniformity.

This paper includes our findings on how navigation is currently supported and hindered by architecture and proposes ways to better support blind navigators and their accompanying technologies through architectural changes. While accessible architecture may be seemingly unfamiliar to technologists, they are familiar to architects and those in universal design who have paid attention to this special population. Conversely, the benefits of accessible designs on both the pedestrians and their technologies are not seen within architecture research. Thus we also include a call for more collaboration amongst many applicable communities – including the blind community, architects, policy makers, and technologists.

2 Related Work

People with and without disabilities navigate within the same spaces; thus environments need to accommodate any pedestrian. Confident and safe independent travel for people with vision impairments results from legislated accommodations, specialized training, and commercial technology. Standardized structural accommodations include Braille labels on doorway entrances and audible pedestrian signals at busy intersections. Many of these features are a result of regulations specified in the Americans with Disabilities Act of 1990 (ADA 1990). "The skills needed to move safely and confidently through an environment are developed through instruction in Orientation and Mobility (O&M)." (MASB) O&M skills include *sensory development* (using non-visual senses for awareness), *white cane techniques* (how to glide or tap a cane to gain information as well as detect obstacles), and *utilizing landmarks* (turning sensory information into usable landmarks). If a person chooses to use a guide dog, they complete additional extensive training to learn how to give commands and understand body language (e.g., Guide Dogs for the Blind at: welcome.guidedogs.com/). Lastly, the most popular supplemental navigation technologies include GPS-based handheld devices such as the Trekker Breeze (store.humanware.com/hus/trekker-breeze-plus-handheld-talking-gps.html) and smartphone applications such as the Ariadne app (www.ariadnegps.eu/).

Independent travel is successfully implemented by blind people everyday, but there are still hindrances and hazardous (as discussed in our findings). For one, the ADA regulations have only two that directly address the needs of people with vision impairments as opposed to other physical disabilities - raised and Braille signage found primarily in Section 703. (Note that even the word "Braille" is misspelled in the regulations as having a lowercase "b".) Similar to the findings of Havik et al. (2012) who studied accessible "shared spaces" created in the Netherlands and Gomez et al. (2014) who studied workplace environments, our research has found that accessible architectural designs neglect or interfere with blind pedestrians. Also, while many blind navigation technologies have been proposed in research, only a few solutions are available and widely used commercially. There are any number of reasons why certain technologies are not widely adopted; however, one difference in the widely adopted technologies is government support and backing. GPS (www.gps.gov/) is a government-regulated technology with associated standards and technical support. Grassroot efforts to have businesses voluntarily outfit their structures or technologies attempting to detect information with no environmental consistency have proven more difficult to implement. Based on these current outcomes, it appears that higher-order organizational standards would not only help with O&M training but also with technology advancement.

Assistive technology has not been ignored in universal/inclusive design efforts. Chapters in "Universal Design" (Steinfeld et al. 2012) and "Inclusive Design" (Newell in Clarkson et al. 2003), for instance, not only report on architectural features that would benefit people with vision impairments but also review the latest technologies at the time of their publishing. However, these compilations do not readily integrate technology *with* architecture. Consistency in architectural features can aid in the reliability of technological detection as much as physical detection with a mobility aid or other senses. Thus we hope to inspire consensus and additions to regulations such as the ADA to improve independent blind navigation as well as the potential technologies that would support it.

3 Exploratory Navigation Studies

We conducted four exploratory studies with 46 participants total (25 female, ages 23-75); note four people participated in two studies (such as interview and observation). All had O&M training and used a mobility aid. We conducted *phone interviews* with 30 participants (14 female, ages 23-75) regarding O&M training, challenges in current navigation, and their use of navigation technology. We *observered* five participants (three female, ages 25-63) on diverse everyday tasks including a neighborhood stroll, mall shopping, and commuting home during an evening rush hour. We convened two *focus groups;* one group of eight (six female, ages 31-63) met once a month for six months in Washington, D.C. and the other group of seven (four female, ages 30-66) met once in Atlanta, Georgia. Focus group discussions expanded the interview topics. Focus group participants also submitted *diary entries* the month after the session(s). Diaries captured additional navigation experiences relayed upon further reflections. Findings from these studies were combined with research on O&M training to create a view of how navigation is currently accomplished.

4 Current Navigation Strategies and Obstacles

Following we present findings on how tactual, auditory, and olfactory cues are used to understand and navigate an environment. We also present ways in which sensory cues are unavailable or impeded.

4.1 Outdoor and Indoor Strategies

A white cane mobility aid provides both tactual and audible information; one can create informative echoes, determine boundaries, and identify the presence of a physical object (at least at ground level). One interview participant uses echoes to "tell how many feet away a wall is in a big building which sighted people find amazing". Differing cane techniques taught in O&M, such as gliding it along the ground or tapping it side-to-side, are used in differing environments. For instance, one interview participant explained "if it's a narrow sidewalk then I'll slide it continuously to make sure I'm not veering, but if it's a wide sidewalk then I'll tap." Veering is an important concept to note; people with vision impairments cannot walk straight without a tactual boundary as a guide.

Canes are for obstacle detection, guide dogs are for obstacle avoidance. While cane users intentionally tap objects to get information, dogs use their vision to avoid obstacles along the route. The tangible feedback from the dog's movement is then used to walk more freely in space. Dogs act upon owner command for turns and when to stop, intelligently overriding commands in face of danger (such as oncoming car). However, as one dog owning observation participant cautioned, "Good travelers still need good tehniques from O&M specialists. There's no shortcuts, you still need foundations like lining up in the street, listening to cars, and o'clock orientation." This means both guide dog and cane users are continually using information from other senses.

Sidewalks themselves are counted for travel (i.e., a location is 2 blocks away) but cues along the structure also help create a mental layout, inform and confirm a route, and set a safe walking boundary. Tactile cues included large and small stationary items (e.g., hydrants and bike racks) and changes in terrain (e.g., going up hill) used as landmarks. Cane users need tactile borders to walk straight and these were either designed structures (e.g., retaining walls) or created (e.g., using the difference in texture from grass to concrete). When available, the sidewalk's edge/curb is also a tangible feature used to keep from veering. Auditory cues included echolocation created by a tongue-click and/or white cane as well environmental sounds for landmarking. Sounds included distinct noises from businesses (e.g., a car wash), traffic noise (e.g. loud in industrial setting vs. quiet in residental setting), and people (e.g., kids playing near one observation participant wife's school). Olfactory cues primarily identified businesses such as bath product stores and coffee shops. Guide dogs are also attuned to smells; one diary participant's chiropractor also runs a cat rescue and he's knows he's near when his dog goes into "hunt mode" at their scent.

Intersections require a lot of concentration to navigate safely and avoid serious injury. For cane users, often corners are confirmed by poles (e.g. stop signs posts) and/or the curb cut. If an audible pedestrian signal is present this is certainly used to provide additional reassurance of when to start crossing. Participants explained that aligning at corners has changed with the addition of curb cuts but generally is to the left or right of the curb cut if it is placed in the center of the corner. Audible cues from traffic and other people help confirm when to cross (for instance, traffic should be moving parallel) but they also help to set a boundary against veering since painted crosswalks can't be seen (if traffic is moving closer or further then that indicates which direction you may be veering). Participants did not have formal techniques to address turning cars, however. An interview participant expressed a common sentiment that crossing is generally dangerous because "you can't make eye contact with the drivers".

Once inside, typically there is an initial open space encountered such as lobbies and main entrances. For these areas there are not many tactual cues available except perhaps a carpet by the doorway (a feature one diary participant found very helpful when present). Assessing what's around is primarily based on audible cues such as listening for elevator chimes or people talking at an information desk to understand the layout and how to navigate. Walking along closed spaces such as hallways is easier because of the physical boundaries and more prevalent auditory information. For instance, in a hallway it is possible to hear and feel doorways along the corridor and hear sounds from people inside the rooms. Rooms are also equipped with Braille labels and raised lettering for tactual location confirmation. To change floors, elevators are equipped with audible signals per the ADA requirements to announce their arrival and floors traversed. Escalators have an unintentional "hum" that many participants used to locate them, and used their hands on the railing or cane on the stairs to determine its direction. Detecting stairs was difficult if they were not out in the open or known to be behind a closed door.

While Braille labels would be available for stairwells, one has to know signage is there to know to look for the labels.

4.2 Obstacles That Impede Successful Navigation

Pedestrian navigation for people with vision impairments is well informed by O&M training and improved by accommodations such as audible pedestrian signals. Nevertheless, participants expressed numerous instances of lacking accommodations and environmental barriers.

Mobility aids provide a plethora of information but have limitations; most well-known is the inability to detect overhead objects because both a white cane and guide dog are ground-facing. It is unreasonable to constantly hold up one's hand so participants spoke of the constant hazard of hitting signs and tree branches. We also learned that waist-high objects with space underneath for wheelchairs, such as phone booths and water fountains, are easy to miss with a cane.

Construction is also a major obstacle for which mobility aids, one's senses, and even technology are ill-equipped to provide assistance. For cane users there are many obstacles including a lack of warning indicators (i.e., a non-visual equivalent for bright orange objects), caution tape is easy to miss, hitting an orange cone is not distinguishable from other objects (thus not conveying danger), and cones do not give an indication of which direction to move to avoid the obstacle (thus one may walk *into* construction rather than around). Even though guide dogs walk around construction, dog as well as cane users still need to understand the construction boundaries and if they need to use a different route at that time and in the future. Also, as one interviewee explained, although her dog once walked her around a hole (and a sighted person pointed it out as well) she was still very nervous because of the potential chance of falling. A focus group participant recounted falling into a man hole that was not bordered and he missed with his cane. Construction is also particularly difficult because it can either be silent (thus there are only visual indicators) or it is noisy (interfering with the use of auditory cues and potentially causing disorienting echoes).

Uneven sidewalk pavement and holes in the ground can be difficult to detect beforehand, causing a tripping hazard. Using changes in ground texture to keep from veering isn't always available if the textures don't change or if it's cold and grass feels hard like concrete. Using the curb as a boundary is not available if cars are parked or driving along the adjacent street and can also be difficult if it places a person along oncoming foot traffic. Where sidewalks are available but not "90 degree angles and straight paths", as one interview participant explained, routes quickly become complicated and require extensive memorization to navigate. They also become difficult to describe to others when needing to be dropped off by transit, as explained and experienced on one of our observations. Some areas do not have sidewalks (for instance in rural areas) or do not have raised sidewalks (only flat terrain visually distinguished by colors). For our participants that experienced these instances, they memorized their routes as much as possible and used GPS to alert of turns. GPS does not cover many of the off-road areas that have the complex or lacking sidewalk structures, however, such as college campuses and open shopping areas making independent navigation even more difficult if not impossible to do safely and reliably.

Audible pedestrian signals at intersections are not always available, do not have consistent audio interfaces, and do not indicate how much time is available for crossing. There are no alternatives to detect veering aside from other people or traffic noise making it more difficult to cross in quiet areas. Curb cuts do not provide a warning and the tactile pavement on the curb cut is not always discernible depending on footwear and walking speed. One diary participant noted he crossed a street once without even knowing it. Curb cuts also often interfere with a precise angle for street crossing alignment, often requiring multiple strategies for differing corners on a route. Designated crosswalks to use for systematic street crossing are also not always available, especially in open areas such as open shopping centers and parking lots. This was an area of grave concern for all of our participants because there were no reliable techniques available to confirm safe traversal.

Unlike doors inside, there are no Braille labels on outdoor signage and houses and GPS is not accurate to the exact door location. While there are strategies for learning open spaces indoors, all participants lamented that open areas are the hardest to navigate because they do not provide enough cues (tactual, audible, or olfactory) to be easily navigated. Closed spaces are easier to explore but using touch to learn detailed information is not always desirable or acceptable. For instance, feeling along public restroom walls for paper towel dispensers is "gross" (as one diary participant put it) and feeling for an open seat on a bench (and thus touching those seated) is not socially acceptable. Elevator chimes make changing floors easier but it has to be in-use to hear the audio cue and chimes are difficult to discern in a bank of elevators. One focus group participant expressed great frustration with the eight elevators at her workplace that "ding randomly" and do not allow enough time to arrive at the doors before they close and are dispatched elsewhere. Escalators and stairs in open areas do not have consistent tactual indicators before approaching them. The exit for elevators may exit a building at a different location than stairs and escalators, causing orientation issues.

5 Architecture Benefitting People and Technology

Focusing our findings on architecture as a navigation tool helped us realize how architectural and environmental accommodations would aid in the challenging scenarios as well as benefit navigation technologies. Accommodations and standardization could alleviate the need for technology all-together, help confirm technology output when used, and make the technology itself more accurate. In the following table we itemize specific significant challenges found in our exploratory studies, propose solutions based on user feedback and general design ideas and projected benefits for both people and technology.

Table 1 Navigation challenges, proposed solutions, and benefits to pedestrians with vision impairments and potential supplemental technologies

Obstacle	Proposed Architectural Change	Pedestrian Benefits	Technology Benefits
Lack of warning before curbs and stairs/escalators	Tactile warning strips	Safer and more reliable early detection	Aid computer vision to identify drop-offs
Veering during crossing highly undetectable	Ridged groove in crosswalk	Use cane in ridge to walk straight	Alleviate complex technology need
No crosswalks in open areas (e.g., shopping centers)	Require/Build crosswalks from street to sidewalk	Can use O&M proper techniques	Use structures to aid mapping and safe route detection
Audible pedestrian signals not universal & exclude timing	Mandate same audible feedback & time countdown	Eliminate memorization & know crossing time	Alleviate complex technology need
Audible signals not always present	Tactile indicator on poles or ground (e.g., to know if 2/3/4-way stop)	Independent determination of crossing structure	Detect corner landmark using indicator location
Medians in crosswalks not consistently designed	Clear crosswalk area or, if needed, use ramp rather than break in pavement	Remove potential tripping hazard	Alleviate complex technology need
Room layouts (esp. open areas) difficult to discern	Accessible directories & layout guides (e.g., floor tactile markers)	Quickly and independently understand layouts	Aid indoor mapping and eliminate privacy issues (e.g., in restrooms)
Detecting & navigating around construction and openings (e.g., cellar doors) is difficult	Require more & larger indicators in standard layout with tactual and/or audible info.	Safer detection and ability to avoid	Detect indicators more accurately
No accessible signage on outdoor structures	Braille and raised text on homes and businesses	Confirm location prior to entering	Find and read addresses more accurately
Restroom signage is not universal	Require/Design universal signage	More easily detect restrooms	More accurate detection
Stairs, escalators, elevators may exit at differing locations	Require/Regulate same exit locations	Alleviate dis-orientation, esp. in emergencies	Aid indoor mapping accuracy

6 Discussion

When we asked our D.C. focus group, "What do you use to help you navigate?", the entire group unanimously and emphatically answered, "Everything!" We certainly sought to gain more specific information to this question through our studies but after reviewing our findings we found the participants were not exaggerating much. It appears that while O&M Specialists do the best they can to teach clients how to utilize their environment to gain information, the strategies used in real-life often end up being haphazard and not very reliable. One observation participant explained that navigation is a "chicken and egg" problem where you need to use unique landmarks along every route but since you can't see them in a distance you have to know enough to know to look for it; each route must be recalled because recognizing a landmark is not sufficient. Another interview participant said that the "raw level of data is exhausting in urban settings; walking around is just no fun."

One Atlanta focus group participant particularly sparked our interest in inclusive architecture. He has traveled solo to several European and Asian countries and found it easier and much less stressful to navigate than in his U.S. home. Tactual features such as ridges in the ground mapping out train stations from door to train and audio features such as universally consistent audible pedestrian signals available at each street corner were items he said were desperately needed in the U.S. With that, we felt it important to explicitly list environmental-related obstacles and architectural design suggestions such as those he cited because these are items not seen in navigation technology research.

The Atlanta focus group participants, upon hearing what the international traveler relayed, longed for such accommodations but were insistent that architectural-related changes would not come without a strong and unified voice from the blindness community. We believe that not only should architects and blind navigators work together to make improvements, but technologists should join with them given the significant benefits to the technology and end users. Often times it appears that architectural changes are associated with people with mobility impairments, a group ironically not well represented in the ADA regulations. Even the common disability symbol in the U.S. is a wheelchair icon. As our research and much of the accessible architecture literature has shown, however, people with vision impairments need to be considered when designing for mobility and navigation because there are potentially severe consequences including tripping or falling, colliding with overhead or waist-level obstacles, and disorientation.

The need for standards is seen in a related navigation field – automotive innovations. Predecessors to the self-driving car such as blind-spot detection are currently commercially available. Consistency in the infrastructure (e.g., what a "car" and "road" looks like) is one aspect of how a teechnology can successfully learn and detect objects with enough accuracy to be approved for commercial use. Without consistent structures on sidewalks and buildings, will we as technology designers be able to build complex blind navigation devices that work successfully enough to be deployed for commercial use? We feel the answer is no.

7 Conclusion

For people with vision impairments, being able to walk independently and safely in complex outdoor and indoor environments has been tremendously improved by the formalization of O&M training, accommodations created by landmark legislation such as the ADA, and navigation technology such as GPS. However, there are still challenges and hindrances to completely safe and independent travel often presented by architectural designs. While exploring current navigation strategies before designing a navigation technology, we observed many of these hindrances firsthand. Accessible architecture and inclusive design literature include many design specifications for people with vision impairments but these designs are not present in real world environments. Additionally, we have not seen where technologists have shown the connection between architectural changes and the technology improvements that would result. Thus we first detailed our findings on how people with vision impairments currently navigate (often in a haphazard fashion despite the best efforts of O&M training). We then offered suggestions for architectural improvements beneficial to people with vision impairments and potential supplemental navigation technologies. We lastly presented a case for technologists to join in efforts with architects and the blindness community to advocate for policy changes and standardization in architectural regulations.

References

ADA (1990) Americans with disabilities act of 1990. Available at: www.ada.gov/archive/adastat91.htm (Accessed in November 2015)

Cang Y, Soonhac H, and Xiangfei Q (2014) A co-robotic cane for blind navigation. IEEE International Conference on Systems, Man and Cybernetics (SMC): 1082-1087

Folmer E (2015) Exploring the use of an aerial robot to guide blind runners. SIGACCESS Accessibility Computing Newsletter 112: 3-7

Gomez JL, Langdon PM, Bichard JA, Clarkson PJ (2014) Designing accessible workplaces for visually impaired people. In: Langdon PM, Lazar J, Heylighen A, Dong H (Eds.) Inclusive designing - Joining usability, accessibility, and inclusion. Springer

Havik EM, Melis-Dankers BJ, Steyvers FJJM, Kooijman AC (2012) Accessibility of shared space for visually impaired persons: An inventory in the Netherlands. British Journal of Visual Impairment 30(3): 132-148

MASB (n.d.) Orientation and mobility. Minnesota State Academy for the Blind. Available at: www.msab.state.mn.us/Programs/orientationmobility/ (Accessed in November 2015)

Newell A (2003) The future for ICT. In: Clarkson J, Coleman R, Keates S, Lebbon C (Eds.) Inclusive design: Design for the whole population. Springer

Steinfeld E, Maisel JL (2012) Universal design: Creating inclusive environments. Wiley & Sons, NJ, USA

Part VI
User Profiling and Visualising Inclusion

Assets, Actions, Attitudes: Hearing and Vision Impaired Mobile Technology Personas

J. T. Morris and J. L. Mueller

Abstract: Designers and engineers utilize personas and user profiles to give life and substance to user research findings. The pace of development and diffusion of mobile wireless technologies make modeling of consumer profiles ever more critical, especially for people with disabilities, for whom mobile technology can be either empowering or disenfranchising. Fueled by global competition and government policy in the US and elsewhere, inclusive design has become a priority for wireless device manufacturers, software engineers, and service providers. This paper discusses the development and use of personas as a critical tool to help stakeholders (the technology industry, regulators, designers and students) understand the needs and preferences of customers with disabilities, and to raise awareness of the importance of designing for people with disabilities – in short, to visualize inclusion. The paper presents data from the biennial Survey of User Needs, a national survey in the United States conducted by the Rehabilitation Engineering Research Center for Wireless Technologies (Wireless RERC). Data are presented on the assets, actions/activities and attitudes of 4 groups of survey respondents: blind, low vision, deaf and hard of hearing. These data inform the development of a user type for each group. Regular interaction with wireless customers with disabilities has enabled us to "flesh out" these user types to help its industry partners better understand their customers with disabilities.

1 Introduction

For people of all ages and abilities, independence and social inclusion are fundamental to health of both body and mind. As mobile wireless technology evolves, equitable access becomes increasingly essential to personal independence, social inclusion and employability. Many consider access to mobile wireless technology a basic human right. Indeed, the United Nations (2006) Convention on the Rights of Persons with Disabilities (CRPD) states that parties to the convention agree to: "undertake or promote research and development of, and to promote the availability and use of new technologies, including information and

J. T. Morris (✉) · J. L. Mueller
Rehabilitation Engineering Research Center for Wireless Technologies, Atlanta, GA, USA
email: john_morris@shepherd.org

P. Langdon et al. (eds.), *Designing Around People*,
DOI 10.1007/978-3-319-29498-8_26

communications technologies, mobility aids, devices and assistive technologies, suitable for persons with disabilities, giving priority to technologies at an affordable cost" (Article 4).

This article discusses the development and use of personas to guide designers and engineers in developing solutions for people with sensory limitations: blindness, low vision, deafness and/or hard-of-hearing. Personas are presented for each limitation, based on data from the Survey of User Needs (SUN), a national survey in the United States on use and usability of mainstream mobile wireless technology by people with disabilities, conducted by the Rehabilitation Engineering Research Center for Wireless Technologies (Wireless RERC).

2 Personas and Mobile Technology

In his book on designing for users, The Inmates are Running the Asylum (2004), Alan Cooper described how effective personas can be when used in the product development process, and how dismally design can fail when users are denied a voice in the product development process. Cooper described a fundamental difference between designing for "users" and designing for personas: Users have few demands and are expected to be "elastic" – to "bend and stretch" to accommodate the design. Personas, on the other hand, are clear, specific expressions of users' characteristics and demands, so that the design can be adapted to meet these needs.

Because personas are compilations of many real people, their presence in the design process is personal and engaging. Designers pay attention to the needs expressed by personas, rather than assuming their customers will simply adapt to their designs. Personas focus on real users and their needs, so that designers do not fall into the common trap of designing only for themselves. Since few designers have disabilities, this focus is especially important in designing mobile wireless products that acommodate the needs of customers with disabilities.

Over the years social science researchers and technology marketers have identified user types and personas of mainstream consumers in various ways. Some have been based on a technology platform, others on the operating system, such as Blackberry, iOS, Android (Morris and Mueller 2014). Others start with the brand of smartphone (e.g., iPhone), and try to identify personal qualities of owners. One wry, but apt, typology identifies seven iPhone user types, including: Fanboy, Unappreciative, Over User, Desk Job, Hacker, Senior Citizen and Complainer (OMG Mugshots 2014).

A study by the Pew Research Center (2007) went beyond devices and operating systems to identify several distinct technology user types based on its own survey research. Development of these user types began with technology ownership and use (referred to as "assets), adding activities that users engage in with their technology ("actions"), as well as their perceptions of how technology impacts their work, family and leisure pursuits ("attitudes").

The Pew's typology of technology users in the general population comprises three general categories (Elite users, Middle-of-the-road users, and Few Tech

Table 6 Attitudes: Most common single word descriptors for your wireless device, by disability type

	Most common	**2nd**	**3rd**	**4th**	**5th**
Deaf (none 6%)	Great, awesome, addicted, all encompassing (20%)	Functional, handy, helpful, useful (15%)	Survival, safety, emergencies, confident (15%)	Important, irreplaceable, necessary (8%)	Underused, just a device, does bare minimum (8%)
Hard of hearing (none 5%)	Fantastic, miracle, amazing, wonderful (14%)	Convenient, handy, helpful, useful (14%)	Vital, needed essential, important, lifeline (13%)	Good, fair, satisfactory, okay, adequate (10%)	Complicated, annoying, frustrating (4%)
Blind	Great, amazing, wonderful, (40%)	Useful (33%)	Frustrated (7%)	Accessible (7%)	Decent (7%)
Low vision (none 8%)	Amazing, fantastic, magical, addicted, love (23%)	Frustrating, challenging limited, shortsighted (9%)	Essential, necessary, needed (7%)	Handy, useful (7%)	Adequate, satisfied, okay, reasonable (7%)

4.1 Vision and Hearing Impaired User Types and Personas

Here we summarize the survey research data on assets, actions and attitudes presented above into a single broad user type for each of the four disabilities discussed:

- **Deaf: Pragmatic omnivores (omni-mobiles?)**–Many have difficulty being understood when speaking; very high rate of ownership of smart devices; highest ownership of tablets. Though they state that their devices are easy to use, respondents report lowest satisfaction among the four groups – likely a result of deaf users' ability and desire to do even more with their devices. Despite lowest rates of usage for work, many regard devices as tools, including for safety and security.
- **Hard of Hearing: Hearing technology integrators/selective users**–Highest mean age in sample; most have hearing aids or cochlear implants; lower use of smart devices than blind and deaf users; lowest rate of usage for work. Like low vision users, these users have the lowest rates of use of top 5 device functions.

- **Blind: Mobile dependent enthusiasts**–Few of these users report other disabilities. All have wireless devices: 100% own smartphones and use screen reader technology, but have lowest ownership of tablets among this group. Use of the top five functions are the highest among the four groups; lowest rate for ease of use, but highest satisfaction (likely resulting from recognition of the critical role of technology in supporting their independence); strong positive feelings for devices.
- **Low Vision: Multiply challenged selective users**–This group has by far the highest rates for having other physical, emotional and cognitive difficulties among the four groups; low rates of use of top five device functions similar to hard of hearing users; high rate of usage for work, second to blind users; highest rate of non-response to singe-word descriptor for device (21%).

Other demographic and contextual characteristics can significantly impact use of mobile technology. We apply these additional chracteristics to "flesh out" the user types into recognizable personas. Table 7 presents one persona for each user type based on conversations with participants in our focus group research.

The user types and personas presented here offer a unique – but not exclusive – perspective on the needs, hopes, challenges, feelings and frustrations of individuals representing four disability types. Additional segmentation of the respondents in each group would offer still more sharply defined personas.

5 Conclusion

User types and personas must necessarily change as technology evolves. For example, wireless pagers represented an important mobile communications innovation for deaf users in the 1990s and early 2000s. A decade later, they had all but disappeared from the technology landscape. Simple mobile phones (referred to as "feature phones" by the U.S. wireless industry) still hold some market share, with a number of companies offering them as solutions for seniors (e.g., Tracfone, GreatCall Jitterbug, Doro PhoneEasy 626). But these simple phones have long since ceded their hold on the general market and public consciousness.

Initially, smartphones posed challenges to people with certain limitations. Until the advent of Apple's VoiceOver and Android's TalkBack screenreaders, blind users struggled with the tactilely featureless surface of touchscreens. Users with low sensitivity in their fingertips or limited hand control struggled to adjust to the precision of touchscreen interfaces. At the same time, some people with developmental disabilities gravitated toward touchscreen tablets, particularly Apple's iPad, which provided the platform for low cost speech generation for those with complex communication needs or limited motor function.

Table 7 Hearing and vision impaired mobile technology personas

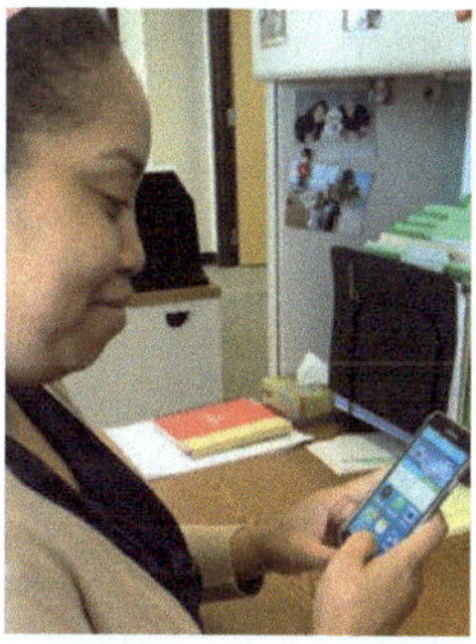	**SAMANTHA** is deaf. She works as an administrator at a primary school for deaf children. She considers wireless access essential to her lifestyle. She lives in the city, has a wide circle of friends, and stays active in local community affairs and events. Sam relies on her smartphone for communication at work – video calls, text messaging, email. She owns a Samsung Galaxy S5 mobile phone because of its large screen and relative affordability among high-end smartphones. In her leisure time, Sam enjoys watching YouTube and other videos on her tablet.
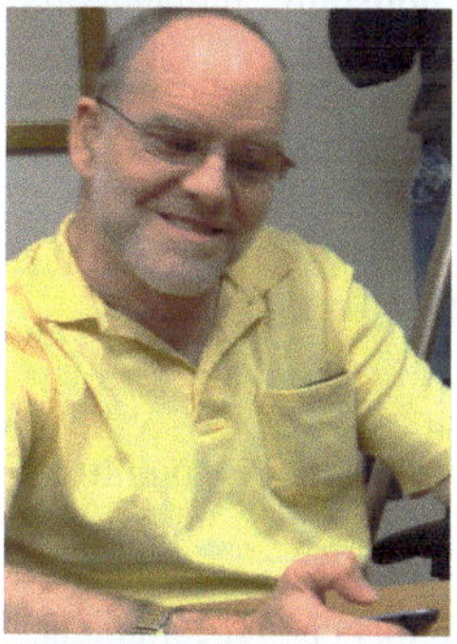	**KURT** is hard of hearing. He has uses bilateral hearing aids and corrective lenses for age-related loss of visual acuity and hearing. He is retired after a long career in the federal government. Kurt finally bought his first smartphone many years after they came to dominate the marketplace. He likes the many features. But he mainly uses just voice and text-based communications. Kurt loves music and has a large collection, but prefers to listen on his powerful home system.
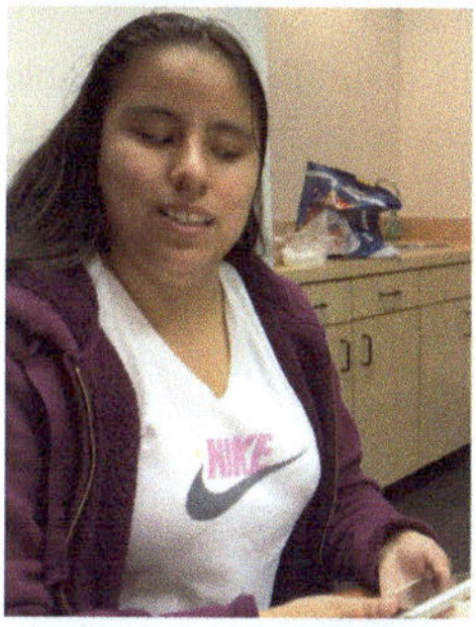	**LORENA** is 24 years old and has been blind since a young age. She is studying to be a voice-writing court stenographer and will work as an independent service provider upon graduation. She's an avid book reader, using mobile app on her on her "amazing" iPhone 5s. Lorena uses VoiceOver to navigate her iPhone's touchscreen, which has enabled her to listen to her music library on iTunes, surf the web, send/receive text messages/emails, check weather, read news, navigate the city, and request/track location of paratransit buses provided by the city transit agency.
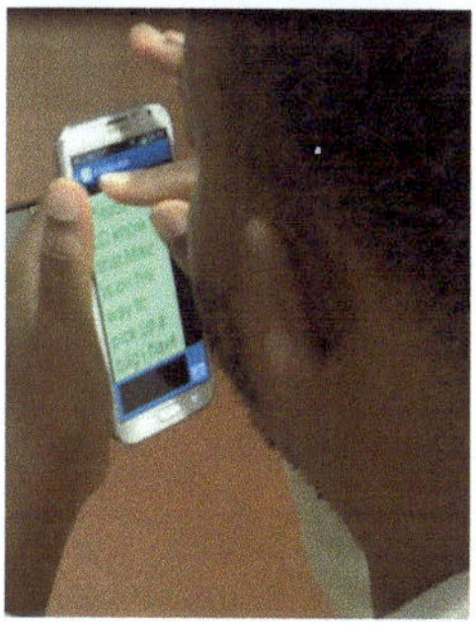	**HOWARD** is a 30 year old social worker and is legally blind due to diabetic retinopathy, which also causes him glare sensitivity. Diabetes has also limited the sensivity in his fingers. Although his vision loss, which began in his late teens, slowed his educational progress, he is currently studying to be a lawyer. Howard uses an Android-based smartphone with a 6-inch screen, on which he uses large-text and reverse contrast display options. Though he can use all functions on his smartphone at work, he prefers his tablet and laptop for leisure activities requiring vision.

The wireless landscape continues to change in evolutionary as well as disruptive ways. Amid this changing landscape, personas will continue to be an effective vehicle for directing industry focus to real customers with and without disabilities. The Wireless RERC continues to adapt the personas described in this paper to assist designers and engineers in meeting the challenges and opportunities presented by new technology and an increasingly inclusive society.

References

CDC (n.d.) Centers for Disease Control and Prevention. National health interview survey. Available at: www.cdc.gov/nchs/nhis.htm (Accessed in November 2015)

Cooper A (2004) The inmates are running the asylum. SAMS Publishing, Indianapolis, IN, USA

Mueller J (2004) Getting personal with universal. IDSA INNOVATION 23: 21-28

Mueller J, Jones M, Broderick L, Haberman V (2005) Assessment of user needs in wireless technologies. Assistive Technology 17: 57-71

Morris J, Mueller J (2014) Blind and deaf consumer preferences for Android and iOS smartphones. In: Langdon PM, Lazar J, Heylighen A, Dong H (Eds.) Inclusive Designing: Joining usability, accessibility and inclusion, pp 69-79. Springer

OMG Shots (2014) The 7 different types of iPhone users – Which one are you? Available at: omgshots.com/2328-the-7-different-types-of-i-phone-users-which-one-are-you.html (Accessed in November 2015)

Pew Research Center (2007) A typology of information and communication technology users. Available at: www.pewinternet.org/2007/05/06/a-typology-of-information-and-communication-technology-users/ (Accessed in November 2015)

United Nations (2006) Convention on the rights of persons with disabilities. Available at: www.un.org/disabilities/convention/conventionfull.shtml (Accessed in November 2015)

United States Census Bureau (2014) American community survey. Available at: www.census.gov/programs-surveys/acs/ (Accessed in November 2015)

Preliminary Findings from an Information Foraging Behavioural Study Using Eye Tracking

J. Chakraborty, M. P. McGuire and G. Pandey

Abstract: Cognitive overload can be a serious impediment in the assimilation of information for all types of users. Research has demonstrated the usefulness of adaptive interfaces in reducing cognitive overload by providing an interface that automatically reacts to the end users' information foraging behavior. In order to understand and compare behaviors and patterns (between sighted and low vision users), it is necessary to understand the information seeking behavior of sighted users for any patterns that may exist as a baseline. These findings can then be compared to data on low vision users in a future study. In this study, eye tracking is used to explore information seeking behavior of visual users. In particular, we compare the gaze patterns of users when using both a traditional interface and complex interface to identify current events of interest. The eye tracking data was analyzed using kernel density statistics and correlation analysis to determine if relationships exist between information seeking behavior, task completion and accuracy. Results show that information seeking behavior tends to be more efficient and accurate when using the traditional interface and that a more complex interface introduces additional cognitive overload.

1 Introduction

With the increasing popularity of social and news media, analyzing information has become very challenging for all users. Various sorting algorithms applied to the interfaces in social and news media websites are meant to assist end users with sorted views of information under classifications such as World News or Business News. These pre-sorted topics are typically found in structured menus on the left, top or bottom of interfaces depending on regional or cultural preferences. As a result of extended interactions with these structured interfaces, end users have become conditioned to set information foraging behaviors. However, the information processing steps are much less efficient for low vision users who rely on screen magnification. Zooming into various areas of the screen amplifies the

J. Chakraborty (✉) · M. P. McGuire · G. Pandey
Towson University, Towson, MD, USA
email: jchakraborty@towson.edu

P. Langdon et al. (eds.), *Designing Around People*,
DOI 10.1007/978-3-319-29498-8_27

risk of cognitive overload. As a result, low vision users tend to process information less efficiently in comparison (Conradie et al. 2015, Fung et al. 2015).

There is a need for improved interfaces for categorizing and visualizing topics and entities and their semantic relationships based on the users' preferences and abilities. Several research studies have shown that adaptive interfaces specifically designed for an end user can ultimately be more effective and efficient (Norcio and Stanley 1989, Pirolli and Card 1999, Salvucci and Anderson 2000, Pirolli 2005, Pirolli 2007). In situations where information is moving fast and the misinterpretation of information can be costly, it is even more important to have the ability to visualize communications in an effective and efficient manner. Data gathered using eye tracking equipment and analyzed for possible patterns can be a useful tool for interface designers tasked with developing interfaces for exploring large amounts of information. The use of such techniques can offer the ability to understand how an end user interprets a visualization to find useful information, thereby promoting the goals of universal and inclusive design (Fletcher et al. 2015, Waller et al. 2015). These goals include the design of a wide range of accessible tools or interfaces for the elderly and people with different abilities. The development of adaptive interfaces can meet these user requirements.

The aim of this pilot study is to collect baseline data of sighted end users' efficiency and effectiveness of information foraging behavior through comparisons of search patterns on a structured news site versus an unstructured news site using eye tracking. We aim to run a second similar study using low vision end users to compare our findings. We define a structured news site as one containing a fixed number of news categorizations such as World News, Business News and Sport News and arranged in grid-like menus typically found at the top, left or bottom of the website. These sites would also have a limited selection of font sizes and colors in the links. We identified Google News (news.google.com) as a good example of an English speaking, structured news site as it met all the criteria. We define an unstructured news site as one that does not contain a pre-fixed number of news categorizations arranged in any particular order such as menus at the top, left or bottom of the website. The font sizes as well as the colors of the links would vary across the website. We identified Newsmap (www.newsmap.jp) as a good example of an English speaking, unstructured news site as it too met all the criteria.

Spatio-Temporal data mining techniques are used to analyze users' gaze patterns and Kernel Density plots are compared. Users' efficiency and effectiveness of foraging for information will be collected. This study will be replicated using low vision users engaged with these structured and unstructured website at a later time. The data will be compared against the baseline reading from this study to determine whether there are significant differences between sighted and low vision users when using Google News and Newsmap. The findings from the comparative study can be used to develop a software engineering understanding of the necessary accessibility requirements to enable low vision users equal opportunities in information foraging.

The remainder of this paper is as follows. Section 2 provides a brief summary of the literature in adaptive interfaces and data mining. Section 3 outlines the experimental design carried out using vision users engaging with the eye tracking equipment. Sections 4 and 5 discuss the data analysis techniques and the Kernel Density results from the eye tracking study. Section 6 discusses the implications of our findings. Finally, sections 7 and 8 draws some conclusions from our study, including some of the limitations of this research, and suggest some future directions based on the findings.

2 Background

Adaptive interfaces have been proposed as a solution to deal with cognitive overload (Norcio and Stanley 1989) and information gathering (Pirolli and Card 1999, Pirolli 2005, Pirolli 2007, Putze et al. 2013). Research applying Miller's (1956) principles has shown promise in increasing information comprehension (Denenberg et al. 2005). The analysis of human eye movements has historically been used in human computer interaction research to evaluate the design of interfaces and numerous eye tracking metrics have been used (Jacob and Karn 2003). Over the last few decades, a great deal of progress has been made in the analysis of human-computer interfaces using eye tracking technology (Duchowski 2007). However, limited research has been carried out to understand user preferences of low vision end users using eye tracking technology. Bonavero et al. (2015) developed an algorithm, Non-dominated Sorting Genetic Algorithm II (NSGA-II) to be tested on specific webpages to assist low vision users in adapting to web pages. Aziz et al. (2015) developed a conceptual design of an Assistive Courseware for Low Vision (AC4LV) through expert review and prototyping to assist low vision learners use assistive technology.

3 Experiment Design

Ten Computer Science students aged 18-22 were recruited as sighted participants for this pilot study through advertisements around the Computer and Information Sciences department at Towson University. The students responded to the advertisement and were invited to participate in the study. Of these students, six were male and four were female. Each participant met with the principal investigator individually in the lab for the experiment. The study was carried out in a PC based computer lab with one installation of the Tobii X2 eye tracking equipment.

Each participant signed an IRB permission form after the study was explained carefully. For the first stage of the study, each user was required to go through a calibration exercise using the Tobii eye tracker. Upon successful calibration, the user was ready to begin the experiment and the Tobii X2 studio was started to record their eye gaze. The user was asked to open the Mozilla browser on the desktop and browse to a news website. Five users were asked to first browse to news.google.com (Figure 1) and the other five were asked to browse to www.news-map.jp (Figure2). Upon arriving at the first website, the user was asked to search through the site and identify the top three stories in the categories of World News, Business News and Sports, in the user's opinion, and share the answers aloud with the investigator. The answers were recorded from P2-P11 by the investigator and checked for correctness against the corresponding news categories on the website.

P1 was a pilot study for whom the data was not counted.

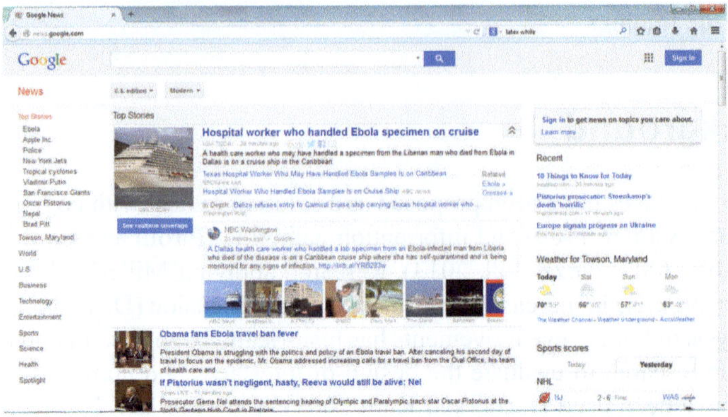

Fig. 1 Google News user interface (http://news.google.com)

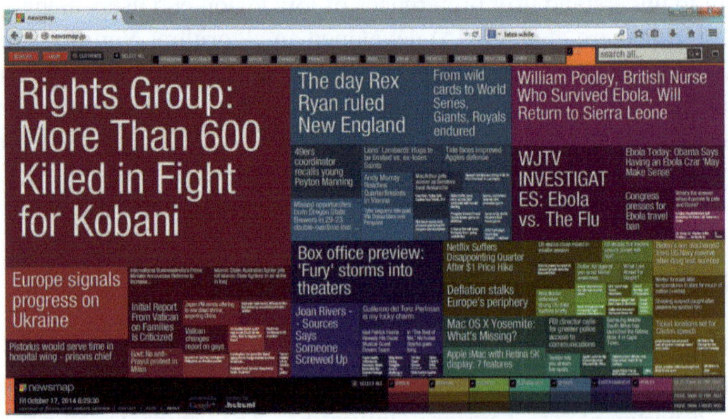
Rights Group: More Than 600 Killed in Fight for Kobani
The day Rex Ryan ruled New England
From wild cards to World Series, Giants, Royals endured
William Pooley, British Nurse Who Survived Ebola, Will Return to Sierra Leone
WJTV INVESTIGATES: Ebola vs. The Flu
Europe signals progress on Ukraine
Box office preview: 'Fury' storms into theaters
Deflation stalks Europe's periphery
Mac OS X Yosemite: What's Missing?
Joan Rivers - Sources Says Someone Screwed Up
newsmap

Fig. 2 Newsmap user interface (http://Newsmap.jp)

Upon completion, the user was asked to browse to the alternate website (from Google News to Newsmap or Newsmap to Google News) to identify the top three stories in the categories of World News, Business News and Sports, in the user's opinion. As with the first website, the answers were said out loud and were recorded by the investigator who checked for their correctness using the color coded news categorization used by the website

At the end of each of participants' experiment session, the recording on the Tobii Studio was stopped and participant data was saved for analysis. All ten participants successfully navigated through both the websites and provided answers to the investigator. The correct answers were not shared with the participants.

4 Data Analysis

The eye tracking data in this study included the following measurements: time stamp, gaze point classification (fixation, saccade, and unclassified), gaze point duration, gaze point x coordinate, and gaze point y coordinate. The gaze point classification was calculated using the I-VT filter available in the Tobii Studio software. The eye tracking data was analyzed using both statistical and data mining methods. Statistical methods including two dimensional (spatial) and one dimensional kernel estimation statistics were used to assess the density of gaze points in the eye tracking data for each participant. Spatio-Temporal clustering was then used to provide a finer grained analysis of the data.

Gaze point density was estimated using one dimensional and two dimensional kernel density estimation. One dimensional kernel density was also calculated individual for the x and y dimension of the screen. This estimate gives a finer grained analysis of the data where we can see the kernel density estimate for each user and determine where in either the x or y dimension their gaze is focused. The one dimensional kernel density estimator for the x dimension is given by the following equation:

$$k_{h(x)} = \frac{1}{2\pi h_x} exp\left[-\frac{1}{2}\left(\frac{x - x_i}{h_x}\right)^2\right]$$

Where K denotes the kernel function and h is the bandwidth parameter. In this study the Gaussian kernel function is used. The two dimensional or spatial kernel density used in the study calculates the density of the gaze points in a neighborhood around the same feature. It is an extension of the one dimensional kernel density calculation above and can be used to find the density of a set of spatial points. The spatial kernel density estimator is given by the following equation:

$$k_{h(x)} = \frac{1}{2\pi h_x h_y} exp\left[-\frac{1}{2}\left(\frac{x - x_i}{h_x}\right)^2 - \frac{1}{2}\left(\frac{y - y_i}{h_y}\right)^2\right]$$

5 Results

Kernel density statistics were calculated for the eye tracking results for each participant for each interface. To do this, the gaze points for Google News were separated from the gaze points for Newsmap and the kernel density was calculated separately for each file. In this section, the spatial kernel density will be presented for each user to show the overall gaze pattern.

5.1 Spatial Kernel Density

The spatial kernel density for Google News is presented in Figure 3. The figure shows that the participants largely focused on the left portion of the screen for Google News. Participants 7, 9, and 11 largely focused on two areas on the left portion of the screen whilst the rest of the participants focused on one area. This difference might be produced by different scrolling patterns of the participants. Also, participants 7, 9, and 11 show an additional gaze focus on the very left side of the screen. This is where the context menu is located on Google News. These participants were observed using the context menu to aid in finding stories under each of the three categories.

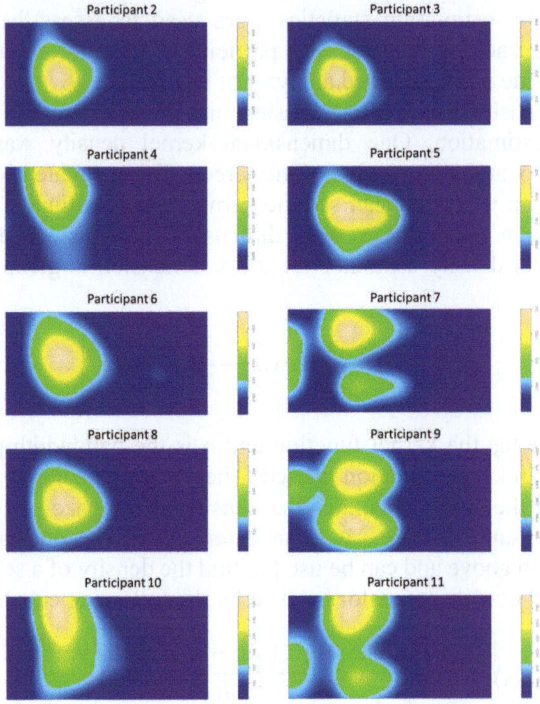

Fig. 3 Two dimensional kernel density for Google News

The spatial kernel density results for Newsmap are presented in Figure 4. This figure shows a strikingly different search pattern than that shown in Google Maps where participants tended to focus on different parts of the screen. Participants 2, 4, 5, and 6 focused on the right side of the screen. This could be due to the smaller font in the News Map interface for stories shown in this area and these participants could have placed more effort in reading these less important stories. Participants 8 and 9 showed a much more dispersed pattern of gaze. These users may have been confused by the interface and were not able to initially find the information that they were seeking causing them to focus on multiple areas.

In comparing the spatial kernel density between Google News and Newsmap, a very different type of visual search is shown. The pattern for Google News shows that the participants were able to focus on one area of the screen and use scrolling to find the information that they were looking for. Then, when presented with Newsmap which is a more complex interface that attempts to show the news in a single screen, the participants had to search more of the screen to find the information that they were looking for. This resulted in a more unconventional search pattern and therefore results were highly variable across participants.

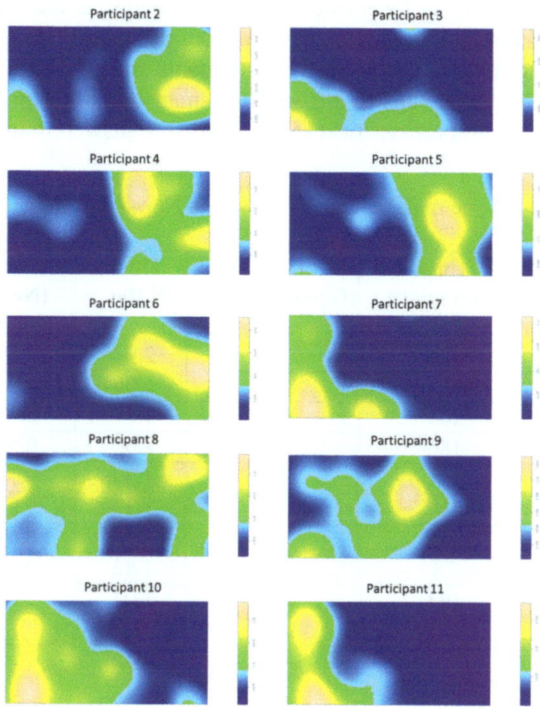

Fig. 4 Two dimensional kernel density for Newsmap

5.2 Assessment of Time to Complete Task and Accuracy

During the experiment, the time to complete task the task and the accuracy of the participant were also measured. The time and accuracy are presented in Table 1. The table includes measurements of the time to complete the task in seconds for both Google News and Newsmap, the time ratio which is time to complete the task for Newsmap divided by the time to complete the task for Google News. During the experiment, it was also noticed that participants 3, 7, 10, and 11 found the context menu in the bottom right portion of the Newsmap interface. This aided them to accurately find stories under the desired categories and therefore their accuracy was much higher for Newsmap.

The time to complete the task for Newsmap was generally longer than that for Google News with the exception of participant 11. Also, the participants were generally more accurate in identifying the appropriate news stores with Google News. It is notable that the participants who found the context menu in Newsmap were all 100% accurate. The time ratio is comparatively lower for participants who were able to figure out the menu on both Newsmap and Google News. They had a perfect accuracy in terms of correctly dividing the news as per the categories. Participant 5 took the longest time to answer the questions with Newsmap as compared to that of Google News and still had the most inaccurate answers. This suggests that this participant had a higher level of cognitive overload than the other participants. Also, participant 5 answered Google News questions in the 70 seconds which is faster than average time (115.7s) taken by participants and got the perfect accuracy. On the other hand, s/he took 186s to answer Newsmap queries which was longer than the average time for all participants (156.1s) and still answered only 3 out of 9 questions correctly.

Table 1 Time ratio for Google News and News Map and impact on accuracy

Participant #	Time (Newsmap)	Time (Google News)	Time Ratio	Accuracy (News Map)	Accuracy (Google News)
2	226	109	2.07	0.89	1
3	129	121	1.06	1	1
4	164	120	1.37	0.67	1
5	186	70	2.65	0.33	1
6	167	120	1.39	0.78	1
7	94	76	1.27	1	1
8	219	156	1.4	0.67	0.89
9	78	55	1.42	0.89	1
10	193	180	1.07	1	1
11	105	150	0.7	1	1

6 Discussion

The results indicate that by using Google News end users were able to achieve higher rates of accuracy in their searches than using Newsmap. The Kernel density plots indicate that users on Google News searched for the top three stories (World News, Business News and Sports News) by primarily searching through the tables on the left column of the website (www.news.google.com). When the plots are compared to the Newsmap website (www.newsmap.jp), the Kernel density plots are not as closely defined, implying that the users' had to conduct searches not primarily based on any part of the screen but rather on personal search patterns. The results also suggest that by using Google News users' found answers to their searches faster than by using Newsmap. The Kernel density plots of both sets of searches support this finding as well. Users' spent more time on the left column of Google News searching for answers while users spent more time searching all over Newsmap for answers.

The findings from this study suggest that end users could potentially benefit from the use of adaptive interfaces that are structured and unstructured. By offering more customizable interface design options towards the end users' preferences and abilities, it is possible to improve efficiency and effectiveness in search behavior. These adaptive interfaces could potentially reduce cognitive overload and thereby reduce costly errors.

7 Conclusions and Limitations

The aim of this research was to collect a baseline of visual user behaviors when conducting searches using a structured versus an unstructured news site and compare the findings from a future study using users with low vision. We collected eye gaze data from ten computer science students using eye tracking and used Tobii Studio to search for gaze patterns. Our findings showed that visual end users performed better with structured news sites.

However, although users performed better with the structured website than the unstructured website, we cannot attribute the level of performance solely to the structure of the website. It could be argued that the end users' search pattern was a result of conditioned behavior based on experience with structured websites. In addition, it can be seen that nearly all users were able to find correct answers using both websites. This suggests that given time to familiarize with an unstructured interface, users could adapt and develop efficient and effective search patterns.

The findings from this study indicate that the participants, computer science students aged 18-22, were able to use the structured website more easily than the unstructured website to conduct searches. Unfortunately, this sample size is not a representation of the general 18-22 year population or computer science students. It could be argued that users with limited internet browsing and searching experience could find unstructured websites more effective tools as the users would not be inhibited by any conditioned behavior. Conversely, one could argue that users with extensive internet browsing and search experience could also find unstructured websites more effective tools as a result of their conditioned behavior.

Other limitations of the study could be memory recall. The participants' response to the top three news stories in the categories of World News, Business News, and Sport for each website (Google News and Newsmap) could have been affected by the order in which they used the websites. For example, the users who went the Google News first could have simply been searching for the world, business, and sport news that were identified in by the categorizations in Google News. Conversely, the users that went to Newsmap first could have been searching for similar stories on Google News. The sample size used in this study was not large enough to try a randomized ordering.

8 Future Directions

With the increasing popularity of social and news media, analyzing information has become very challenging. This problem is acutely experienced by users who have limited vision. Low vision users are heavily reliant on standardized equipment such as a magnified screen with limited customization options, in comparison to blind users with no residual vision who can only use audio or tactile output. As a result, partially blind users will often deal with sensory overload as they try to engage with various standardized interfaces using magnification only. It would be very interesting to measure efficiency and effectiveness in information foraging using Google News and Newsmap with low vision users. Using the findings from this study as a baseline, we can compare the user behaviors of sighted and low vision participants. As a continuation of this study, we will use participants who self-identify as low vision and familiar with internet searches to replicate the study using the Tobii eye tracker. We hope to collect Kernel Density points of data from these users information foraging behavior to compare against the baseline data. Based on the findings of user preferences, we can begin to develop a software engineering understanding of the necessary usability/accessibility requirements to enable low vision users equal opportunities in information foraging.

References

Aziz N, Mutalib AA, Sarif SM (2015) Conceptual design model of assistive courseware for low vision (AC4LV) learners. In: Proceedings of the 2014 International Conference on Advances in Education Technology, Bandung, Indonesia

Bonavero Y, Huchard M, Meynard M (2015) Reconciling user and designer preferences in adapting web pages for people with low vision. In: Proceedings of the 12th Web for All Conference, Florence, Italy

Conradie P, De Marez L, Saldien J (2015) Participation is blind: Involving low vision lead users in product development. In: Proceedings of the International Conference on Software Development and Technologies for Enhancing Accessibility and Fighting Info-exclusion, Sankt Augustin, Germany

Denenberg DA, Hansen L, Czarnota N, Chakraborty J, Norcio AF (2005) The effects of color and layering on comprehension of multi-layered email messages. In: Proceedings of the Human Computer Interaction International, Las Vegas, NV, USA

Duchowski A (2007) Eye tracking methodology: Theory and practice. Springer

Fletcher V, Bonome-Sims G, Knecht B, Ostroff E, Otitigbe J, Parente M et al. (2015) The challenge of inclusive design in the US context. Applied Ergonomics 46: 267-273

Fung CH, Igodan U, Alessi C, Martin JL, Dzierzewski JM, Josephson K et al. (2015) Human factors/usability barriers to home medical devices among individuals with disabling conditions: In-depth interviews with positive airway pressure device users. Disability and Health Journal 8(1): 86-92

Jacob RJ, Karn KS (2003) Eye tracking in human-computer interaction and usability research: Ready to deliver the promises. Mind 2(3): 4

Miller GA (1956) The magical number seven, plus or minus two: Some limits on our capacity for processing information. Psychological Review 63(2): 81

Norcio AF, Stanley J (1989) Adaptive human-computer interfaces: A literature survey and perspective. IEEE Transactions on Systems, Man and Cybernetics 19(2): 399-408

Pirolli P (2005) Rational analyses of information foraging on the web. Cognitive Science 29(3): 343-373

Pirolli P (2007) Information foraging theory: Adaptive interaction with information. Oxford University Press, New York, NY, USA

Pirolli P, Card S (1999) Information foraging. Psychological Review 106(4): 643

Putze F, Hild J, Kärgel R, Herff C, Redmann A, Beyerer J et al. (2013) Locating user attention using eye tracking and EEG for spatio-temporal event selection. In: Proceedings of the 18th International Conference on Intelligent User Interfaces, Santa Monica, CA, USA

Salvucci DD, Anderson JR (2000) Intelligent gaze-added interfaces. In: Proceedings of the SIGCHI conference on Human Factors in Computing Systems, The Hague, The Netherlands

Waller S, Bradley M, Hosking I, Clarkson PJ (2015) Making the case for inclusive design. Applied Ergonomics 46(Part B): 297-303

Reducing Exclusion in Future Cars Using Personas with Visual Narratives and Design Anthropology

M. Kunur, P. M. Langdon, M. D. Bradley, J.-A. Bichard, E. Glazer, F. Doran, P. J. Clarkson and J. J. Loeillet

Abstract: This paper presents the use of picture scenarios in a narrative form to portray aspects of car use, currently and for the near future. The scenarios are based on user personas and design anthropology. It aims to enable automotive engineers and designers to empathise and understand the experiences of different car users in diverse purposes, places and usage situations. Persona profiles are mapped from the ethnographic interviews that have been conducted with car users from different parts the world. These personas then are used in scripts, which are translated into a sequential visual language that provides insight for the development of Human Machine Interface (HMI) design concepts. Narrative visualisation provides a powerful tool for portraying cultural trends and individual differences, exploring different situations, describing personal reactions and feelings, and evaluating the usability of vehicle functions. This project has shown the value of using visual tools to analyse, compare and explore diverse personas, and cultural attributes based on ethnographic case studies to scenario-based HMI tasks applied to future car designs. Such picture scenarios can help engineers and designers explore driver and passenger behaviours, expectations, emotions and motivations. The realistic visual details of each persona lead to an improved understanding of the user needs such as for visually impaired, people with disabilities, children, parents, seniors, technophobic or technophilic people. A series of iHMI potential design concepts for future cars will emerge for selection and development.

1 Introduction

This project between the Inclusion Unit of the Cambridge Engineering Design Centre (EDC) at the University of Cambridge, Department of Engineering, and the

M. Kunur (✉) · P. M. Langdon · M. D. Bradley · P. J. Clarkson
Cambridge Engineering Design Centre, University of Cambridge, Cambridge, UK

J.-A. Bichard · E. Glazer · F. Doran
Helen Hamlyn Centre for Design, Royal College of Art, Kensington Gore, London, UK

J. J. Loeillet
Jaguar Land Rover, Human Machine Interface, HMI Project, International Digital Lab, University of Warwick, Coventry, UK

P. Langdon et al. (eds.), *Designing Around People*,
DOI 10.1007/978-3-319-29498-8_28

Helen Hamlyn Centre for Design at the Royal College of Art in London focuses on the future inclusive Human Machine Interface (iHMI) concepts in vehicle design. With the collaboration between anthropologists, psychologists, engineers, vehicle designers and visualisers potential design concepts through the understandings of people's experience with a car have been examined. Vehicle models differ from each other regarding how they accommodate drivers and passengers who have varying physical, mental and cognitive abilities, as well as varying in their age, gender and culture. Ethnographic research investigates people from different countries with different experiences, lifestyles and needs. Visual representation of such ethnographic findings is a powerful tool that provides a good understanding of users' behavioural patterns to the designer. Personas set in scenarios (environments and situations) within the context of the persona's response are used in the design process to represent user archetypes.

The exploration of creative and realistic inclusive HMI ideas for future cars requires an understanding of how people around the world drive, travel and use cars of today. Tools of scenario visualisation based on ethnographic studies on diverse personas, narratives, and user experience are proven to be beneficial for automotive engineers and designers for creating innovative ideas and developing realistic automotive iHMI concepts. Rapid growth in ageing increasingly requires the inclusion of participants from older age groups as well as disabled and less-abled users in the design process. This rise in activity and profile has been catalysed in part by the ten year i~design programme of research (2000-2010) funded by the EPSRC and led by the EDC in partnership with the Helen Hamlyn Centre for Design at the Royal College of Art. Scenarios set out for the research are benefiting from the experience of i~design 3 project that has promoted active living through more inclusive design (Waller et al. 2010).

2 Inclusive Design

The need for inclusive design is increasing in an ageing developed world due to the relationship between ageing and capability loss. Currently, half of the adult population in the UK are over the age of 45, a large proportion of these individuals have some form of significant capability loss, whether it is, for example, physical, visual, auditory or cognitive. The iHMI approach assumes that any human user can be impaired (disabled) in their effectiveness by characteristics of their environment, the task, and the design of the user interface they are presented with (Rosson and Carroll 2002, Bichard et al. 2007). Such impairment may take the form of perceptual, cognitive and physical movement functional limitations that then translate into inability. It can arise out of capability limitation or from excessive demands of new technology interfaces. This project aims the reduction of such user exclusion in future vehicles in HMI as well as layout, seating, access and egress through persona based user experience embedded in visual narratives and design anthropology.

2.1 Role of Anthropology

Anthropology-grounded research aims to understand the *lived experience of people* from their direct *real world viewpoint.* It approaches participants without judgment or pre-conceived notions in order to understand their own interpretation (Malinowski 1922). The research is by nature qualitative, as it sets out to grasp the subtleties and details of people's everyday routines. It is concerned with personal experiences, daily rituals, and individuals' understandings of the world set in the broader socio-cultural context (Geertz 1973).

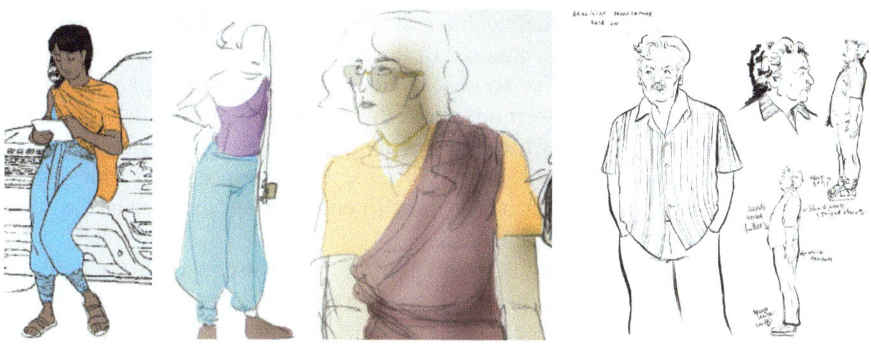

Fig. 1 Initial sketch studies of the personas based on the ethnographic research

2.2 The Use of Personas

Personas are fictional characters but they are based around people's experiences, actions and desires learned from ethnographic interviews that focus on understanding user lifestyles, aspirations, motivations and needs. They are used in the design process to represent user archetypes.

Personas are often coupled with scenarios (environments and situations) to set the context of the persona's response. The primary aim of a persona is to illustrate the user's behaviour patterns to the designer, it should be believable and can work to both stimulate new design concepts and help to validate them.

Pruitt and Grudin (2003) suggest that the use of ethnographic data help in developing realistic personas. Personas require a certain amount of detail that should not be based just on the designer's own assumptions and experience. Hence wider engagement from users through ethnographic methods is strongly encouraged to develop the richness and diversity of the persona (Cooper 1999).

Character illustrations provide the viewer with a detailed look of the persona, facial expression, personal appearance and the clothing. In most cases the photographs provide work to help the visualiser draw as realistic image of the persona as possible, perhaps capturing the important details more effectively than the photographs. It is very important that the personas should not be based just on the designer's own assumptions and experience. Personas require proper details of the users through ethnographic methods that enable to draw out the richness, diversity and nuances of real life experience.

Although it is argued that the use of personas may be considered 'too arty' (Pruitt and Grudin 2003) for science and engineering based enterprises yet cite the power of fictional characters to engage. It is made even stronger when the narrative is placed alongside visual representations. Especially, captions and speech bubbles used in storyboard frames prove to be very informative. The geographical place and climate, built environment and surroundings, and the road and traffic situation in which the persona carries out the narrated tasks set the context of the persona. This provides a key set of actions that the persona can undertake. These narratives are known as scenarios and offer a 'sketch of use' in the design process. Present time storyboard frames inspire believable and stimulating new design concepts that are further illustrated in future sequences of the storyboard to help validate them. It is more effective and informative to observe a human face rather than looking at abstract data for the user. It says more about the person rather than just a number. Scenarios provide the story in which the persona is set, and a sequence of actions that the persona undertakes. They provide the opportunity for wider communication of the user's possible actions. In engineering, the scenario is set as a list of steps and known as a 'usage case'.

In order to gain the most relevant information from the car user such as the daily life and routines, needs and desires, experiences and inspirations, questions need to be pre-structured by the interviewer to help build a realistic picture of the participant as a persona. Davies (1999) tells us that research based mainly on semi-structured interviewing has become a very popular and important form of qualitative research across the social sciences, especially in anthropology, sociology, psychology and other applied social sciences.

The approach taken here developed the persona and usage cases based on interviews with people representing that particular context. Based on these and because of resource limitations a new deliverable format of a 'doculet' was proposed. Each persona generated a small document/pamphlet consisting of professionally printed set of around 30 pages. Content consisted of general introductory material on inclusion and future HMI and the persona description with some illustrations. Key HMI elements of the usage cases were then illustrated with relevant text from user interviews, HMI and the proposed design response. This was accompanied by images in the form of photographs, schematics, interior vehicle sketches illustrating future HMI and the inclusive audit comparisons.

During this research, interviews are transcribed and analysed for keywords and related descriptions; fieldwork generates detailed diary entries on observations of participants (Bichard and Gheerawo 2010) Ethnographic research conducted in strategically targeted different parts of the world within Brazil, USA, Europe, India and China looks for answers for the most likely and diverse personas linked to major car user locations in the world. Each persona appeared in a narrative for a typical present day scenario that happens in one geographical place. Every present day scenario is overlapped by the future vision of the same scenario, with the innovative HMI concepts likely to change the way cars are being driven or used by the user. Narrative scripts are visualised in storyboard format for the flow of user actions and movements.

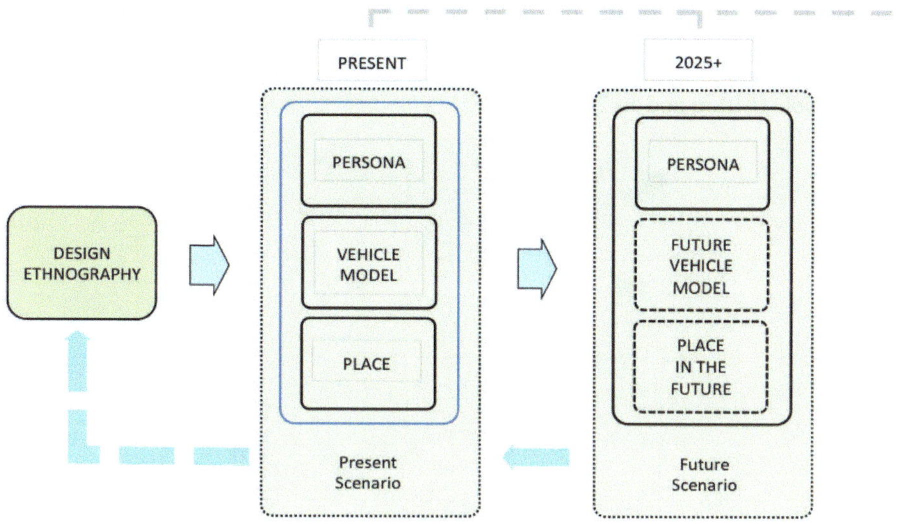

Fig. 2 Diagram of current user-centred scenario leading to future scenario based on design ethnography

One of the advantages of using storyboards is the quick changes and additions to the visual flow of the narrative build-up. Therefore it is a powerful tool as narrative sequences can be seen altogether; present and future scenarios can be compared almost instantly whether the storyboard frames are laid on the table or stuck on the wall, allowing the project participants to use sticky notes either creating more storyboard frames or moving around or removing them where necessary. At this stage visualisers may help capturing ideas by drawing very quick sketches and diagrams that is part of the research phase storyboarding. Thus, during this visual process, each user experience or interaction within the scenario can be broken into its more specific components over time, which allows the group to analyse more closely. Therefore, this visual brainstorming prompts attendees to come up with inspiring and innovative ideas that can be further captured in the future storylines:

> *'A storyboard is a visual narrative of an interaction scenario. With origins in cinema, it is a story-telling device that describes characters, the activities they engage in, the objects that they need and/or use, their motivations, emotions and reactions to interactions, and an environment for those interactions.'*
>
> (Van der Lelie 2006)

After completing the initial storyboards through design thinking workshops conceptual ideas emerge. These ideas are drawn in more detailed storyboards to represent the design details as well as the user interactions to reflect the user's action, experience, emotion, feelings and thoughts in many ways leading to storyboard prototypes. Sections of the storyboard that relate to each design idea are discussed within the group. The final working designs that the users would take to overcome the needs or the problems are selected through this decision process. Each project prototype solution becomes a tangible design module used in the overall automobile design. The user remains as the main character to interact with the vehicle (Sirkin and Ju 2014).

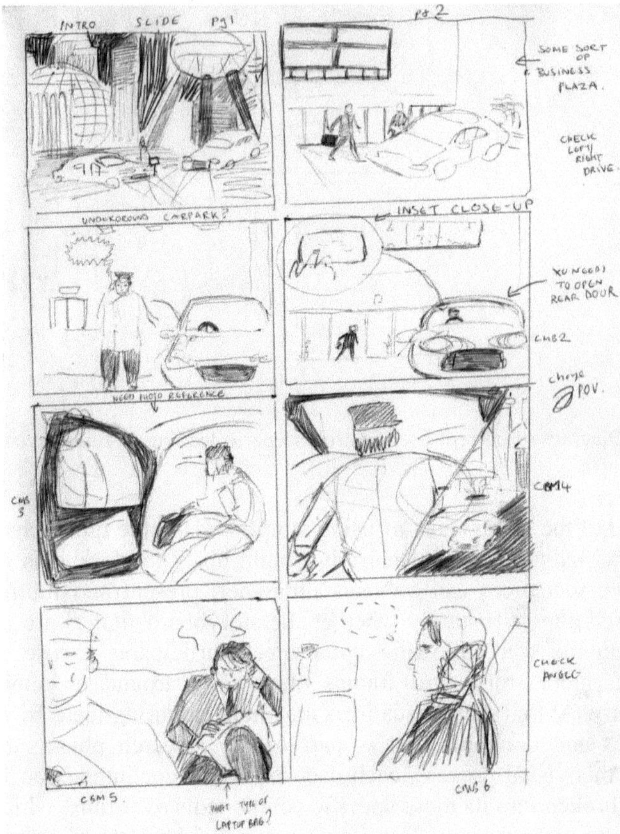

Fig. 3 Quick storyboard sketches show frame to frame sequence that is developing the narrative with proposed iHMI design ideas for a specific car model

2.3 User-centred Design Cases Developed from Personas

Final stage sequential visual work provides design solutions throughout the visual scenario in more detailed and coloured drawings focusing on how the user interacts with the car in a specific environment and reveals the experience of certain users due to their age, ability, gender, personality and culture. Thus, engineers and designers have better understanding of creating innovative and inspiring automotive designs that are more inclusive. Conceptual design drawings derived from the sequential story frames open up to different ways of design thinking and development amongst the stakeholders.

Each persona, either a driver or a passenger is considered to be associated with an existing car model during the design thinking interaction workshop. Key project engineers, researchers and visualisers discuss and build a realistic storyline around the persona, car, place and environment in a set of tasks and situations.

2.4 The iHMI "Pipeline" to Concepts

The realistic details on the character illustrations of each persona are essential for better understanding of the users' including older people, the visually impaired and wheelchair users, child and parent, technophobic or technophile persons. Each HMI concept can be sketched as required in task sequences, with detail and scaled paper model produced for detailed step-by-step design.

The required interactions can be observed, photographed and captured on video for in-depth design thinking workshops. A series of HMI working design concepts for future cars will emerge from this pipeline for prototyping and engineering.

The iHMI "pipeline" is a research approach, which allows developing key concepts that take into account the needs of real customers. This approach includes the following steps:

- persona selection,
- identification of user needs and usages (anthropology interview),
- understanding of the current product (inclusive audit),
- current scenario based on anthropology and inclusive outputs,
- future scenario,
- selection of key concepts.

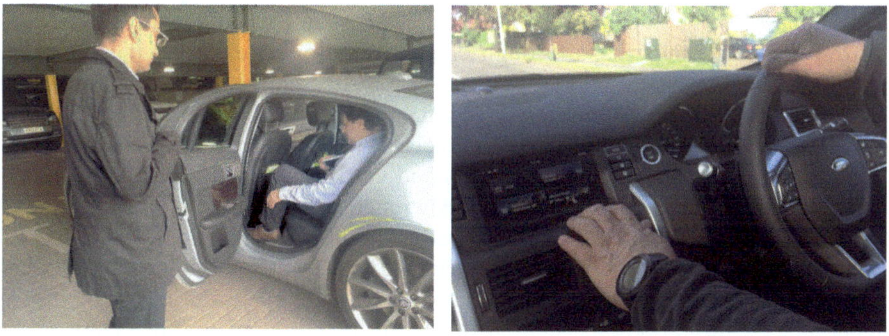

Fig. 4 Exploring an executive saloon car from the business user perspective and capturing the sequence of tasks that can be evaluated as potential HMI concepts to be later illustrated in scenario storyboards. Researchers here act as observer-participants.

2.5 Validity of the Concepts through Visual Narratives

Visual narratives are quick to draw and the sequence of storyboards can be rearranged and changed where necessary either in the early stages with paper and pencil sketching or scanned digital images on screen in developing stages. Details in drawings, colour, line quality, view angles, pan movements, speech bubbles and other explanatory texts within the storyboards are in continuous progress to capture the most realistic iHMI design ideas that can be well understood and executed by the design engineers. Therefore, the final presentation provides valid design proposals integrated in visual future narratives that are easy to follow. One of the benefits of storyboarding is to understand how technology reshapes human activity and influences the understanding of the reaction to a system (Truong et al. 2006). The team analyses the final presentation of visual scenarios and develop further conceptual sketches of iHMI ideas through design thinking and user journey mapping activities. Where necessary paper prototypes and 3D models are produced to provide better feedback from the project team where ethnography and iHMI researchers review the final validation of realistic design proposals.

Sequential narrative frames executed to date are in two parallel timelines: current scenarios where the persona is interacting with an existing vehicle and environment, and future scenarios where the same persona is visually tested against an expected future car. Storyboards mainly focus on two elements: (1) user perspective that portrays the characteristics of the user including age, gender, profession, cultural background and disability, and (2) the vehicle perspective that combines components and devices within the vehicle where the user interacts with the interface of controls and displays. This parallel layout of the current and future storyboard lines allow the team some potentially useful participatory workshop in order to resolve the issues; whether through redesign of the interface, or perhaps through changing the order of tasks. It is expected that more investigation will be required for better understanding of the user's expectations of the right interior arrangements and right location of controls and displays as well as other components, such as: seats, storage, arm, head and foot rests, cup holder, sound, light, air units and work stations. The usage cases will be matched to design using inclusive design metrics (Langdon et al. 2013).

Each case study illustrated the users' relationship with the vehicle and the surrounding environment. The success of the approach was highlighted through the feedback from the company automotive engineers and during the company technology exhibition. This demonstrated the potential of visual techniques in relating user needs to engineered technology and design.

3 Conclusion

Storyboard techniques are a fast and effective way of visually presenting, communicating and sharing scenarios with designers and engineers as well as other stakeholders. This project finalised visual material as a series of booklets that are self-explanatory brief documents each focusing on one persona case, design sketches and drawings of the future design ideas and interfaces. It included future vehicle design ideas detailing of the interiors, door apertures, seating, driver and passenger areas emerged from the set of persona case studies within each scenario. The sequential drawings illustrated how each user interacts with the vehicle and its environment. These may differ inclusively from each other due to different needs and expectations. A consistent visualisation for a number of inclusive design based personas using vehicles with future HMI interfaces were generated. The outcome from these workshops will be analysed and further reviewed for potential design projects.

References

Bichard J-A, Coleman R, Langdon PM (2007) Does my stigma look big in this? Considering acceptability and desirability in inclusive design of technology products. In: Stephanidis C (Ed.) Universal access in HCI. Springer-Verlag, Berlin

Bichard J-A, Gheerawo R (2010) The designer as ethnographer: Practical projects in industry in design anthropology object culture in the 21st century, pp. 45-55. Springer, Wien, New York, USA

Cooper A (1999) The inmates are running the asylum. SAMS/MacMillan, Indianapolis, IN, USA

Davies CA (1999) Reflective ethnography: A guide to researching selves and others, pp.169-170. Routledge, London, UK

Geertz C (1973) Available light: Anthropological reflections on philosophical topics, pp. 11-17. Princeton University, NJ, USA

Langdon PM, Johnson D, Huppert F, Clarkson PJ (2013) A framework for collecting inclusive design data for the UK population in applied ergonomics. Applied Ergonomic 46(Part B): 318-324

Pruitt J, Grudin J (2003) Personas: Practice and theory. In: Proceedings of the 2003 Conference on Designing for User Experiences, San Francisco, CA, USA

Rosson MB, Carroll JM (2002) Scenario-based design. In: Jacko J, Sears A (Eds.) The human-computer interaction handbook: Fundamentals, evolving technologies and emerging applications, pp. 1032-1050. Lawrence Erlbaum Associates

Sirkin D, Ju W (2014) Using embodied design improvisation as a design tool. In: Proceedings of the International Conference on Human Behaviour in Design 2014, Ascona, Switzerland

Truong KN, Hayes GR, Abowd GD (2006) Storyboarding: An empirical determination of best practices and effective guidelines. In: Proceedings of the 6th Conference on Designing Interactive systems, University Park, PA, USA

Van der Lelie C (2006) The value of storyboards in the product design process. Personal and Ubiquitous Computing 10(2): 159-162

Waller SD, Langdon PM, Clarkson PJ (2010) Using disability data to estimate design exclusion. Universal Access in the Information Society 9(3): 195-207

Author Index

P. Langdon et al. (eds.), *Designing Around People*,
DOI 10.1007/978-3-319-29498-8

MIX
Papier aus verantwortungsvollen Quellen
Paper from responsible sources
FSC® C105338

If you have any concerns about our products,
you can contact us on
ProductSafety@springernature.com

In case Publisher is established outside the EU,
the EU authorized representative is:
Springer Nature Customer Service Center GmbH
Europaplatz 3, 69115 Heidelberg, Germany

Printed by Libri Plureos GmbH
in Hamburg, Germany